CURRENT PROBLEMS IN SOCIOBIOLOGY

CURRENT PROBLEMS IN SOCIOBIOLOGY

EDITED BY
KING'S COLLEGE SOCIOBIOLOGY GROUP,
CAMBRIDGE

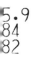

CAMBRIDGE UNIVERSITY PRESS

Cambridge

London   New York   New Rochelle

Sydney   Melbourne

Published by the Press Syndicate of the University of Cambridge
The Pitt Building, Trumpington Street, Cambridge CB2 1RP
32 East 57th Street, New York, NY 10022, USA
296 Beaconsfield Parade, Middle Park, Melbourne 3206, Australia

© Cambridge University Press 1982

First published 1982

Printed in Great Britain at the
University Press, Cambridge

Library of Congress catalogue card number: 81–10129

British Library Cataloguing in Publication Data

Current problems in sociobiology.
1. Social behavior in animals – Addresses,
essays, lectures
I. King's College
Sociobiology Group
591.5   QL775

ISBN 0 521 24203 7 hard covers
ISBN 0 521 28520 8 paperback

Contents

List of Participants

S.D. ALBON, *Research Centre, King's College, Cambridge, England, and Department of Zoology, Large Animal Research Group, 34A Storeys Way, Cambridge, England*

P.P.G. BATESON, *Sub-Department of Animal Behaviour, University of Cambridge, Madingley, Cambridge, England*

B.C.R. BERTRAM, *Research Centre, King's College, Cambridge, England and Zoological Society of London, Regent's Park, London, NW1 4RY, England*

N.A. CHAGNON, *Department of Anthropology, Pennsylvania State University, University Park, Pennsylvania 16802, USA*

T.H. CLUTTON-BROCK, *Research Centre, King's College, Cambridge, England and Department of Zoology, Large Animal Research Group, 34A Storeys Way, Cambridge, England*

N.B. DAVIES, *Department of Zoology, University of Cambridge, Downing Street, Cambridge, England*

R. DAWKINS, *Department of Zoology, University of Oxford, South Parks Road, Oxford, England*

R.I.M. DUNBAR, *Research Centre, King's College, Cambridge, England and Sub-Department of Animal Behaviour, University of Cambridge, Madingley, Cambridge, England*

P.H. HARVEY, *School of Biological Sciences, University of Sussex, Falmer, Brighton, Sussex, England*

P.J. JARMAN, *School of Natural Resources, University of New England, Armidale, New South Wales 2351, Australia*

N. KNOWLTON, *Department of Biology, Yale University, P.O. Box 6666, New Haven, Connecticutt 06520, USA*

A. ŁOMNICKI, *Institute of Environmental Biology, Jagiellonian University, ul. Karasia 6, 30-060 Krakow, Poland*

G.A. MACE, *Department of Zoology, University of Newcastle upon Tyne, England*

J. MAYNARD SMITH, *School of Biological Sciences, University of Sussex, Falmer, Brighton, Sussex, England*

P. O'DONALD, *Department of Genetics, University of Cambridge, Downing Street, Cambridge, England*

G.A. PARKER, *Department of Zoology, University of Liverpool, Brownlow Street, Liverpool, Lancashire, England*

D.I. RUBENSTEIN, *Research Centre, King's College, Cambridge, England and Department of Biology, Princeton University, Princeton, New Jersey 08540, USA*

E.A. THOMPSON, *Department of Mathematical Statistics, University of Cambridge, Mill Lane, Cambridge, England*

R.W. WRANGHAM, *Research Centre, King's College, Cambridge, England and c/o Dr I. Devore, Department of Anthropology, Harvard University, Boston, Mass. USA*

Preface

The papers in this volume were originally presented at a conference held at King's College, Cambridge on 4–6 July 1980, to mark the culmination of the King's College Sociobiology project. For this conference, all those who had been closely involved with the project were invited to submit papers concerned with unsolved problems in sociobiology.

In order to understand how the King's Sociobiology group came to be formed it is necessary to understand that Cambridge Colleges are relatively independent of the University and some have great wealth of their own. Every so often a college that is rich enough can behave like a Renaissance patron and do something that a British university, largely dependent on State support, could rarely do. My own College, King's, decided in the mid-sixties to use some of its considerable resources to help subjects that looked exciting but did not have an adequate toehold within the University. It established a Research Centre in which a group of people within the same subject could hold Fellowships. Each programme was to last up to five years and, in addition to themselves, members could draw in short-term visitors, research assistants and graduate students. The idea was that a lively group would give sufficient impetus to their subject to keep it going in Cambridge after the project had ended in the Research Centre.

Early in 1975 Nick Humphrey and I, as Fellows of King's, suggested to the College that the Research Centre should establish a project in behavioural ecology. During the sixties and early seventies the fruits of numerous field studies of animals were starting to suggest coherent explanations for the ways in which social behaviour might be related to ecological conditions. The ideas were brought together by the increasingly powerful use of evolutionary theory. A mass of seemingly unrelated evidence started to make sense and the subject looked exceptionally promising. King's decided to support behavioural ecology and, once it had done so, the Convenor of the Research Centre, Donald Parry, took over the job of organising the project. Along with running a busy University Department of his own, he handled with consummate efficiency every stage from advertising the Fellowships to administering the most active phase of the programme. A lot of its subsequent success was due to his efforts.

After the project had been running for a year, its title was changed from Behavioural Ecology to Sociobiology since we wanted to include functional studies of social behaviour which were not necessarily ecological in character. The term 'Sociobiology' had been in use since the late 1940s; indeed, the present-day American Animal Behavior Society had grown out of a section of the Ecological Society of America and the American Society of Zoologists called 'Animal Behavior and Sociobiology'. However, we should, perhaps, have been quicker to realise how much opinion would be polarized by the recent attempts to inject a particular brand of biology into the social sciences. The lacerations resulting from the ensuing ideological conflict have not yet healed, and in many places 'Sociobiology' is either a battlecry or a term of abuse. Fortunately, the Research Centre project was unaffected, largely because the people who were appointed to the group were strongly committed to empirical research. Nobody who knew their work could accuse them of doing bad science. Furthermore, they would tolerate neither sloppy argument nor extravagant generalisations from studies of animals to humans.

After two years of recruiting the Sociobiology Group had four Fellows with longer-term appointments: Brian Bertram, Tim Clutton-Brock, Dan Rubenstein and Richard Wrangham. They were joined by Robin Dunbar who had been awarded one of the much prized Science Research Council Advanced Fellowships. During the course of the project Adam Łomnicki and Geoff Parker each came for one year while on sabbatical leave from their Universities. Peter Jarman, Nancy Knowlton and Napoleon Chagnon worked for shorter periods in the Research Centre and, while they did not hold Fellowships, played vigorous parts in its intellectual life. In addition, Elizabeth Thompson, who was already a Fellow of the College, brought much needed mathematical skills to bear on some of the problems that were being discussed, and Steve Albon collaborated throughout with Tim Clutton-Brock on their study of red deer. Of the numerous other people who, by their talks and discussions, contributed so much to making the years of the project exciting and enjoyable, Nick Davies, Richard Dawkins, Paul Harvey, John Maynard Smith and Peter O'Donald were especially influential.

One of the most important aspects of the Research Centre's work was the weekly seminar. The talks and the discussions they generated were excellent and, what proved crucial, attracted a regular audience from groups scattered throughout Cambridge and East Anglia. People from different Departments and research groups suddenly found that they had interesting things to say to each other. The Research Centre was operating exactly as it should do and providing a focus for discussion and an impetus for further research. After four productive years which culminated in the conference from which this book has been produced, the Sociobiology Group has now dispersed. What remains behind is a widespread enthusiasm for studies of the evolution of behaviour and behavioural ecology and, at the same time, cool sanity about the issues. That legacy, along with each member's personal contribution to research, is the lasting achievement of the King's Sociobiology Group.

October 1980   Patrick Bateson

Acknowledgments

It is a very real pleasure to thank the Provost and Fellows of King's College for their interest, help and support in the Sociobiology Project over the last five years. For all of us, our time in the Research Centre provided opportunities for research and collaboration which would have been unavailable elsewhere. We are particularly grateful to Pat Bateson and Nick Humphrey for instigating the project; to Donald Parry and Herbert Huppert who administered the Research Centre together with the board of managers, for their help, sympathy and toleration in dealing with our various needs; to Hazel Clarke, the Research Centre's administrative secretary, for secretarial help and unflagging good humour; and to the staff of King's College for their part in making King's a pleasant place to work. We are also grateful to the staff of the Department of Zoology, the Sub-department of Animal Behaviour, and the Computer Centre, all of which provided us with specialized facilities unavailable in the Research Centre. Finally, we should like to thank the large number of colleagues who participated in the Research Centre's activities and whose stimulating interest and encouragement were the spur for so many of our activities.

The Editors

Acknowledgments

Introduction

JOHN MAYNARD SMITH

The papers in this volume are concerned with two main topics – the concepts of sociobiology, and the ways in which hypotheses can be tested.

Much of the discussion of concepts takes the form of arguments about the meanings of words – fitness, altruism, replicator and so on. I do not think these arguments are purely semantic. Certainly, some difficulties have arisen because words have been used in different senses by different people; for example, the phrase 'group selection' has been used in such different ways that it has become almost meaningless. However, our difficulties could not be solved merely by an agreement to use words in particular ways. The trouble is, of course, that we would not agree on appropriate meanings. The reason would not be obstinacy on our part. It would be that words are the means whereby we order our thoughts. Consequently, if two scientists see the world in different ways, they will want to use words differently to describe it.

In this introduction I want to suggest that two main concepts have dominated the study of the evolution of social behaviour during the past fifteen years, but that in the last four years a third idea, not in fact a particularly new one, has been increasingly prominent.

Of the two dominant concepts, the first, tracing back primarily to the work of John Crook, is that social systems should be seen as ecological adaptations. The second, which we owe mainly to W.D. Hamilton, is that the evolution of behaviour is influenced by the fact that the genes of relatives may be identical. The latter idea has had an extraordinary fascination for biologists. Theoreticians have been attracted by its intellectual elegance, and by the fact that it offers an explanation for what would otherwise by an anomaly – the existence of behaviour patterns which do not increase the classical fitness of the individual displaying them. Field workers have been impressed by the observation that, far more often than not, societies do consist of relatives. There may be another reason for the fascination; students of Hamilton would not be surprised to find that scientists are obsessed by kinship.

I do not doubt that biologists have been right to be excited by these two concepts. However, I think that an interest in kinship may have blinded some of us to a third idea. This is the very obvious one that two animals may cooperate because it pays both of them to do so. This is not a new idea, and it has not been wholly missing in discussions of sociobiology, but its importance may have been underrated. The process has usually been called 'mutualism'. When writing my own chapter in this book, I had some reservations about the term, because it has usually been used by ecologists to refer to interactions between members of different species. On reflection, however, I can see little danger in its use; the term competition is used both for inter- and intraspecific interactions, so why not mutualism? It will always be possible to add a qualifying adjective when there is any possibility of confusion.

It seems likely, then, that the immediate future of sociobiology will be concerned with the joint effects of mutualism and of kin selection on the evolution of societies, subject to particular ecological constraints. This future is clearly foreshadowed in this volume.

The testing of hypotheses has become a sensitive subject among sociobiologists. Who wants to be accused of telling Just So stories? Perhaps the most promising thing that has happened – also reflected in this volume – is the recognition that the statistical analysis of comparative data calls for just as much care and sophistication as the analysis of experimental results. However, in one field that interests me – that of sex ratio – our difficulty is not that we can think up a variety of hypotheses to explain the data and are unable to decide between them, but that we are unable to think of any adequate hypothesis. This is a disturbing state of affairs, but at least it suggests that if we can formulate a hypothesis which makes quantitative predictions, we ought to be able to test it.

It is hard to think about animal societies without wondering what light they may shed on human ones. Although only one chapter in this book is specifically concerned with man, the question is certainly in the minds of several of the contributors. I cannot answer it, but I will make some comments. The first is a very general one. The explanations of animal societies offered by biologists are essentially reductionist. That is, they attempt to explain the structure of societies as a consequence of the properties of the individuals which compose them. By no means all sociological or anthropological theories are of this kind. Theories in economics are reductionist; even Marxist theories of capitalist economic systems assume that individuals behave so as to maximise their profits, or the return on their labour, although Marxists would insist that the particular goals of individuals are socially determined. But many sociological theories are not reductionist even in this limited sense. The properties of individuals are seen as produced by society, and even as serving the purposes of that society, and not the other way round. If sociobiologists are to persuade sociologists that their ideas and methods are relevant to man, the first thing they must establish is that reductionist theories of *some* kind are relevant; it is a further, and to my mind more doubtful, step to persuade them that the concept of inclusive fitness is appropriate to human behaviour.

While reading about human sociobiology during the past few years, one thing has struck me very forcibly. The works which I have found most interesting have not been those which, whether for or against, have dealt with general or philosophical issues, but those which discuss specific societies, as do, for example, Dickeman, Irons and Chagnon. There is, however, a question which often remains unanswered by those who apply sociobiological concepts to man. What *kind* of explanation are they offering? I can think of at least two answers to this question, but I suspect that there are many more. The first would be that they are seeking an explanation of why particular social systems are associated with particular ways in which people obtain the necessities of life – i.e. with particular ecologies. This would be analogous to the first problem of sociobiology – why do particular animal social systems evolve in particular ecological circumstances?

There is, however, a second kind of explanation. One could accept the rules and customs of a society as given, and ask whether the actions of different people in that society – rich and poor, old and young, male and female – are those which would be predicted if each individual is behaving, subject to the rules, in the way which would maximise his or her inclusive fitness. In the same vein, one could also ask whether, if people do act in such a way, the results of their actions will preserve the society or transform it. It may be that few sociobiologists think that inclusive fitness can be applied in such a direct manner. If so, it would help if they told us what they do think. It cannot merely be that human behaviour is influenced by kinship, and that kinship has something to do with genetic relationship, because surely, despite some very odd remarks by anthropologists, that is uncontroversial?

I

Natural selection and sociobiology

Edited by
R.W. WRANGHAM

It is a remarkable tribute to Darwin that ideas whose seeds he planted more than a hundred years ago are still developing with enormous vigour. Sociobiology is a prime example. Since 1964 it has blossomed into a rapidly changing discipline growing along several different branches. As with any such endeavour, this process brings not only excitement but also a danger of overextension: the beauty of new ideas can obscure their proper interpretation. In acknowledgment of sociobiology's sudden growth, therefore, the essays in Section 1 are directed to taking stock of issues at the root of the discipline.

First, Dunbar examines the nature of evolutionary explanations. He takes up the familiar accusation that Darwinism is tautological, arguing that although the accusation is wrong it is useful because it draws attention to limitations in the ways evolutionary theory should be used. The intuitive appeal of sociobiological explanations hides a number of traps, and Dunbar discusses how some of them can be avoided. Among other things he calls for a more careful use of language, undoubtedly a necessary step on the path to a strong science and one which is overdue in the present instance.

The second chapter concerns altruism, a subject of central importance in the modern development of sociobiology. In 1964 Hamilton provided the first satisfactory explanation for its evolution, and here Maynard Smith discusses subsequent theoretical advances. The diversity of recent proposals concerning the evolution of altruism is more than enough to cause confusion, and we are still a long way from a coherent theory. Maynard Smith clarifies the field by identifying five mechanisms by which altruism might be favoured, and by pointing out their different assumptions and implications. Kin selection has traditionally been the most important and it is given special attention here because two distinct methods have been proposed for analysing its effects. By outlining the merits of each Maynard Smith shows how they can be reconciled. His chapter thus points the way to an integration of the mechanisms of social evolution more sophisticated than is currently available.

The recent focus on altruism has been accompanied by extensive discussion of the level at which natural selection is supposed to act. The mid-1960s saw a solid attack on group selection theory, leading ultimately to a reconsideration of individual selection, and the concept of the selfish gene. The debate concerns the merits of groups, individuals and genes as 'units of selection'. These have sometimes been treated as similar kinds of 'unit', a view which Dawkins devotes chapter 3 to rejecting. He shows that two distinct arguments are involved in discussions of the level at which selection acts, and holds that the conflict between 'individual-selectionists' and 'gene-selectionists' is more apparent than real because the processes which they describe are complementary. Sociobiology's reductionism is therefore seen as a tool for understanding complexity rather than as a dismissal of the importance of individual characteristics. Dawkins' essay should do much to clear up a major source of misunderstanding.

In the final chapter of this section O'Donald discusses one of the most important questions in the logical structure of kin-selection theory: what is the basis for the idea that natural selection leads to the maximisation of inclusive fitness? Given the widespread acceptance of Hamilton's theory it is perhaps surprising that this needs to be asked at all. There is a variety of outstanding difficulties, however. For instance, the original proof lacks generality: the assumptions it makes about population structure mean that for many species its conclusions are invalid. Another problem concerns the use of words. Many authors use the term 'inclusive fitness' to refer to actual personal fitness plus the fitness of relatives devalued by the coefficient of relationship. Though this definition is helpful because it allows inclusive fitness to be measured easily, it is not what Hamilton showed to be maximised. O'Donald discusses a third issue. He argues that the classical methods of population genetics are inadequate for modelling the spread of genes which influence the fitness of kin. In particular, it is necessary to take gene frequencies into account in new ways when calculating subsequent changes in gene frequency. O'Donald argues that when this is done inclusive fitness values can still be regarded as independent of gene frequency. Like Maynard Smith he goes on to conclude that so long as the effects of a given behaviour are small the spread of genes responsible for it can be modelled accurately by simple methods. In other cases, however, they cannot. His analysis brings a valuable level of precision to models of the evolution of social behaviour and illustrates how carefully sociobiology must proceed.

1

Adaptation, fitness and the evolutionary tautology

R.I.M. DUNBAR

'... for it was a kind of cloud that overshadowed knowledge for a while and blew over.'
(Francis Bacon, *De Augmentis Scientiarum*, 1623.)

Introduction

As the major unifying force in biology, Darwin's theory of evolution by natural selection remains virtually unchallenged by serious contenders after more than a century of debate. Yet, it frequently stands accused of being tautologous by both philosophers of science (Smart, 1963; Manser, 1965; Popper, 1972) and biologists (Birch & Ehrlich, 1967; Peters, 1976) alike. Although a number of philosophers (Ruse, 1973; Hull, 1974) and biologists (Maynard Smith, 1969; Thompson, 1981) have argued against this criticism, many biologists are inclined to dismiss it as either vacuous or at best irrelevant to the way in which they conduct their research. Such a response, of course, leaves the main thrust of the criticism unanswered, a fact that would be of only passing significance were it not the case that the criticism, if true, leaves evolutionary biology based on such weak foundations that its pursuit as a serious scientific discipline becomes a trivial exercise in dogmatism in the worst sense (cf. Feyerabend, 1963).

In this chapter, I will try to show that the criticism of circularity is ill-founded because it rests on a mistaken view of the structure of Darwinian explanations. I will argue that although a correct formulation of Darwinian explanations resolves the circularity without issue, it does so at the expense of placing some significant restrictions on the metaphysical framework within which most sociobiologists operate. These restrictions have more important consequences than the original criticism.

The structure of evolutionary explanations

The Darwinian formula

Darwinian explanations are conventionally conceived as involving a three-step argument (see Maynard Smith, 1969; Williams, 1970; Hull, 1974). Lewontin (1978), for example, states that three steps (or principles as he calls them) are 'necessary and sufficient to account for evolutionary change by natural selection', namely,

> 'Different individuals within a species differ from one another in physiology, morphology and behaviour (the principle of variation); the variation is in some way heritable, so that on average offspring resemble their parents more than they resemble other individuals (the principle of heredity); different variants leave different numbers of offspring either immediately or in remote generations (the principle of natural selection)'.

Unfortunately, it is this formulation that lies at the very root of the criticism of circularity, for it offers us no necessary reason why different variants should leave different numbers of offspring other than the fact that they do indeed do so.

The problem, in a nutshell, is this: if the criticism is valid, then evolutionary explanations are reduced to mere descriptions of observed fact. Statements that appear to offer explanations for the evolution of particular characters turn out on closer analysis to be no more than restatements in definitionally equivalent form of the facts that they purport to explain. More specifically, if the terms 'survival' and 'fittest' in Darwin's unfortunate catch-phrase 'the survival of the fittest' can only be defined (or at least recognised operationally) in terms of each other, then the phrase merely observes that 'the survivors survive'. Any pretence at genuine explanation dissolves away, since definitions explain nothing. A particularly lucid explanation of this difficulty has recently been given by Brady (1979).

There is a widespread belief that, because each of the three statements can be empirically verified, the formulation cannot be tautological (see for example Connolly, 1966). Unfortunately, this claim misses the point entirely. That the principles can be shown to be empirically true is not in dispute; but the argument so formulated remains a simple description of observed facts, and no amount of empirical evidence will turn it into an *explanation* of those facts (except in the trivial sense that an account of the biochemical bases of heredity is an explanation of *how* evolution is brought about – though it is not an answer to the evolutionary biologist's problem of *why* it is brought about*). The fundamental purpose of science is to

---

*I should stress that, in saying this, I do not mean to belittle the achievements of molecular geneticists, but merely to point out that an explanation at one logical level need not, and often will not, be an explanation at another level. This distinction is commonly blurred, and the resulting obfuscation has made nonsense of an already murky area.

explain, and to be accused of failing to do this when laying claim to offering explanations (and sociobiologists at least certainly make such a claim: see Wilson, 1975) is a very serious matter. Circular definitions remain circular no matter how well founded their empirical content may be.

What is missing from this formulation is the *modus operandi* that specifies why different variants leave different numbers of offspring. This missing element is provided by the notion of *adaptation*, a concept that was central to Darwin's (1859) own conception of the theory (as Lewontin (1978) in fact acknowledges later in the same paper). By incorporating a statement about adaptation, we obtain a specification of the Darwinian formula which (though pared to the bare bones) is, in all fundamental respects, complete:

(1) There is individual variation in particular characters;

(2) Some of this variance is (genetically) inherited;

(3) Some of these variants are better adapted than others;

And, finally, because of the mathematical relations enshrined in the laws of heredity implied in (2), it follows from (3) that

(4) Other things being equal, those variants that are better adapted will contribute more to the species' gene pool in future generations (and their characters will therefore come to dominate).

The fourth statement is the crux of the *evolutionary* argument, since nothing in the three premises necessarily requires that evolution (in the biological sense of the term) should occur. Moreover, it is to (4), and no other statement, that reference is being made when the term 'fitness' is mentioned by population geneticists. This raises the crucially important issue of the distinction between *adaptation* (*sensu* statement (3)) and *fitness* (*sensu* statement (4)).

Definitions

The concepts of adaptation and fitness have always been unusually difficult to define, partly because fundamental theoretical concepts are invariably problematic when defined with respect to the real world (see Ghiselin, 1966) and partly because these particular terms have often been used by biologists in quite startlingly different ways. In the present context, however, it will be necessary to attempt fairly precise definitions in order to clarify their relationship.

Adaptation. Strictly speaking, *adaptation* refers to some 'problem set by nature' and entails the notion of a solution that permits the organism to overcome that problem efficiently (see for example Ghiselin, 1966; Williams, 1966; Lewontin, 1978). The criterion term 'efficient' here conveys the notion of 'design for a purpose', which I take to mean that a solution can be shown to be the most effective in terms of first principles (cf. Maynard Smith, 1978). A character is said to be 'better adapted' than any of its alternatives (*qua* competitors) when it permits its possessor to achieve the immediate objectives set by that problem more rapidly, or at less cost energetically, or with greater frequency, or by whatever criterion is most appropriate to that problem.

A formal definition of a biological adaptation would have to look something like this: 'An attribute that permitted the possessor to accomplish those immediate objectives that it must achieve in order to survive and reproduce successfully'. Note that the function of the latter phrase is to delimit the kinds of problems that are to count as relevant to *biological* adaptations: it is not in itself part of the definition of an adaptation as such.

The idea of *function* is implicitly involved, and, indeed, questions about adaptation may be considered to be questions about function. We can, however, ask about the function of a particular character at several different levels. We may, for example, ask about the functions of a given type of feeding behaviour in relation to food ingestion, in relation to day-to-day survival, in relation to mating activities and in relation to rearing offspring. Naturally, the behaviour in question will have more direct evolutionary significance at some levels than at others, but the important point is that each level is contributory to successful solutions at higher levels (where by 'higher' is meant closer causal proximity to the animal's ultimate problem of contributing offspring to the next generation). There is, in other words, a nested hierarchy of problems leading up to this ultimate problem, and although in general, when referring to adaptation, we refer to the immediately relevant problem, the global functional context should not be overlooked.

The difficulty of recognising adaptations in practice has sometimes led to their being defined operationally in terms of their effects on reproductive success or on fitness (e.g. Williams, 1966; Clutton-Brock & Harvey, 1979): thus, an adaptation is whatever increases fitness. The poverty of operationalism is amply demonstrated by such a strategem, since by defining adaptation in this way the very circularity we wish to avoid is neatly reinstated. In consequence, we either beg the central question of *how* adaptations increase fitness or make any statements about adaptations redundant. Similar problems are encountered with another common operational definition, namely that an adaptation is a correlation between an animal's characters and its environment. This, of course, is the basis of the comparative method, the single most powerful tool we have for identifying adaptations in nature. It is not, however, an adequate definition since a correlation *per se* is not sufficient evidence of 'design for a purpose'. Great care needs to be taken to avoid confusing a theoretical construct with the means we employ to recognise it in practice.

One further point of confusion should be noted. The word adaptation is used to refer both to the process of adaptation and to the end product of this process. I refer here only to the first: that is, the sense in which we speak of a character being more or less adapted (sometimes, even *pre-adapted*) to solving a particular biological problem (i.e. to the way in which an adaptation works). It remains the case that, as a result of changes in fitness, an adaptation (*qua* end product) comes to be. For completeness, we might have considered the addition of a fifth statement to this effect in the Darwinian formulation on p. 11, though for convenience in the present context I have chosen to subsume it under (4). Such a statement provides the evolutionary loop back through statement (3) that lies at the heart of the evolutionary process.

Finally, it is worth noting in conclusion that it is to adaptation, and *not* fitness, that Darwin's term 'fit' (or 'fittest') refers (see Maynard Smith, 1969). It is precisely this confusion that has generated so much of the acrimony over the tautological status of Darwin's theory.

Fitness. The term *fitness* has come to be used in population genetics to refer to relative changes in gene frequency (Falconer, 1960; Dobzhansky, 1970; Cavalli-Sforza & Bodmer, 1971). Fitness is a measure of the *rate of spread* of a given gene, and it is usually defined with reference either to the 'normal' (i.e. wild type) or the fastest-spreading allele: in either case, the reference allele is defined as having unit fitness, and is used as a yardstick against which to assess the viability of the alternative alleles (as measured by their rates of spread) (Wilson & Bossert, 1971). It should also be noted that fitness is strictly environment-specific: the same genotype can have high fitness in one habitat and low fitness in another (Fisher, 1930; Maynard Smith, 1969; Wright, 1969).

Considerable confusion has, perhaps, been created by the fact that fitness (as understood by population geneticists) is an abstraction that is virtually unmeasurable (Wright, 1968). Consequently, a variety of indices of fitness have been used, both in practice and in theoretical models, in order to render applications of the mathematics of gene frequency changes to real world situations more tractable (Wright, 1969). Fitness has, for example, been equated with lifetime mating success (Gadgil, 1972), lifetime reproductive success (Falconer, 1960; Maynard Smith, 1969; Cavalli-

Sforza & Bodmer, 1961), the number of descendents at some arbitrarily distant future time (Ricklefs, 1973), the Malthusian parameter *m* (Fisher, 1930; Wright, 1969; Crow & Kimura, 1970) and the rate of spread of a gene (Fisher, 1930; Wright, 1969), all of which may be expressed in terms of absolute values or relative to the contributions of other units of interest (Wright, 1969; Crow & Kimura, 1970). Nonetheless, the consensus is clearly that, strictly speaking, the term fitness is meaningful only when it is understood as measure of success relative to that of other specified genotypes. We can see this most clearly in the anomalous case of a declining population, where the fitness of a particular allele may be both increasing (as its frequency in the species' gene pool increases relative to the frequency of other *alleles* at the same locus) and declining (as the species' numbers decline relative to those of other *species*).

In the final analysis, a very clear distinction has to be made between the *concept* of fitness (*qua* notional construct in theoretical models) and the *measures* (or indices) of fitness (as used in practice to interpret the implications of these models in the real world)*. If the distinction between these two is blurred, we are led either to suppose that fitness is reproductive success (cf. Howard (1979) who seems to use the two terms interchangeably) or by further slippage to suppose that fitness and adaptations in general are synonymous. That fitness is not the same as reproductive ability was noted by Dobzhansky (1970) who observed that a genotype in a completely lethal environment will have zero fitness even though it may be both viable and fertile. Reproductive success is a necessary but not a sufficient condition for fitness; indeed if 'inclusive fitness' (*sensu* Hamilton, 1964) has any force as an evolutionary factor, it may not even be a necessary condition.

Evolutionary biology and population genetics

We have, in the Darwinian equation, a statement with two distinct levels of explanation: first, the observable 'facts' are interpreted in terms of adaptations, and these adaptations are then interpreted in their turn in terms of fitness and the evolution of genes. This duality is perhaps not surprising. Owing to the length of time required to bring about genuine

---

* Some confusion is introduced here by the often colloquial use of the term fitness. Falconer (1960), for example, refers at one point to fitness as an accumulation of the individual's developmental and physiological processes (p. 332). This seems only to mean that it is a collection of adaptations. It is worth stressing, however, that geneticists in general do not always use population-genetic terminology with the same rigour as population geneticists: Falconer is writing primarily as an applied geneticist with the aim of providing a theoretical background to animal breeding experiments.

changes in gene frequency by selection, it is seldom possible to see evolution at work (though we may see phenotypic evidence that is consistent with such an interpretation, for example toe reduction in the equids or melanism in Kettlewell's (1961) moths). This, together with the fact that an important component is readily susceptible to mathematical analysis, has given rise to a divergence between the two component disciplines. While biologists have continued to remain interested mainly in the diversity of characters and their adaptive significance, population geneticists have been concerned primarily with the gene frequency changes themselves and the ways in which these occur as Mendelian (or neo-Mendelian) processes.

Nonetheless, there is an important sense in which the two concepts are closely related. If the Darwinian equation is to carry the full weight of Darwin's original notion, we find that adaptation only acquires its full *Darwinian* connotation when seen in the light of changes in gene frequencies. Indeed, the difficulty of explaining evolution on the basis of adaptation alone without recourse to an underlying genetic basis is indicated by the fact that Darwinism fell into disrepute towards the end of the last century because it lacked a convincing hereditary basis. It was only subsequently rescued from oblivion and re-established as a legitimate subject for study by serious scientists as late as the 1930s as a result of the developments that had in the meantime taken place quite independently in genetics (Huxley, 1942).

Fitness, on the other hand, is predicated on the existence of adaptations. Strictly speaking, fitness is a consequence of adaptation, but it is not a part of the notion of adaptation even though changes in gene frequency (i.e. increases in fitness) may result in the appearance of better-adapted populations. Such changes occur not because changes in fitness produce better adaptations (in individuals), but because those individuals that are less well adapted fail to contribute so often to the species' gene pool. The distinction turns on the two senses of 'adaptation' alluded to earlier.

If adaptations did not exist, then any changes that occurred in gene frequencies would not imply fitness in the Darwinian sense: rather, we would ascribe the changes in frequency to genetic drift, neutral mutations or some similar process operating outside of natural selection. In fact, in the unlikely event of adaptations being shown not to exist, population geneticists might be hard-pressed to talk about the Darwinian fitness of anything. This is not, however, to say that they would not be able to continue discussing population genetic models in exactly the same form as they do now. Population genetics is essentially a self-contained logico-deductive system, a fact that is made perfectly clear by Williams' (1970) successful axiomatisation of it. It thus bears the same relationship to biological phenomena as Newtonian mechanics or Euclidean geometry bear to the physical world. They are formal mathematical systems that happen (more or less) to describe real world phenomena. That the geometry of the universe is in fact Riemannian is not grounds for rejecting Euclidean geometry out of hand: to all intents and purposes, the world *is* rectilinear in so far as most everyday Euclidean applications are concerned. Precisely the same relationship holds in the case of population genetics: there is no necessary reason why there should have to be anything in the universe to which this particular system of equations applies. But, so long as they continue to yield useful predictions and can be modified to take account of anomalous observations without destroying their fundamental structure, then they serve a valuable heuristic function.

One further point emphasises the disjunction between the two disciplines. The theory of evolution by natural selection stands or falls by a demonstration of *both* adaptation and consequent (correlated) changes in gene frequencies. Disproof of the laws of population genetics would not constitute disproof of evolutionary explanations as a whole, but only disproof of evolutionary explanations of a particular kind. We would still be able to discuss adaptations, though we would be obliged to find an alternative explanation for their maintenance through time (for example, in terms of learning or perhaps Lamarckian inheritance). This observation underscores the point that the relationship between fitness and adaptation is not a simple one-to-one translation. Dobzhansky (1970) goes so far as to assert that we cannot draw inferences about fitness from a knowledge of adaptation, nor of adaptation from a knowledge of fitness. Indeed, Fisher (1930), in one of the first major works on population genetics, devotes only a few pages to a discussion of adaptation, while Wright (1969), in what is perhaps the major treatise on the subject, fails to mention the word even once, though he makes oblique reference to those facets of an organism that provide the underlying basis for differential gene production. For theoretical population genetic analyses, we need to know *only* that there is differential reproduction, not *why* it occurs.

Are Darwinian explanations circular?

The relationship between the concepts of adaptation and fitness might seem to confirm the worst fears of the anti-Darwinians. Each appears to depend on the other in a way that makes them virtually inseparable. It is, however, crucial to appreciate that they are not *definitionally* interdependent: adaptation is not *defined* in terms of fitness, nor vice versa. Adaptation (and hence reproductive success) is defined with reference to *individuals*, whereas fitness is defined with reference to genes and is thus a characteristic of populations. Although these two levels do bear an obvious relationship to each other, this relationship is probably only one-to-one in asexually reproducing species (and then only under limited circumstances). This point is highlighted by Prout's (1969) proof that an exact estimate of fitness requires a minimum of five generations (and probably more, depending on the number of parameters that have to be estimated from the pedigrees) in sexually reproducing species, but only one transition (i.e. two generations) in asexually reproducing species, *providing* all selection occurs within one generation. If selection is spread across several generations, then correspondingly more generations are required to obtain a valid estimate of fitness (Prout, 1965).

The crucial point is that each concept takes on a new *significance* when they are juxtaposed in the Darwinian formula. This is particularly easy to see in the case of adaptation. Things may be adapted for all manner of reasons: a hammer is adapted to hitting nails in precisely the same sense that an anteater's tongue is adapted to feeding on ants. The distinction between these two examples is that in the second we would wish to add a fitness-statement, whereas in the first we would not. By so doing, the two sentences acquire quite different implications, even though the uses of the term 'adaptation' in each sentence are in principle not only identical, but also remain essentially unchanged by whether or not we add a fitness-statement. What *is* altered is the *theoretical context within which they are to be interpreted*, and, as a consequence of this, we alter the implications that each statement carries. The second becomes a subject of interest to evolutionary biologists; the first remains of interest only to technologists and craftsmen.

What, however, are we to make of the relationship between adaptation and fitness in so far as each presupposes the existence of the other within the well-constructed Darwinian formula? Although it is clear that the two concepts are not defined circularly, the fact that they are interdependent for their wider significance (as opposed to definitional *meaning*) might still be taken as evidence of some kind of circularity, or at the very least of an inherent weakness in this direction.

Such a criticism can only be taken seriously if we ignore the quintessential nature of scientific theories. Theories (*qua* models of the universe) are inevitably built upon assumptions that, by tacit agreement among the practitioners, remain unchallenged and above proof (Kuhn, 1970; Lakatos, 1978). Were we to do otherwise, we would be forced to treat the sciences in linear order (and even that assumes that we could rise beyond more fundamental problems in the philosophy of science). As such, we operate within metaphysical systems that unavoidably colour our interpretation of the world by providing observed events with a significance that they do not in themselves otherwise possess (Feyerabend, 1963; Hamlyn, 1970; Harré, 1972). So much so, in fact, that the same set of 'facts' have often been given quite different interpretations by conflicting theories at times of crisis in science (for some examples in physics, see d'Abro, 1951). Theories provide a conceptual framework within which we operate, and this framework may presuppose as given more fundamental sciences.

The significance of this in the present context is that we do not need to recount in detail the full theory underlying the assumed element in evolutionary explanations. In other words, giving an explanation about how a biological adaptation works does not require us to recount the whole of population genetics theory. Instead, an explanation in terms of the adaptive significance of a trait raises a flag which, in effect, refers us to population genetics by implying that the evolutionary part of the account will have a detailed explanation along the lines suggested by population genetics. By the same token, a population-genetic argument about fitness raises a similar notional flag which refers us to the nature of biological adaptations.

It is worth pointing out here, perhaps, that population genetics makes similar kinds of assumptions about the relationship between Mendelian genes and the biochemistry of molecular genetics: the one is not *necessarily* related to the other in any kind of one-to-one relationship, nor can the one be reduced to the other (in the technical sense of theory reduction) (Hull, 1974). That population geneticists make explicit assumptions that cannot in a strict sense be reconciled with what we know of the biochemistry of heredity does not mean that we should dispense with population genetics altogether.

Some implications for sociobiological explanations

I have argued that much of the controversy over the supposedly tautological nature of evolutionary explanations is a consequence of an inadequate formulation of their structure. The distinction between adaptation and fitness has been drawn by, among others, Williams (1966), Hull (1974) and Thompson (1981). I have sought to make this distinction explicit with respect to the structure of Darwinian explanations and to place the argument in its broader context in order to show how the components relate to each other. In this section, I draw attention to some of the consequences of this distinction, with particular reference to sociobiological explanations (though the points apply equally to all evolutionary explanations). These consequences are mainly in the form of logical traps for the unwary: they are not necessarily inevitable, but they are, I believe, commonly perpetrated (albeit unintentionally) and may result in serious error if pursued beyond legitimate bounds.

The gene as metaphor

Sociobiological arguments are commonly phrased in terms of genes, these often being ascribed intentional or purposive-like characteristics (e.g. the 'selfish gene', Dawkins, 1976). Such statements are essentially metaphorical in that, by providing a familiar analogy or a simple means of expression, we capture the essence of a complex phenomenon and are thereby able to come to grips with it more easily. The use of metaphor is common practice even in the most theoretical disciplines. In physics, for example, the elementary particles known as quarks are ascribed properties such as *colour*, *strangeness* and *beauty* which are collectively known as *flavours* (Mulvey, 1979), but these terms are not taken literally by particle physicists.

So long as we remain clear about the metaphorical status of these terms, they serve a valuable psychological function. The practice becomes problematic only when the practitioners begin to confuse the metaphor with the real world. This, of course, is not a new problem for, in so far as all theories ultimately possess only metaphorical status, the history of science is littered with instances in which the real world and the theory have been confused. Newtonian physics itself is the paradigm example (d'Abro, 1951).

The term 'gene' is used in four quite different senses by geneticists, none of which can be intertranslated without difficulty (Whitehouse, 1973). Since sociobiology follows population-genetic usage in defining genes as units of selection, they assume a genetic basis for behaviour though the actual biochemistry of inheritance is seldom (if ever) known. Moreover, the models used invariably assume single-locus effects, even though few biological phenomena owe their origin to a single gene (Wright, 1969; Whitehouse, 1973). This need not necessarily be a serious problem: population genetics has, after all survived the better part of a century on similar assumptions. Nonetheless, we should exercise caution in making unnecessarily naive assumptions when generating predictions to be tested in the field, the more so when the test relates to the adaptiveness of characters and is thus one step removed from the changes in gene frequency to which the models actually refer. Such models are not meant for testing in the conventional sense: rather, they are meant to assess the plausibility of a specific explanation (see below).

It is, perhaps, worth adding in this context, that a metaphorical use of the term 'fitness' as a generic shorthand to refer to an individual's reproductive and/or survival abilities is likewise quite admissible. In making such a statement, we usually make implicit *ceteris paribus* (i.e. 'other things being equal') assumptions about the relationship between adaptations and fitness. A problem arises only when subtle shifts in usage give a false sense of legitimacy to conclusions drawn from data. There is little to be gained from false claims to theoretical authenticity other than confusion, though it would be a pity to discourage a useful shorthand for this reason alone.

At this point, we might ask whether it is necessary to make any assumptions *at all* about an underlying genetic basis. In so far as the notion of adaptation makes no presumptions about the ontogenetic origins of the adapted character, the answer will probably be in the negative. Although a heritability assumption is given in the second premiss of the well-formulated Darwinian explanation on page 11, strictly speaking this does not necessarily imply genetic inheritance (hence the parentheses round the qualifier 'genetically'). Nonetheless, if Darwinian explanations are to mean what they say, then the final fitness-statement implies that either there must be a genetic basis or, at the very least, whatever non-genetically inherited adaptations occur must have predictable consequences for future gene frequencies. In this sense, it is reasonable to suppose that a genetically programmed ability to make (flexible) behavioural decisions that have the ultimate consequence of influencing fitness would be selected for, even though the behaviour itself was not being actively selected in the genic sense. This notion of programming for adaptability does raise a major conceptual issue, namely what is the basis on which the animal makes its decision.

Levels of explanation

The purposive-like 'behaviour' of genes can lead to more serious problems when the distinction between adaptation and fitness is blurred. In this event, animals (and more especially humans) may get credited with the ability to choose their lifetime strategies deliberately in order to maximise their fitness (see Durham, 1979). Such an interpretation is plausible precisely because even animals can legitimately be viewed as choosing behaviours that allow them to achieve specific biological objectives, including, for example, feeding in order to feel less hungry or mating in order to satisfy sexual needs. These specific objectives are, naturally, correlated with fitness and will surely have a more or less direct effect on changes in gene frequency over time. But this fact is not evidence that animals (or even humans) deliberately seek to maximise their *fitness.*

The case of reproductive success is perhaps the most obviously confusing, since reproduction has the most direct bearing on fitness. To confuse these two, however, is to commit the most serious of all category mistakes in the form of a confusion of levels of explanation (in this case, proximate and ultimate explanations). As Tinbergen (1963) has pointed out, biologists can ask four quite different kinds of causal questions about a given biological phenomenon, each demanding an explanation at a different conceptual level, and all of which may be asked and answered simultaneously without conflict. In the present context, we may ask quite legitimate questions about (a) how a character has evolved in a phylogenetic sense, (b) why it has evolved in an adaptive (functional) sense, (c) what motivational mechanisms make that adaptation possible, and (d) how it has evolved in the sense that some genetic process underlies it. Each of these questions may be relevant and important, and, although sociobiologists will in general be concerned mainly with (b) and (c), only with respect of (c) is there likely to be any cognitive content to the answer.

Heuristical traps

Williams (1966) argued that biologists should concentrate on the problem of function (or 'teleonomy' as he termed it) and not on the question of evolution *per se*: 'The central biological problem', he wrote, 'is not survival as such, but *design for survival*' (my italics). Birch & Ehrlich (1967) made a similar plea for greater emphasis on the biology in connection with the excessive evolutionary content of ecology in the 1960s. They argued that field biologists should concentrate more of their attention on the immediate factors influencing a species' numbers, and less on speculations as to how any such adaptations might have evolved.

The problem is that fitness-oriented questions will tend to encourage an emphasis on outcomes and a concomitant tendency to ignore the complex chain of events that gives rise to these behavioural end-products. This is not of itself necessarily serious, providing the biology is sufficiently well understood to permit the right end-product to be identified (though in practice this is probably rarely the case). The real problem is that several different mechanisms might give rise to the same predicted outcome, with the consequent risk that a match between observed predicted outcomes will be assumed to be proof of the validity of the theory ostensibly being tested. Strictly speaking, we are only entitled to conclude that the theory in question has not been excluded as a possible explanatory candidate. Examples of cases in which different theoretical explanations yield indistinguishable outcomes are by no means uncommon in biology. They include such cases as learned versus genetically determined changes in behaviour (Pringle, 1951) and density-dependent versus frequency-dependent selection (Clarke, 1972), while, on a finer scale, Seyfarth (1977) has offered an elegant demonstration that the same distribution of grooming partnerships would result among female monkeys whether they chose their partners on the basis of kin selection or in order to promote the formation of defensive coalitions to their own personal advantage.

Distinguishing between possible explanations for an observed phenomenon will invariably require us to understand in detail the biological mechanisms that brought the phenomenon about. In this respect, the sophistical desert into which Learning Theory was driven in the 1940s and 1950s precisely because researchers assumed the theory and ignored the biology should stand as a cautionary tale (see for example Thompson, 1981).

In a more recent case, Kurland (1977) set out to test the relevance of Hamilton's theory of kin selection to primate behaviour by examining the distribution of certain theoretically relevant behaviours. One of these was grooming, which was taken to be altruistic on the grounds that a benefit was conferred on the recipient. Hamilton's (1964) theory, however, demanded that altruistic actions also incur a cost to the performer: having committed himself to the altruism of grooming, Kurland was forced to speculate as to the possible costs of grooming. In so doing, he not only ignored the many positive gains to the performer (for example, in terms of coalition formation: see Seyfarth, 1977, 1980; Dunbar, 1980), but was also led to attribute costs to the behaviour which will not merit close biological scrutiny.

Emphasis on evolutionary considerations as a guiding principle may thus result in research questions being formulated to emphasise supposed correlates of fitness that may not be relevant to the actual biological significance of the phenomenon under study. To the extent that biological questions are questions about adaptation, those phrased in terms of fitness and its immediate correlates may lead to a misinterpretation of the biological phenomena whenever these are concerned with solving a logically prior problem that is not directly correlated with fitness in the way presumed. Animals may be prepared to trade some loss of efficiency in terms of immediate biological problems for longer-term gains in overall reproductive output (Dunbar, 1980).

Ceteris paribus *traps*

If we make a prediction based on some theoretical argument, but the data do not support the prediction, we may conclude either that the theory is wrong or that the behavioural measure chosen was an inappropriate test, but we have no good grounds for preferring one explanation rather than the other. This situation will inevitably tend to encourage either rubrics of the kind 'Accept the result if it fits your expectations; search for a "better" behavioural measure if it does not' or a resort to *ad hoc* attempts to explain away anomalous results through the invocation of confounding variables. More often than not, this reflects a state of ignorance about the underlying biology, combined with a 'super-Kuhnian' reluctance to dispense with the theory at all. The inevitable historical component in both evolutionary and adaptationist explanations makes this problem especially acute.

We might, for example, want to test predictions about the fitness of males of different sizes, and we might take the number of females to which the male controls access as an adequate index of his reproductive output. Choice of such an index obviously assumes that a great many other things are equal (for example, that females do not interfere adversely with each other's fecundability as their density increases, that the survivorship of males is not inversely related to harem size, that harem size is not a function of a male's age, and so on). Although Howard (1979) found that a variety of indices of seasonal reproductive success in bullfrogs correlated well with the actual number of hatchlings produced, the correlations were by no means perfect. In such circumstances, the researcher is obliged to rely on hope that the effect under investigation is large enough to swamp any errors in measurement. *A fortiori*, even though short-term indices of reproductive success may correlate well with each other, we have no guarantee that seasonal reproductive output will bear any consistent relationship to lifetime reproductive success. Seasonal reproductive success will be a reasonable estimate of lifetime reproductive success if, *and only if*, survivorship is not negatively correlated with seasonal reproductive success *and* reproductive success does not vary consistently with age. If the fact of obtaining high seasonal success imposes a high cost on the male (due to, say, increased risk of dying while fighting), then males with very low seasonal success could in principle gain as high a lifetime output as the seasonally most successful males (Gadgil, 1972; Dunbar, 1982). Similarly, if instantaneous (or seasonal) reproductive success varies in any way consistently with age, then *all* males will achieve approximately the same net lifetime output despite wide variation among males during any one season. Beyond this, the relationship to fitness remains unfathomable.

It may be worth pointing out in conclusion that *ceteris paribus* clauses are a normal component of all scientific disciplines, from physics to biology. The problem is not that biology is unusual in this respect, but rather that such clauses are more obtrusive in the life sciences.

Prediction versus postdiction

Scriven (1959) has argued that evolutionary biology is necessarily postdictive rather than predictive, these being regarded as two equally legitimate ways of going about science. There is much to be said for this view, but we do need to differentiate between at least three different kinds of predictions that evolutionary biologists might be tempted to make. First, we might wish to make predictions about the future course of evolution (i.e. future gene frequency changes); second, we might wish to predict the morphology or behaviour of a species about which we had some (limited) background knowledge together with some general (statistical) principles relating the relevant variables; and third, we might wish to predict the behaviour of an animal on a particular occasion, given a good deal of knowledge about the animal's biology together with some theoretical rules thought to govern the particular behaviour in question.

There can be little doubt that predictions of the first kind are vacuous, since future gene frequency changes necessarily depend on the degree of environmental stability in the future, and this can never be known with any certainty. The best we could do, therefore, is to make predictions that are so heavily festooned with *ceteris paribus* clauses that we would never know in the event of a mismatch whether the theory was at fault or whether one of the *ceteris paribus* clauses had failed.

Predictions of the second type might at first sight seem more likely candidates for a predictive biology. However, even predictions in this sense can only be at best trivial (i.e. predictions *can* be made, but without any real justification for supposing that they are much better than random guesses). This is a consequence of the historical component that necessarily makes every species unique because it has evolved under its own peculiar set of conditions. Although it is possible to generate general rules relating sets of environmental variables to sets of organismic variables, these rules are necessarily statistical. Consequently, it will seldom be possible to predict with any precision where on the graph any one particular species will lie, since a large variety of other factors may result in deviations from predicted values. This much is evident from the often large variance round regression lines in eco-correlate analyses (see for example Clutton-Brock & Harvey, 1977*a*, *b*). Statistical rules can only be tested against other distributions, though even here it remains unclear whether we would in fact be in a position to assert that the biological assumptions demanded by the hypotheses were precisely fulfilled for any given taxon. The folly of this situation is underlined by the fact that strict adherence to Popperian principles would require us to reject what might actually be a perfectly sound hypothesis simply because one species operated on a different set of rules (though there are good grounds for believing that Popper's principles are far too strict: see Lee, 1969; Lakatos, 1978).

In practice, most explanations of this kind are necessarily postdictive. This is not a resort to *ad hoc* explanations (*pace* Lewontin, 1979), but rather recognition that 'predictions' of this type are not predictions at all, but historical explanations in disguise (see also Lee, 1969). Historical explanations should not be confused with historical descriptions: postdictive explanations seek to make sense of the observed phenomena by attempting to provide an account of why they have evolved to the state they have in the light of our current understanding of evolutionary processes using the rules and generalisations then available.*

The final possibility is less ambitious since it asks simply whether sensible predictions can be made about the behaviour of individual organisms under specific conditions in the light of specifiable evolutionary rules. In such cases we might, for example, assess the extent to which animals conformed to predictions derived from certain optimality criteria, these being presumed to underlie the particular evolutionary process relevant to the situation in hand (e.g. Maynard Smith, 1978). In this sense, it is quite legitimate to argue that biologists make predictions, even though they are not evolutionary predictions of the kind that would usually be associated with Darwinian theory. Nonetheless, they derive from evolutionary theory in that they are set firmly into a Darwinian framework. As such, they are not tests of that framework as a whole, but they do test components of it that may subsequently have to be modified or rejected in the light of the results. In other words, we test specific hypotheses about the way in which animals are adapted, while assuming that those that are better adapted will have higher fitness (i.e. that their genes will come to dominate in due course). It is important to note that we are able to make *bona fide* predictions in this case precisely because we are dealing with adaptations and not

---

*There is a longstanding belief among scientists in general that predictive explanations are somehow more powerful than postdictive explanations, even though this view has long since been abandoned by philosophers of science because it presupposes an asymmetry between observation and explanation that cannot be shown to be logically necessary (see for example Lakatos, 1978).

with fitness, a possibility that would clearly be lost if these two concepts were definitionally equivalent.

Summary

1. A proper formulation of Darwinian explanations shows that there are two quite distinct explanatory components, namely statements about adaptations and statements about gene frequency changes (i.e. fitness). Conflation of these two concepts has in the past led to accusations of tautological reasoning.
2. The biologist's task lies in understanding the nature of adaptations, while the evolutionary problem of fitness changes is properly the domain of population geneticists. The two domains are mutually dependent in that each provides the theoretical context or rationale for the other.
3. Failure to distinguish clearly between these components may result in a number of unnecessary errors being perpetrated. These are mainly of two kinds: those that make excessive claims about the significance of observations, and those that attempt to make predictive tests that are quite inappropriate.

I am indebted to Nicholas Thompson for first drawing my attention to this issue many years ago. This paper has benefitted from a great many discussions with both him and my other colleagues at Bristol University (Department of Psychology) and, more recently, my colleagues at Cambridge. The paper was written while I was in receipt of a Science Research Council (UK) Advanced Fellowship.

References

Birch, L.C. & Ehrlich, P.R. (1967). Evolutionary history and population biology. *Nature, London*, **214**, 349–52.

Brady, R.H. (1979), Natural selection and the criteria by which a theory is judged. *Systematic Zoology*, **28**, 600–21.

Cavalli-Sforza, L.L. & Bodmer, W.F. (1961). *The Genetics of Human Populations*. San Francisco: Freeman.

Clarke, B. (1972). Density-dependent selection. *American Naturalist*, **106**, 1–13.

Clutton-Brock, T.H. & Harvey, P.H. (1977a). Primate ecology and social organisation. *Journal of Zoology, London*, **183**, 1–39.

Clutton-Brock, T.H. & Harvey, P.H. (1977b). Species differences in feeding and ranging behaviour in primates. In *Primate Ecology*, ed. T.H. Clutton-Brock, pp. 557–84. Academic Press: London.

Clutton-Brock, T.H. & Harvey, P.H. (1979). Comparison and adaptation. *Proceedings of the Royal Society, London*, B, **205**, 547–65.

Connolly, K. (1966). A comment on papers by Mr. Manser and Professor Flew. *Philosophy*, **41**, 356–7.

Crow, J.F. & Kimura, M. (1970). *An Introduction to Population Genetics Theory*. Harper and Row: New York.

d'Abro, A. (1951). *The Rise of the New Physics, its Mathematical and Physical Theories.* Dover: New York.

Darwin, C.H. (1859). *The Origin of Species.* Murray: London.

Dawkins, R. (1976). *The Selfish Gene.* Oxford University Press: Oxford.

Dobzhansky, T. (1970). *The Genetics of the Evolutionary Process.* Columbia University Press: New York.

Dunbar, R.I.M. (1980) Determinants and evolutionary consequences of dominance among female gelada baboons. *Behavioural Ecology and Sociobiology,* **7,** 253–65.

Dunbar, R.I.M. (1982). Intraspecific variations in mating strategy. In *Perspectives in Ethology,* vol. **5,** ed. P.G. Bateson & P.H. Klopter. New York: Plenum Press.

Durham, W.H. (1979). Towards a coevolutionary theory of human biology and culture. In *Evolutionary Biology and Human Social Behaviour: an Anthropological Perspective,* ed. N.A. Chagnon & W. Irons, PP.39–59. Duxbury Press: North Scituate, Mass.

Falconer, D.S. (1960). *Introduction to Quantitative Genetics.* Longmans: London.

Feyerabend, P.J. (1963). How to be a good empiricist – a plea for tolerance in matters epistemological. In *Philosophy of Science, the Delaware Seminar,* vol. **2,** ed. B. Baumrin, pp.3–39. Interscience Publishers: New York.

Fisher, R.A. (1930). *The Genetical Theory of Natural Selection.* Clarendon Press: Oxford.

Gadgil, M. (1972). Male dimorphism as a consequence of sexual selection. *American Naturalist,* **106,** 574–80.

Ghiselin, M.T. (1966). On semantic pitfalls of biological adaptation. *Philosophy of Science,* **33,** 147–53.

Hamilton, W.D. (1964). The genetical theory of social behaviour, I, II, *Journal of Theoretical Biology,* **7,** 1–52.

Hamlyn, D.W. (1970). *The Theory of Knowledge.* Macmillan: London.

Harré, R. (1972). *The Philosophies of Science.* Oxford University Press: Oxford.

Howard, R.D. (1979). Estimating reproductive success in natural populations. *American Naturalist,* **114,** 221–31.

Hull, D.L. (1974). *Philosophy of Biological Science.* Prentice – Hall: Englewood Cliffs, N.J.

Huxley, J.S. (1942). *Evolution: The Synthetic Theory.* Allen and Unwin: London.

Kettlewell, H.B.C. (1961). The phenomenon of industrial melanism in Lepidoptera. *Annual Review of Entomology,* **6,** 245–62.

Kuhn, T.S. (1970). *The Structure of Scientific Revolutions.* University of Chicago Press: Chicago.

Kurland, J.A. (1977). *Kin Selection in Japanese Monkeys.* Contributions to Primatology, vol. **12.** Karger: Basel.

Lakatos, I. (1978). *The Methodology of Scientific Research Programmes.* Cambridge University Press: Cambridge.

Lee, K.K. (1969). Popper's falsifiability and Darwin's natural selection. *Philosophy,* **44,** 291–302.

Lewontin, R.C. (1978). Adaptation. *Scientific American,* **239,** 157–69.

Lewontin, R.C. (1979). Sociobiology as an adaptationist program. *Behavioural Science,* **24,** 5–14.

Manser, A.R. (1965). The concept of evolution. *Philosophy,* **40,** 18–34.

Maynard Smith, J. (1969). The status of neo-Darwinism. In *Towards a Theoretical Biology,* vol. **3,** ed. C.H. Waddington, pp.82–9. Edingburgh University Press: Edinburgh.

Maynard Smith, J. (1978). Optimization theory in evolution. *Annual Review of Ecology and Systematics,* **9,** 31–56.

Mulvey, J. (1979). The new frontier of particle physics. *Nature, London,* **278,** 403–9.

Peters, R.H. (1976). Tautology in evolution and ecology. *American Naturalist,* **110,** 1–12.

Popper, K.R. (1972). *Objective Knowledge: An Evolutionary Approach.* Clarendon Press: Oxford.

Pringle, J.W.S. (1951). On the parallel between learning and evolution. *Behaviour*, **3**, 174–215.

Prout, T. (1965). The estimation of fitnesses from genotypic frequencies. *Evolution*, **19**, 546–51.

Prout, T. (1969). The estimation of fitnesses from population data. *Genetics*, **63**, 949–67.

Ricklefs, R.E. (1973). *Ecology*. Nelson: London.

Ruse, M. (1973). *The Philosophy of Biology*. London: Hutchinson.

Scriven, M. (1959). Explanation and prediction in evolutionary theory. *Science*, **130**, 477–82.

Seyfarth, R.M. (1977). A model of social grooming among adult female monkeys. *Journal of Theoretical Biology*, **65**, 671–98.

Seyfarth, R.M. (1980). The distribution of grooming and related behaviours among adult female vervet monkeys. *Animal Behaviour*, **28**, 798–813.

Smart, J.J.C. (1963). *Philosophy and Scientific Realism*. Routledge Kegan Paul: London.

Thompson, N.S. (1981). Towards a falsifiable theory of evolution. In *Perspectives in Ethology*, vol. **4**, ed. P.P.G. Bateson & P.H. Klopfer, pp. 51–73. Plenum Press: New York.

Tinbergen, N. (1963). On the aims and methods of ethology. *Zeitschrift für Tierpsychologie*, **20**, 410–33.

Whitehouse, H.L.K. (1973). *Towards an Understanding of the Mechanism of Heredity*. Arnold: London.

Williams, G.C. (1966). *Adaptation and Natural Selection*. Princeton University Press: Princeton, N.J.

Williams, M.B. (1970). Deducing the consequences of evolution: a mathematical model. *Journal of Theoretical Biology*, **29**, 343–85.

Wilson, E.O. (1975). *Sociobiology: The New Synthesis*. Belknap Press: Cambridge, Mass.

Wilson, E.O. & Bossert, W.H. (1971). *A Primer of Population Biology*. Sinauer: Sunderland, Mass.

Wright, S. (1968). *Evolution and the Genetics of Populations*, vol. 1, *Genetic and Biometric Foundations*. University of Chicago Press: Chicago.

Wright, S. (1969). *Evolution and the Genetics of Populations*, vol. 2, *The Theory of Gene Frequencies*. University of Chicago Press: Chicago.

2

The evolution of social behaviour – a classification of models

J. MAYNARD SMITH

By an 'altruistic' trait is meant a trait which, in some sense, lowers the fitness of the individual displaying it, but increases the fitness of some other members of the same species. A number of qualitatively different processes have been proposed whereby genes determining such traits can increase in frequency. This essay attempts two things. First, I propose a classification of these processes, and second, I discuss different ways in which one of them, kin selection, can be modelled mathematically.

A classification of mechanisms

The purpose of classifying mechanisms is as follows. Different mechanisms depend on different assumptions about population structure, and also about the way in which selection is acting. A classification should bring out these differences as clearly as possible, so that the possible relevance of the various mechanisms to particular cases is likewise made clear.

My first attempt at a classification (Maynard Smith, 1964) aimed at distinguishing a process which Wynne Edwards (1962) had proposed to explain the regulation of animal numbers and which he called 'group selection', and a process proposed by Hamilton (1964) to explain the evolution of social behaviour. I suggested the term 'kin selection' for the latter in the hope that the existence of two terms would help to distinguish two processes which seemed to me quite different. The essential difference between them is that the former requires the existence of groups (demes) which are in large measure reproductively isolated from one another, whereas the latter can operate in a single random-mating population provided that relatives interact.

Since that time, two things have happened which force a reconsideration of that classification. The first is that new processes have been suggested which are qualitatively different from either of the two above. These include Trivers'(1971) suggestion of 'reciprocal altruism', and a process which might be called 'synergistic selection' or 'trait-group selection' – i.e. that the fitness of all the members of a temporary (non-reproductive) group increases with the proportion of altruists in the group (Wilson, 1975; Matessi & Jayakar, 1976). The latter process differs from reciprocal altruism in that it does not depend on learning or memory, and from group selection as understood by Wynne Edwards and described in my 1964 paper in that it does not require reproductively isolated groups.

The second reason for requiring a new classification is a semantic one. Several authors, notably Wilson (1975) and Uyenoyama (1979) have used the term 'group selection' to describe models in which no reproductively isolated groups occur (and, in Wilson's case, in which no groups even of a temporary nature need occur). This seems to me a pity. but it cannot be undone. The only way now to avoid hopeless semantic confusion is to abandon the term 'group selection' altogether, or to use it only with some qualifying word (e.g. trait-group selection, group-extinction selection) which will make clear which of several wholly different mechanisms is intended.

I think it is useful to distinguish the following processes:

(1) *Individual selection.* Not involving selection for altruistic traits.
(2) *Interdemic selection.* Reproductively isolated groups exist: A depending on differential production of migrants (Wright, 1945); B depending on group extinction (Wynne Edwards, 1962).
(3) *Kin selection.* Reproductively isolated groups need not exist, but interactions occur between relatives (Hamilton, 1964).
(4) *Synergistic selection.* Interactions occur between non-relatives (Cohen & Eshel, 1976; Wilson, 1975; Matessi & Jayakar, 1976).
(5) *Reciprocal altruism* (Trivers, 1971).

Particular models may include more than one of these processes; for example, the models of Wilson (1975) and Matessi & Jayakar (1976) include processes (3) and (4).

Individual selection

Hamilton (1971) pointed out that animal aggregates could arise if each individual behaves so as to reduce its own chances of being taken by a predator, even if the result of aggregation was to increase the total rate of predation. In such cases, apparently social behaviour is explained solely in terms of individual advantage.

Alexander (1974) has suggested that eusocial behaviour may have evolved by 'parental manipulation'. That is, offspring behave in an apparently altruistic manner because their behaviour is controlled by their parents. If altruistic acts between sibs increase the number of surviving reproductives, genes in the mother causing such behaviour will spread. However, models of this process should also take into account selection on genes expressed in the offspring; if so, kin selection is also relevant (Craig, 1979).

In treating parental manipulation as an example of individual and not of kin selection, it will be apparent that I am distinguishing between actions which ensure the survival of an individual's own offspring and those ensuring the survival of collateral relatives. I recognise that there are advantages in emphasising the similarity between these two processes, but on balance it seemed to me better to separate them in the above classification.

Interdemic selection

This term was used by Wright to describe a component of his 'shifting balance' theory of evolution, first proposed fifty years ago (Wright, 1931) and recently summarised in Wright (1970). Although he was not primarily concerned with the evolution of altruistic traits, it will be helpful briefly to summarise his ideas.

His starting point was the existence of separate 'adaptive peaks' separated by 'valleys'. The essence of this idea can be stated for a haploid with two loci (although Wright did not imagine that adaptive peaks were separated only by alleles at two loci). Suppose that the present state of a population is ab, but that the genotype AB would be superior (i.e. a higher adaptive peak). If genotypes Ab and aB are inferior to ab, a large random-mating population could never make the transition $ab \rightarrow AB$. However, if the species is subdivided into a number of small and partially isolated populations, the transition can occur. One population will make the transition by chance. Then, by virtue of the greater fitness of AB genotypes, this one population will send out more migrants than others, and these migrants will increase the probability that other local populations will evolve to AB.

The relevance of Wright's model has been much debated, partly because it is uncertain how often evolving populations have to cross adaptive valleys, and partly because no detailed mathematical analysis of the proposed crossing of an adaptive valley has been undertaken. The nearest is perhaps Lande's (1979) analysis of the establishment of a chromosome translocation which is deleterious when heterozygous. Lande supposes that the new structure is fixed in a single deme by genetic drift, and then in the species by random extinction and splitting of demes.

Later, in a review of Simpson's *Tempo and Mode in Evolution*, Wright (1945) suggested that his model could explain the spread of an altruistic trait determined by alleles at a single locus. His model is shown in Fig. 2.1*a*. The idea is that a gene *A*, for 'altruism', would be replaced by its allele *a* by natural selection within a single group, but that the number of migrants produced by a group increases with the frequency of allele *A* in that group. If *A* is to increase in frequency, there must be differences in the frequency of *A* in different groups. Wright argued that such differences would arise by chance if the groups were small enough. He also argued that the process required that the rate of migration be low, but it is not clear why he thought so.

Wright did not give a mathematical analysis of his model in his 1945 review. Uyenoyama (1979) has recently analysed what she refers to as Wright's model. However, she does so only for a case in which 100% of individuals migrate to join a random-mating pool in every generation. Thus no 'demes' in Wright's sense of the word exist in her model, which turns out to be a variant of a model, discussed below, by Matessi & Jayakar (1976).

It is not clear whether or in what circumstances a model of the kind shown in Fig. 2.1*a* could lead to the spread of a gene for altruism. I suspect that the conditions would be extremely severe. In particular, it is worth pointing out that the conditions would be more severe than for Wright's shifting balance model for the establishment of an inversion or translocation. Thus in the latter cases, once a deme has crossed the valley to a new peak, *AB*, it is proof against invasion by *ab* migrants. In contrast, a deme which is wholly *A* can be converted back to *a* by a single *a* immigrant.

One way in which interdemic selection models can be altered so as to make the spread of an altruistic gene more likely is by introducing periodic extinction of demes, and their replacement by the splitting of existing demes, or by a few founders from existing demes (Fig. 2.1*b*). If demes with a high proportion of *A* alleles are less likely to go extinct, or more likely to provide the founders of new demes, this will favour the spread of *A*. Models of this kind have been analysed mathematically by Maynard Smith (1964), Levins (1970), Boorman & Levitt (1973), Levin & Kilmer (1974), Gilpin (1975) and Eshel (1972), and experimentally by Wade (1977). The general conclusion is that such models can lead to the spread of altruistic genes, but only if there exist demes with very little genetic interchange, which either are of small size or arise from a few founders.

Fig. 2.1. Population structure for different models of the evolution of altruism. *a*, interdemic selection depending on differential migration; *b*, interdemic selection depending on group extinction; *c*, synergistic selection.

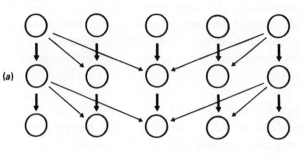

(a)

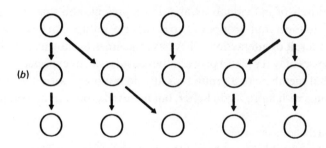

(b)

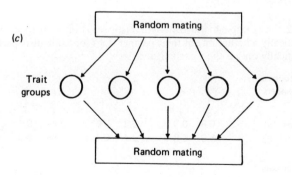

(c)

Trait groups

Kin selection

Hamilton (1964), building on earlier suggestions by Fisher (1930) and Haldane (1932), argued that genes determining altruistic traits can increase in frequency if the interacting individuals are genetically related. An essential difference between this process and those discussed above is that kin selection can be effective in a random-mating population provided that relatives interact with one another. Models of kin-selection are discussed later.

Synergistic selection

I now turn to models in which there is no reproductive isolation between demes, and no genetic relationship between interacting individuals (Fig. 2.1c). However, selection is supposed to act on groups of interacting individuals – 'trait groups' in Wilson's (1975) terminology.

The essential features of such models are illustrated in Fig. 2.2a. Suppose that two kinds of individuals, A and a, are present, and that they assort randomly to form trait-groups of two (of course, groups can be larger than this). As a result of interactions, they have the fitnesses shown in the figure; these fitnesses may represent probabilities of survival, or expected breeding success, but members of a group typically do not breed with one another. Thus groups with more As do better, but in mixed groups as do better than As.

Three conclusions emerge:

(i) It is possible for As to be fitter on average than as. Thus if A and a are equally frequent, as shown, then 2.2 A individuals survive out of 4, but only 2 a individuals out of 4. It is easy to choose fitness values which have this consequence.

Fig. 2.2. An example to illustrate synergistic selection. a, altruists perform altruistically whether or not their partner does so; b, altruists perform altruistically only if their partner does so.

Trait groups of two members	A	A	A	a	a	a
	↓	↓	↓	↓	↓	↓
Fitnesses (a)	0.8	0.8	0.3	0.6	0.4	0.4
(b)	0.8	0.8	0.4	0.4	0.4	0.4
No. of groups if $p(A) = \frac{1}{2}$		1		2		1
No. of groups if $p(A) = p \ll 1$		0		$2p$		$1 - 2p$

(ii) The system is frequency-dependent. Thus when A is rare, A is less fit than a. As Charlesworth (1979) has pointed out, this leads to difficulties in accounting for the initial spread of genes for altruism in randomly assorting groups. Matessi & Jayakar (1976) do describe cases in which A increases when rare, but these are cases in which the fitness of a single A individual in an otherwise a group is higher than that of a individuals in all-a groups, although lower than the as in its own group.

(iii) Groups must be small. If groups are large and randomly formed, all will have the same proportion of A, so that the only selective effect will be the superiority of a within groups.

All these conclusions were drawn by Matessi & Jayakar (1976); a similar model was analysed by Cohen & Eshel (1976). Wilson (1975) considered a more restricted model of the way individuals interact. He supposed that each A individual acted so as to alter its own fitness by d and that of each other member of the group by r. If trait-groups are randomly formed, it is at once obvious that, whatever the initial frequencies, A will increase in frequency if d is positive and decrease if d is negative. The value of r is irrelevant, because a change in fitness to a random sample of the population cannot alter which of two genotypes is fitter. Indeed, as shown in Fig. 2.3, for this model there is no need to think of 'groups', but only of interactions between neighbours. Thus the random-assortment version of Wilson's model seems to me best regarded as a case of individual selection; Wilson prefers to see it as a case of group selection, because altruists may be less fit than non-altruists in the same trait group, and yet may increase in frequency in the population as a whole.

It is implicit in Fig. 2.2a that in a mixed trait group the non-altruists benefit to some extent from the actions of the altruists. However, this need not be so. The benefits may accrue only when both members of a pair act cooperatively, as in Fig. 2.2b. This could happen either because potential altruists have the intelligence to cease acting altruistically if their acts are not reciprocated, or because benefits require the cooperation of both partners. Obviously, with the fitnesses of Fig. 2.2b, type A always increases. However, the initial rate of increase would be slow unless, through kinship or other reasons, the rare A individuals were brought together more often than would happen by chance.

Fitnesses of the kind shown in Fig. 2.2a, capable of favouring altruism in randomly formed trait-groups, cannot be generated by the scheme of a cost $(-d)$ to each donor and a corresponding gain $(+r)$ to each recipient. The essential feature is that the gain to a pair (or larger group) of interacting altruists is greater than would be predicted from the interaction of an altruist and a non-altruist. For this reason I have suggested the term 'synergistic selection'. The familiar term 'mutualism' may be a better alternative, but in ecology its use has been confined to interactions between members of different species.

Both Matessi & Jayakar (1976) and Wilson (1975) considered what will happen if members of a trait-group are genetically similar, and concluded that this would favour the spread of genes for altruism. If, as would usually be the case, the genetic similarity is a consequence of kinship, this is a straightforward case of kin selection. Wilson points out (as had Hamilton) that there could be genetic similarity for other reasons – for example, membership of a trait group might depend on genetically determined habitat choice or survival of particular selective events. However, this would affect the frequency of the gene A only if the same gene had pleiotropic effects both on altruism and on trait group membership, which does not seem very likely.

Uyenoyama (1979) starts with a model resembling Fig. 2.1a, but sets the migration parameter to unity so that all individuals migrate, ending with a

Fig. 2.3. A model of 'trait-group selection'. 'Ego' is a typical individual carrying gene A, and acts so as to increase his own fitness by d and the fitness of his neighbours by r. Provided his neighbours are a random sample of the population, gene A will increase provided d is positive. The value of r is irrelevant. No 'groups' need exist, since the population can be continuously distributed.

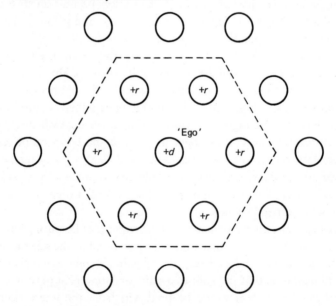

model essentially similar to that of Matessi & Jayakar. She allows the frequency of the gene A to vary between groups either because of small group size, or because selection acts on the A locus differentially between groups; drift proves to be the more important factor unless the variance of selection is large.

Reciprocal altruism

Trivers (1971) points out that if there are repeated opportunities for interaction between the same individuals, then an individual which helps only those which help it in return will be favoured by selection. Such reciprocal altruism can evolve only if the same individuals meet repeatedly, if they are capable of learning and memory, and if the benefits to the individual which is helped are large compared to the costs to the helper. Given these conditions, reciprocal altruism can be evolutionarily stable (see Fig. 2.4).

Of the various processes discussed, interdemic selection seems unlikely to be important, because it depends on very special assumptions about population structure (Maynard Smith, 1976). However, I have argued elsewhere (Maynard Smith, 1978a) that an extreme form of interdemic selection, where 'demes' are represented by species and parthenogenetic varieties, may have played a role in the maintenance of sexual reproduction.

Kin selection is bound to operate wherever relatives interact. It is now widely believed to have been important in the origin of social behaviour both in vertebrates and insects and is relevant to the evolution even of plants (Mirmirani & Oster, 1978) and prokaryotes (Maynard Smith,

Fig. 2.4. A payoff matrix for Trivers' (1971) concept of reciprocal altruism. S is always selfish, A is always altruistic and R is altruistic only to those which are altruistic to it. d is the cost and r the benefit of an interaction. Payoffs are to an individual adopting the strategy on the left against the strategy above. Provided $r > d$, R is an ESS. Note that if R is absent, S is an ESS and A is not.

	S	A	R
S	0	r	0
A	$-d$	$r-d$	$r-d$
R	0	$r-d$	$r-d$

1978*b*). However, it is not always possible to represent the interactions between members of a group as a simple loss of fitness by one of them and a corresponding gain by others, the gains and losses combining additively. Fitness may be a more complex function of the numbers and kinds of individuals in a group. If so, it is possible that cooperation may be selectively favoured even when the interacting individuals are unrelated – i.e. synergistic selection.

The importance of synergistic selection or mutualism in the evolution of the social insects has been emphasised by Lin & Michener (1972) and West-Eberhard (1975, 1978). A few examples will illustrate its potential importance. Vehrencamp (1979, quoting Buskirk, 1975) describes the case of the orb-web spider *Metabus gravidus*, in which groups of 15–20 females may cooperate to build a web spanning a stream where food is particularly abundant. They cooperate only in building the support lines over the river; within this structure each female builds her own orb. Thus a group of females can exploit a resource unavailable to single spiders.

These female spiders are probably unrelated, so that only mutualism is involved. More often, mutualism and kin selection act together (West-Eberhard, 1975). For example, in the tropical wasp, *Metapolybia aztecoides*, a group of females cooperate to found a nest. West-Eberhard (1978) has argued that this is because a single female would have no chance of success. However, when the nest is established, fighting between the females results in one of them becoming queen and the others workers. If they were not related, there would be no selection favouring the losers staying to help. Thus synergistic and kin selection are both involved. A similar example is afforded by cooperation between male lions taking over and defending a pride of females (Bertram, 1976; Bygott, Bertram & Hanby, 1979). The males are usually related, so kin selection is relevant. However, a single male could not acquire a pride, so that the effects of interaction of fitness are of the kind illustrated in Fig. 2.2*a*, rather than a simple transfer of reproduction from a donor to a recipient. Therefore cooperation would be favoured by selection even between unrelated males; in fact, there are occasional cases of unrelated males holding a pride. As a general rule, it seems likely that an analysis of the evolution of social behaviour will require an evaluation of the relative importance of kin selection and of synergistic effects.

Reciprocal altruism is clearly fundamental in human social life. Trivers (1971) showed how it can act in interspecific interactions between cleaning fish and their clients, and Packer (1977) has made a strong case that it can lead to cooperation between baboons.·

Kin selection

The standard method of thinking about kin selection today is to use Hamilton's (1964) formula, $B/C > 1/r$. That is to say, if an interaction occurs in which a 'donor' sacrifices C offspring and a 'recipient' gains an additional B offspring, then the gene causing the donor to act will increase in frequency if $B/C > 1/r$, where r is the coefficient of relatedness of the donor to the recipient. Although (as Hamilton pointed out) the formula is only approximate when selection is strong, and although use of it has led to a luxuriant crop of errors (Dawkins, 1979), the method is the most powerful available to us. I am primarily concerned here to justify its use rather than to propose an alternative. The justification I offer is a simplified version of one due to Charlesworth (in press); it does not differ in principle from that given by Hamilton, although it may be easier to follow.

Consider the following model. Each individual during its life participates in $2n$ pairwise interactions, in half of which it is a 'potential donor' and in half a 'potential altruist'. Each individual is supposed to have an initial fitness, before interaction, of G. In each interaction, the potential donor may, depending on its genotype, perform an 'altruistic act', in which case it decreases its own expectation of offspring by C ($=$ cost) and increases the expected offspring of the potential recipient by B ($=$ benefit).

This model can apply to cases in which an individual participates in only one interaction in its life. Consider for example a *Polistes* species in which pairs of females fight to determine which is dominant, the loser having the choice of helping the winner to raise her offspring, or of departing and raising her own (Orlove, 1975). In this case, $n = 1/2$, and the loser is the 'potential donor'. A given genotype will play the role of potential donor and potential altruist equally frequently.

I suppose that a pair of alleles A and a influence whether a potential donor becomes an actual altruist. This is unaffected by the recipient's genotype, and also by learning (so that there can be no reciprocal altruism). There are two different ways in which one can decide whether A and a will increase in frequency.

(i) 'Inclusive fitness'. One considers all the consequences of the altruistic act, both in costs to the donor and in benefits to the recipient, and asks whether the performance of the act increases the frequency of the gene which caused it.

(ii) 'Neighbour-modulated fitness'. This approach was mentioned by Hamilton (1964), but not pursued because of mathematical difficulties which will appear below. It has recently been developed by Cavalli-Sforza & Feldman, 1978; (see also Orlove, 1975, 1979). It starts from the obvious fact that if we can correctly calculate the expected number of offspring produced by all the genotypes in the population, this is sufficient to determine what will happen, so there is no need to take into account 'vicarious' offspring produced by relatives. However, in calculating the expected number of offspring produced by 'ego', we must allow for any help ego may receive. If ego has genes for 'altruism', his relatives are more likely to have them also, and this must be taken into account in calculating ego's fitness.

Consider first a haploid population, such that genotype A always acts altruistically if it is a potential donor, and a never does. The neighbour-modulated fitnesses are

$$\left.\begin{array}{l} W_A = G - nC + nB[r + (1 - r)p] \\ W_a = G + nB(1 - r)p, \end{array}\right\} \qquad (1)$$

where p is the frequency of allele A and r is the probability that donor and recipient are genetically identical by descent.

Gene A will increase in frequency if $W_A > W_a$; that is, if $Br > C$, or $B/C > 1/r$. Hamilton referred to the term $G - nC + nBr$ as the 'inclusive fitness' of genotype A. The inclusive fitnesses are sufficient to determine the direction of evolutionary change. They do not determine the rate of change, which also depends on the 'diluting effect' $nB(1 - r)p$, common to all genotypes.

Before proceeding to the more difficult case of diploid inheritance, a few points should be made

    (i) The direction of change does *not* depend on the gene frequency p. This feature is preserved in diploid models.

    (ii) A knowledge of the coefficient of relatedness r is sufficient to specify the (neighbour-modulated) fitnesses W_A and W_a. This is not generally true in the diploid case.

If, as is usually the case, r is calculated from a pedigree, equations (1) are exact only when selection is weak. This is because selection alters the probability that an allele will be present in a relative. This difficulty affects both methods alike. The only way round it in most cases is computer simulation (e.g. Orlove, 1975). Fortunately, the inaccuracies introduced seem to be small.

Consider now a diploid model. For simplicity, let the gene for altruism be dominant, so that AA and Aa are altruists and aa is not. Let $P(\bar{A}/X)$ be the probability that a potential donor is an altruist, given that the recipient has genotype X. For simple dominance

$$P(\bar{A}/X) = 1 - P(aa/X),$$

where $P(aa/X)$ is the probability that the potential donor has genotype aa. The neighbour-modulated fitnesses are then:

$$\left.\begin{aligned}
W_{AA} &= G - nC + nB[1 - P(aa/AA)] \\
W_{Aa} &= G - nC + nB[1 - P(aa/Aa)] \\
W_{aa} &= G + nB[1 - P(aa/aa)].
\end{aligned}\right\} \tag{2}$$

Unfortunately, the required conditional probabilities do not depend solely on the coefficient of relatedness, r. To illustrate this, consider two cases: in case 1, donor and recipient are always half sibs; in case 2, they are always double first cousins. These relationships were chosen because both have $r = 1/4$.

The conditional probabilities $P(aa/AA)$ etc. were calculated using the method of Jacquard (1974). There is no need for the reader to follow these calculations, although they are not difficult to do for half sibs. However, it is important to note that they are based on the assumption that no selection is acting. Therefore the conclusion drawn below, that the inequality $B/C > 1/r$ correctly predicts the direction of evolution, is precise only when selection is weak. Cavalli-Sforza & Feldman (1978) give an exact treatment of interactions between full sibs when the altruism allele is rare. An exact treatment of more distant relationships will be very difficult.

Substituting these probabilities gives

Case 1. $$\left.\begin{aligned}
W_{AA} &= G - nC + nB(1 - \tfrac{1}{2}q^2) \\
W_{Aa} &= G - nC + nB(1 + \tfrac{1}{4}q - \tfrac{1}{2}q^2) \\
W_{aa} &= G + nB(1 - \tfrac{1}{2}q - \tfrac{1}{2}q^2)
\end{aligned}\right\} \tag{3}$$

Case 2. $$\left.\begin{aligned}
W_{AA} &= G - nC + nB(1 - \tfrac{9}{16}q^2) \\
W_{Aa} &= G - nC + nB(1 - \tfrac{3}{16}q - \tfrac{9}{16}q^2) \\
W_{aa} &= G + nB(\tfrac{15}{16} - \tfrac{6}{16}q - \tfrac{9}{16}q^2)
\end{aligned}\right\} \tag{4}$$

The first point to note is that the two sets of equations are not the same. This might lead one to fear that the spread of gene A cannot be predicted solely from a knowledge of r, B and C. This fear, however, is groundless. Given the above fitnesses, it is straightforward to find the inequality which must be satisfied if A is to increase in frequency. This inequality turns out to be independent of p, and in fact it is $B/C > 4$ in both cases, as predicted by the inclusive fitness method.

It should now be clear why Hamilton chose to abandon neighbour-modulated fitness and to pursue inclusive fitness. But why does the latter method work? One reasonably general method (following Charlesworth, 1981) of deriving the inequality $B/C > 1/r$ is as follows. Suppose that, in a diploid population in one generation, there are N pairwise interactions in which an altruistic act is performed. A pair of alleles A, a influence (in any way) whether a potential donor performs an altruistic act.

Let p_1 = frequency of allele A in (actual) donors,

$\quad$ p_2 = frequency of allele A in (actual) recipients,

$\quad$ p = frequency of allele A in whole population.

Then, as a consequence of the N acts, the number of A genes present in the next generation is increased by $2NB - 2NC$. Hence the frequency of A among the additional genes is

$$p' = \frac{Bp_2 - Cp_1}{B - C}. \tag{5}$$

Allele A will increase if $p' > p$. The crucial step, due to Hamilton, is to recognise that

$$p_2 = rp_1 + (1 - r)p, \tag{6}$$

where r is the fraction of genes in the recipients which are identical by descent to genes in the donors.

Substituting (6) into (5) gives

$$Br(p_1 - p) > C(p_1 - p).$$

Provided that $p_1 > p$ (that is, the possession of an allele A on average makes an individual more likely to be an altruist), this reduces to

$$B/C > 1/r \tag{7}$$

This result does not depend on any assumption about dominance, and is independent of the gene frequency. This inclusive fitness approach is simpler mathematically, because it is necessary only to calculate the gene frequency in a relative, and not the genotype frequency. It is also intuitively easier to think about all the consequences of the acts of an individual than about the effects on an individual of the acts of his relatives.

However, as Cavalli-Sforza & Feldman (1978) point out, there is no guarantee that the results of social interactions can be represented by a set of costs and benefits which can be combined additively. For example, the classic example of alarm notes in bird flocks is hard to represent in this way (Maynard Smith, 1980). The inclusive fitness method does seem to depend on the possibility of such an additive combination of costs and benefits. In any particular case, it is certainly worth attempting such a representation. Unhappily, the attempt may not succeed. If is does not, there seems no alternative to the more difficult method of calculating neighbour-modulated fitnesses.

Summary

1. By an 'altruistic' trait is meant a trait which, in some sense, lowers the fitness of the individual displaying it, but increases the fitness of some other members of the same species.

2. A number of qualitatively different processes have been proposed whereby genes determining such traits can increase in frequency.

3. This essay attempts two things: first, I propose a classification of these processes, and, second, I discuss different ways in which one of them (kin selection) can be modelled mathematically.

References

Alexander, R.D. (1974). The evolution of social behaviour. *Annual Review of Ecology and Systematics*, **5**, 325–83.

Bertram, B.C.R. (1976). Kin selection in lions and in evolution. In *Growing Points in Ethology*, ed. P.P.G. Bateson & R.A. Hinde, pp. 281–301. Cambridge University Press: Cambridge.

Boorman, S.A. & Levitt, P.R. (1973). Group selection at the boundary of a stable population. *Theoretical Population Biology*, **4**, 85–128.

Buskirk, R.E. (1975). Coloniality, activity patterns and feeding in a tropical orb-weaving spider. *Ecology*, **56**, 1314–28.

Bygott, J.D., Bertram, B.C.R. & Hanby, J.B. (1979). Male lions in large coalitions gain reproductive advantages. *Nature*, **282**, 839–41.

Cavalli-Sforza, L.L. & Feldman, M.W. (1978). Darwinian selection and altruism. *Theoretical Population Biology*, **14**, 268–80.

Charlesworth, B. (1979). A note on the evolution of altruism in structured demes. *American Naturalist*, **113**, 601–5.

Charlesworth, B. (1981). Models of kin selection. In *Evolution of Social Behaviour*, ed. H. Markl. Darlem Konferenzen: Berlin (In press.)

Cohen, D. & Eshel, I. (1976). On the founder effect and the evolution of altruistic traits. *Theoretical Population Biology*, **10**, 276–302.

Craig, R. (1979). Parental manipulation, kin selection, and the evolution of altruism. *Evolution*, **33**, 319–34.

Dawkins, R. (1979). Twelve misunderstandings of kin selection. *Zeitschrift für Tierpsychologie*, **51**, 184–200.

Eshel, I. (1972). On the neighbourhood effect and the evolution of altruistic traits. *Theoretical Population Biology*, **3**, 258–77.

Fisher, R.A. (1930). *The Genetical Theory of Natural Selection.* Clarendon Press: Oxford.

Gilpin, M.E. (1975). *Group Selection in Predator–Prey Communities.* Princeton University Press: Princeton, N.J.

Haldane, J.B.S. (1932). *The Causes of Evolution.* Longmans, Green: London.

Hamilton, W.D. (1964). The genetical evolution of social behaviour. I and II. *Journal of Theoretical Biology*, **7**, 1–16 and 17–32.

Hamilton, W.D. (1971). Geometry for the selfish herd. *Journal of Theoretical Biology*, **31**, 295–311.

Jacquard, A. (1974). *The Genetic Structure of Populations.* Springer–Verlag: Berlin.

Lande, R. (1979) Effective deme sizes during long-term evolution estimated from rates of chromosomal rearrangement. *Evolution*, **33**, 234–51.

Levin, B.R. & Kilmer, W.L. (1974). Interdemic selection and the evolution of altruism: a computer simulation study. *Evolution*, **28**, 527–47.

Levins, R. (1970). Extinction. In *Some Mathematical Problems in Biology*, ed. M. Gerstenhaber, pp. 77–107. The Americal Mathematical Society: Providence, R.I.

Lin, M. & Michener, C. (1972). Evolution of sociality in insects. *Quarterly Review of Biology*, **47**, 131–59.

Matessi, C. & Jayakar, S.D. (1976). Conditions for the evolution of altruism under Darwinian selection. *Theoretical Population Biology*, **9**, 360–87.

Maynard Smith, J. (1964). Group selection and kin selection. *Nature*, **201**, 1145–7.

Maynard Smith, J. (1976). Group selection. *Quarterly Review of Biology*, **51**, 277–83.

Maynard Smith J. (1978*a*) *The Evolution of Sex*. Cambridge University Press: Cambridge.

Maynard Smith (1978*b*). The evolution of behaviour. *Scientific American*, **239**, 136–45.

Maynard Smith, J. (1980). Models of the evolution of altruism. *Theoretical Population Biology*, **18**, 151–9.

Mirmirani, M. & Oster, G. (1978). Competition, kin selection and evolutionarily stable strategies. *Theoretical Population Biology*, **13**, 304–31.

Orlove, M.J. (1975). A model of kin selection not invoking coefficients of relationship. *Journal of Theoretical Biology*, **49**, 289–310.

Orlove, M.J. (1979). Putting the diluting effect into inclusive fitness. *Journal of Theoretical Biology*, **78**, 449–50.

Packer, C. (1977). Reciprocal altruism in *Papio anubis*. *Nature*, **265**, 441–3.

Trivers, R.L. (1971). The evolution of reciprocal altruism. *Quarterly Review of Biology*, **46**, 35–57.

Uyenoyama, M.K. (1979). Evolution of altruism under group selection in large and small populations in fluctuating environments. *Theoretical Population Biology*, **15**, 58–85.

Vehrencamp, S.L. (1979). The roles of individual, kin and group selection in the evolution of sociality. In *Social Behaviour and Communication*, ed. P. Marler, pp. 351–94. Plenum: New York.

Wade, M.J. (1977). Experimental study of group selection. *Evolution*, **31**, 134–53.

West-Eberhard, M.J. (1975). The evolution of social behaviour by kin selection. *Quarterly Review of Biology*, **50**, 1–33.

West-Eberhard, M.J. (1978). Temporary queens in *Metapolybia* wasps: non-reproductive helpers without altruism? *Science*, **200**, 441–3.

Wilson, D.S. (1975). A theory of group selection. *Proceedings of the National Academy of Sciences of the U.S.A.*, **72**, 143–6.

Wright, S. (1931). Evolution in Mendelian populations. *Genetics*, **16**, 97–159.

Wright, S. (1945). Tempo and mode in evolution – a critical review. *Ecology*, **26**, 415–19.

Wright, S. (1970). Random drift and the shifting balance theory of evolution. In *Mathematical Topics in Population Genetics*, ed. K. Kojima, pp. 1–31. Springer–Verlag: Berlin.

Wynne Edwards, V.C. (1962). *Animal Behaviour in Relation to Social Behaviour*. Oliver and Boyd: Edinburgh.

3

Replicators and vehicles

RICHARD DAWKINS

The theory of natural selection provides a mechanistic, causal account of how living things came to look as if they had been designed for a purpose. So overwhelming is the appearance of purposeful design that, even in this Darwinian era when we know 'better', we still find it difficult, indeed boringly pedantic, to refrain from teleological language when discussing adaptation. Birds' wings are obviously 'for' flying, spider webs are for catching insects, chlorophyll molecules are for photosynthesis, DNA molecules are for... What *are* DNA molecules for? The question takes us aback. In my case it touches off an almost audible alarm siren in the mind. If we accept the view of life that I wish to espouse, it is the forbidden question. DNA is not 'for' anything. If we wish to speak teleologically, all adaptations are for the preservation of DNA; DNA itself just *is*. Following Williams (1966), I have advocated this view at length (Dawkins 1976, 1978), and I do not want to repeat myself here. Instead I shall try to clear up an important misunderstanding of the view, a misunderstanding which has constituted an unnecessary barrier to its acceptance.

The identity of the 'unit' of selection' has been controversial in the literature both of biology (Williams, 1966; Lewontin, 1970; Leigh, 1977; Dawkins, 1978; Alexander & Borgia, 1978; Alexander, 1980) and philosophy (Hull, 1981). In this paper I shall show that only part of the controversy is real. Part is due to semantic confusion. If we overlook the semantic element we arrive at a simplistic hierarchical account of the views that have been expressed in the literature. Living matter is nested in a hierarchy of levels, from ecosystem through species, deme, family, individual, cell, gene, and even nucleotide base pair. According to this analysis each one of the protagonists in the debate on units of selection is perched on a higher or a lower rung of a ladder, sniping at those above and below him. Thus Gould (1977) remarks that in the last fifteen years 'challenges to Darwin's focus on individuals have sparked some lively debates among evolutionists. These challenges have come from above and from below. From above, Scottish biologist V.C. Wynne-Edwards raised orthodox hackles fifteen years ago by arguing that groups, not individuals, are units of selection, at least for the evolution of social behavior. From below, English biologist Richard Dawkins has recently raised my hackles with his claim that genes themselves are units of selection, and individuals merely their temporary receptacles.'

At first blush, Gould's hierarchical analysis has a neatly symmetrical plausibility. Much as my sense of mischief is tickled by the idea of being allied with Professor Wynne-Edwards in a pincer-attack on Darwin's individual, however, I reluctantly have to point out that the dispute between individual and group is different in kind from the dispute between individual and gene. Wynne-Edwards's attack from above is best seen as a factual dispute about the level at which selection is most effective in nature. My attack from below is a dispute about what we ought to *mean* when we talk about a unit of selection. Much the same point has been realised by Hull (1981), but I prefer to persist in expressing it in my way rather than to adopt his terminology of 'interactors' and 'evolvors'.

To make my point I shall develop a distinction between *replicator survival* and *vehicle selection*. Anticipating the conclusion, there are two ways in which we can characterise natural selection. Both are correct; they simply focus on different aspects of the same process. Evolution results from the differential survival of *replicators*. Genes are replicators; organisms and groups of organisms are not replicators, they are vehicles in which replicators travel about. Vehicle selection is the process by which some vehicles are more successful than other vehicles in ensuring the survival of their replicators. The controversy about group selection versus individual selection is a controversy about the rival claims of two suggested kinds of vehicle. The controversy about gene selection versus individual (or group) selection has been a controversy about whether, when we talk about a unit of selection, we ought to mean a vehicle *at all*, or a replicator. In any case, as I shall later argue, there may be little usefulness in talking about discrete vehicles at all.

Replicators

A replicator may be defined as any entity in the universe of which copies are made. Replicators may be subclassified in two overlapping ways (Dawkins, 1982, chapter 5). A germ-line replicator, as distinct from a dead-end replicator, is the potential ancestor of an indefinitely long line of descendant replicators. Thus DNA in a zygote is a germ-line replicator, while DNA in a liver cell is a dead-end replicator. Cutting across this classification, an active, as distinct from a passive, replicator is a replicator that has some causal influence on its own probability of being propagated. Thus a gene that has phenotypic expression is an active replicator. A length of DNA that is never transcribed and has no phenotypic expression whatever is a passive replicator. 'Selfish DNA' (Dawkins, 1976, p. 47; Doolittle & Sapienza, 1980; Orgel & Crick, 1980), even if it is not transcribed, should be considered passive only if its nature has absolutely no influence on its probability of being replicated. It might be quite hard to find a genuine example of a passive replicator. Special interest attaches to *active germ-line replicators*, since adaptations 'for' their preservation are expected to fill the world and to characterise living organisms. Automatically, those active germ-line replicators whose phenotypic effects happen to enhance their own survival and propagation will be the ones that survive. Their phenotypic consequences will be the attributes of living things that we see, and seek to explain.

Active, germ-line replicators, then, are units of selection in the following sense. When we say that an adaptation is 'for the good of' something, what is that something? Is it the species, the group, the individual, or what? I am suggesting that the appropriate 'something', the 'unit of selection' in that sense, is the active germ-line replicator. The active germ-line replicator might, therefore, be called the 'optimon', by extension of Benzer's (1957) classification of genetic units (recon, muton and cistron).

This does not mean, of course, that genes or other replicators literally face the cutting edge of natural selection. It is their phenotypic effects that are the proximal subjects of selection. I have been sorry to learn that the phrase 'replicator selection' can be misunderstood along those lines. One could, perhaps, avoid this confusion by referring to replicator survival rather than replicator selection. (In passing I cannot help being reminded of Wallace's (1866) passionate plea to Darwin to abandon 'natural selection' in favour of 'survival of the fittest', on the grounds that many people thought 'natural selection' implied a conscious selecting 'agent' (see also Young, 1971). My own prejudice is that anybody who misunderstands 'replicator selection' is likely to have even more trouble with 'individual selection').

Natural selection does not inevitably follow whenever there exist active germ-line replicators. Certain additional assumptions are necessary, but these, in turn, are almost inevitable consequences of the basic definition. Firstly, no copying process is perfect, and we can expect that replicators will sometimes make inexact copies of themselves, the mistakes or mutations being preserved in future descendants. Natural selection, of course, depends on the variation so created. Secondly, the resources needed to make copies, and to make vehicles for propagating copies, may be presumed to be in limited supply, and replicators may therefore be regarded as in competition with other replicators. In the complicatedly organized environments of eukaryotic cells, each replicator is a competitor specifically of its alleles at its own locus on the chromosomes of the population.

There is a problem over how large or how small a fragment of genome we choose to regard as a replicator. Is it one cistron (recon, muton), one chromosome, one genome, or some intermediate? The answer I have given before, and still stick by, is that we do not need to give a straight answer to the question. Nobody is going to be hanged as a result of our decision. Williams (1966) recognised this when he defined a gene as 'that which segregates and recombines with appreciable frequency' (p. 24), and as 'any hereditary information for which there is a favorable or unfavorable selection bias equal to several or many times its rate of endogenous change' (p. 25). It is clear that we are never going to sell this kind of definition to a generation brought up on the 'one gene one protein' doctrine, which is one reason why I (Dawkins, 1978) have advocated using the word replicator itself, instead of gene in the sense of the Williams definition. Another reason is that 'replicator' is general enough to accommodate the theoretical possibility, which one day may become observed reality, of non-genetic natural selection. For example, it is at least worth discussing the possibility of evolution by differential survival of cultural replicators or 'memes' (Dawkins, 1976; Bonner, 1980), brain structures whose 'phenotypic' manifestation as behaviour or artefact is the basis of their selection.

I have lavished much rhetoric, or irresponsibly purple prose if you prefer, on expounding the view that 'the unit of selection' (I meant it in the sense of replicator, not vehicle) must be a unit that is potentially immortal (Dawkins, 1976, chapter 3), a point which I learned from Williams (1966). Briefly, the rationale is that an entity must have a low rate of spontaneous, endogenous change, if the selective advantage of its phenotypic effects over those of rival ('allelic') entities is to have any significant evolutionary effect. For a replicator such as a small length of chromosome, mutation and crossing over within itself are hazards to its continued replication, in exactly the same sense as are predators and reluctant females. Any arbitrary length of DNA has an expected half-life measured in generations. The world tends to become full of replicators with a long half-life, and therefore full of their phenotypic products. These products are the characteristics of the animals and plants which we see around us. It is these that we wish to explain. Of those phenotypic products, the ones that we, as whole animal biologists, are particularly interested in are those that we see at the whole animal level, adaptations to avoid predators, to attract females, to secure food economically, and so on. Replicators that tend to make the successive bodies they inhabit good at avoiding predators, attracting females, etc., tend to have long half-lives as a consequence. But if such a replicator has a high probability of internal self-destruction, through mutation in its broad sense, all its virtues at the level of whole animal phenotypes come to naught.

It follows that although any arbitrary length of chromosome can in theory be regarded as a replicator, too long a piece of chromosome will quantitatively disqualify itself as a potential unit of selection, since it will run too high a risk of being split by crossing over in any generation. A replicator worthy of the name, then, is not necessarily as small as one recon, one muton, or one cistron. It is not a discrete, all or none, unit at all, but a segment of chromosome whose length is determined by the strength of the 'whole animal level' selection pressure of interest. As Francis Crick (1979) has written, 'The theory of the "selfish gene" will have to be extended to any stretch of DNA'.

It further follows that critics of the view advocated here cannot score debating points by drawing attention to the existence of within-gene (cistron) crossing over. I am grateful to Mark Ridley for reminding me that most within-gene crossovers are, in any case, indistinguishable in their effects from between-gene crossovers. Obviously, if the gene concerned happens to be homozygous, paired at meiosis with an identical allele, all the material exchanged will be identical, and the effect will be indistinguishable from a crossover at either end of the gene. If the gene is heterozygous, but differs from its allele by only one nucleotide, a within-gene crossover will be indistinguishable in effect from a crossover at one of the two ends of the gene. Only on the rare occasions when the gene differs from its allele in two places, and the crossover occurs between the two places, will a within-gene crossover be distinguishable from a between-gene crossover. The general point is that it does not particularly matter where crossovers occur in relation to cistron boundaries. What matters is where crossovers occur in relation to heterozygous nucleotides. If, for instance, a sequence of six adjacent cistrons happens to be homozygous throughout an entire species, a crossover anywhere within the six will be exactly equivalent to a crossover at either end of the six.

The possibility of widespread linkage disequilibrium, too, does not weaken the case (Clegg, 1978). It simply increases the length of chromosomal segment that we expect to behave as a replicator. If, which seems doubtful, linkage disequilibrium is so strong that populations contain 'only a few gametic types' (Lewontin, 1974, p. 312), the effective replicator will be a very large chunk of DNA. When what Lewontin calls l_c, the 'characteristic length' (the distance over which coupling is effective), is only 'a fraction of the chromosome length, each gene is out of linkage equilibrium only with its neighbours but is assorted essentially independently of other genes farther away. The characteristic length is, in some sense, the unit of evolution since genes within it are highly correlated. The concept is a subtle one, however. It does not mean that the genome is broken up into discrete adjacent chunks of length l_c. Every locus is the center of such a correlated segment and evolves in linkage with the genes near it' (Lewontin, 1974, p. 312). In the same spirit, I played with the idea of entitling an earlier work 'The slightly selfish big bit of chromosome and the even more selfish little bit of chromosome' (Dawkins, 1976, p. 35).

I used to think that, in species with asexual reproduction, the whole organism could be thought of as a replicator, but further reflection shows this to be equivalent to the Lamarckian heresy. The asexual organism's *genome* may be considered a replicator, since any alteration in it tends to be preserved. But an alteration in the organism itself is quite likely to have been imprinted from the environment and will not be preserved. It is not replicated. Asexual organisms do not make copies of themselves, they work to make copies of their genomes.

An adaptation is a tool by which the genes that made it have levered themselves through the past, into the present where it demands our explanation. But the tools and levers do not rattle around loose in the world, but come neatly packaged in tool-kits: individual organisms or other vehicles. It is to vehicles that we now turn.

Vehicles

Replicators are not naked genes, though they may have been when life began. Nowadays, most of them are strung along chromosomes, chromosomes are wrapped up in nuclear membrances, and nuclei are enveloped in cytoplasm and enclosed in cell membranes. Cells, in turn, are cloned to form huge assemblages which we know as organisms. Organisms are vehicles for replicators, survival machines as I have called them. But just as we had a nested hierarchy of would-be replicators – small and large fragments of genome – so there is a hierarchy of nested vehicles. Chromosomes and cells are gene vehicles within organisms. In many species, organisms are not dispersed randomly but go around in groups. Multi-species groups form communities or ecosystems. At any of these levels the concept of vehicle is potentially applicable. Vehicle selection is the differential success of vehicles in propagating the replicators that ride inside them. In theory selection may occur at any level of the hierarchy.

One of the clearest discussions of the levels of selection is that of Lewontin (1970), although his paper, like my own first discussion of the matter (Dawkins, 1976), suffers from its failure to make a clear distinction between replicators and vehicles. Lewontin does not mention the gene as one of the levels in his hierarchy, presumably because he rightly regards it as obvious that it is changes in gene frequency that ultimately matter, whatever level selection may proximally act on. Thus it is easy, and probably largely correct, to interpret his paper as being about levels of *vehicle*. On the other hand, at one point he says the following:

> 'The rate of evolution is limited by the variation in fitness of the units being selected. This has two consequences from the point of view of comparison between levels of selection. First, the rapidity of response to selection depends upon the heritability of differences in fitness between units. The heritability is highest in units where no internal adjustment or reassortment is possible since such units will pass on to their descendent units an unchanged set of information. Thus, cell organelles, haploid organisms, and gametes are levels of selection with a higher heritability than diploid sexual genotypes, since the latter do not perfectly reproduce themselves, but undergo segregation and recombination in the course of their reproduction. In the same way, individuals have a greater heritability than populations and assemblages of species' (Lewontin, 1970, p. 8).

This point makes sense only if the units being referred to are would-be replicators; indeed it is the same point as I made a few pages back. This suggests that Lewontin was not entirely clear over whether he was talking about units of selection in the sense of replicators (entities that become more or less numerous as a consequence of selection) or vehicles (units of phenotypic power of replicators). The same is suggested by the fact that he cites M.B. Williams's (1970) axiomatization of Darwin's theory as indicating that 'the principles can be applied equally to genes, organisms, populations, species, and at opposite ends of the scale, prebiotic molecules and ecosystems'. I would maintain that genes and prebiotic molecules do not belong in the hierarchical list. They are replicators; the rest are vehicles.

An organism is not a replicator, not even a very inefficient replicator with a high probability of endogenous change. An organism's *genome* can be regarded as a replicator (a very poor one if reproduction is sexual), but to treat an organism as a replicator in the same sense as a gene is tantamount to Lamarckism. If you change a replicator, the change will be passed on to its descendants. This is clearly true of genes and genomes. It is not true of organisms, since acquired characteristics are not inherited.

The reason we like to think in terms of vehicle selection is that replicators are not directly visible to natural selection. Gould (1977) put it well, albeit he mistakenly thought he was scoring a point against the whole replicator concept: '... I find a fatal flaw in Dawkins's attack from below. No matter how much power Dawkins wishes to assign to genes, there is one thing he cannot give them – direct visibility to natural selection. Selection simply cannot see genes and pick among them directly. It must use bodies as an intermediary.' The valid point being made is that replicators do not expose themselves naked to the world; they work via their phenotypic effects, and it is often convenient to see those phenotypic effects as bundled together in vehicles such as bodies.

It is another matter whether the individual body is the only level of vehicle worth considering. That is what the whole group selection versus individual selection debate is about. Gould comes down heavily in favour of the individual organism, and this is the main one of the would-be units that I shall consider.

Of all the levels in the hierarchy of vehicles, the biologist's eye is drawn most strongly to the individual organism. Unlike the cell and the population, the organism is often of a convenient size for the naked eye to see. It is usually a discrete machine with an internally coherent organization, displaying to a high degree the quality which Huxley (1912) labelled 'individuality' (literally indivisibility – being sufficiently heterogeneous in form to be rendered non-functional if cut in half). Genetically speaking, too, the individual organism is usually a clearly definable unit, whose cells have the same genes as each other but different genes from the cells of other individuals. To an immunologist, the organism has a special kind of 'uniqueness' (Medawar, 1957), in that it will easily accept grafts from other parts of its own body but not from other bodies. To the ethologist – and this is really an aspect of Huxley's 'individuality' – the organism is a unit of behavioural action in a much stronger sense than, say, half an organism, or two organisms. The organism has one central nervous system. It takes 'decisions' (Dawkins & Dawkins, 1973) as a unit. All its limbs conspire harmoniously together to achieve one end at a time. On those occasions when two or more organisms try to coordinate their efforts, say when a pride of lions cooperatively stalks prey, the feats of coordination among individuals are feeble compared with the intricate orchestration, with high spatial and temporal precision, of the hundreds of muscles within each individual. Even a starfish, whose tube-feet each enjoy a measure of autonomy and may tear the animal in two if the circum-oral nerve ring has been surgically cut, looks like a single entity, and in nature behaves as if it had a single purpose.

For these and other reasons we automatically prefer to ask functional questions at the level of the individual organism rather than at any other level. We ask, 'Of what use is that behaviour pattern to the animal?' We do not ask, 'Of what use is the behaviour of the animal's left hind leg to the left hind leg?' Nor yet do we usually ask 'Of what use is the behaviour of that pair of animals to the pair?' We see the single organism as a suitable unit about which to speak of adaptation. No doubt this is why Hamilton (1964*a, b*), in his epoch-making demonstration that individual altruism was best explained as the result of gene selfishness, sugared the pill of his scientific revolution by inventing 'inclusive fitness' as a sop to the individual organism. Inclusive fitness, in effect, amount to 'that property of an individual organism which will appear to be maximized when what is really being maximized is gene survival' (Dawkins, 1978). Every consequence that Hamilton deduced from his theory could, I suggest, be derived by posing the question: 'What would a selfish gene do to maximize its survival?' In effect, Hamilton was accepting the logic of gene (replicator) selection while affirming his faith in the individual organism as the most salient gene vehicle.

Presumably it would, in principle, be possible to imagine a group-level equivalent of individual inclusive fitness: that property of a group of organisms which will appear to be maximized when what is really being maximized is the survival of the genes controlling the phenotypic characters of the group. The difficulty with this is that, while we can conceive of ways in which genes can exert phenotypic power over the limbs and nervous systems of the bodies in which they sit, it is rather harder to conceive of their exerting phenotypic power over the 'limbs' and 'nervous systems' of whole groups of organisms. The group of organisms is too diffuse, not coherent enough to be seen as a unit of phenotypic power.

And yet to some extent the individual organism, too, may be not quite such a coherent unit of phenotypic power as we have grown to think. It is certainly much less obviously so to a botanist than to a zoologist:

> 'The individual fruit fly, flour beetle, rabbit, flatworm or elephant is a population at the cellular but not at any higher level. Starvation does not change the number of legs, hearts or livers of an animal but the effect of stress on a plant is to alter both the rate of formation of new leaves and the rate of death of old ones: a plant may react to stress by varying the number of its parts' (Harper, 1977).

> Harper feels obliged to coin two new terms for different kinds of 'individual'. 'The "ramet" is the unit of clonal growth, the module that may often follow an independent existence if severed from the parent plant' (Harper, 1977, p. 24).

> The 'genet', on the other hand, is the unit which springs from one single-celled zygote, the 'individual' in the normal zoologists' sense. Janzen (1977) faces up to something like the same difficulty, suggesting that a clone of dandelions should be

regarded as equivalent to a single tree, although spread out along the ground rather than raised in the air, and divided up into separate physical 'plants' (Harper's ramets). Janzen sees a clone of aphids in the same way, although Harper presumably would not: each aphid in a clone develops from a single cell, albeit the cell is produced asexually. Harper would therefore say that a new aphid is produced by an act of *reproduction*, whereas Janzen would regard it as having *grown* like a new limb of its parent.

It might seem that we are now playing with words, but I think Harper's (1977, p. 27) distinction between reproduction by means of a single-celled (asexual or sexual) propagule, and growth by means of a multicellular propagule or runner, is an important one. What is more, it can be made the basis of a sensible criterion for defining a single vehicle. Each new vehicle comes into being through an act of reproduction. New parts of vehicles come into being through growth. The distinction has nothing to do with that between sexual and asexual reproduction, nor with that between ramet and genet.

One act of reproduction, one vehicle

I do not know whether Harper had the same thing in mind, but for me the evolutionary significance of his distinction between growth and reproduction is best seen as arising out of a view of development which I learned from the works of J.T. Bonner (e.g., 1974). In order to make complex adaptations at the level of multicellular organs – eyes, ears, hearts, etc., – a complex developmental process is necessary. An amoeba may give rise to two daughters by splitting down the middle, but an eye, or a heart, cannot give rise to two daughter eyes, or two daughter hearts, by binary fission. Eyes and hearts are so complex that they have to be developed from small beginnings, built by orderly cell division and differentiation. This is why insects whose life cycle takes them through two radically different bodies, like caterpillar and butterfly, do not attempt to transform larval organs into corresponding adult organs. Instead development restarts from undifferentiated imaginal discs, the larval tissues being broken down and used as the equivalent of food. Complexity can develop from simplicity, but not from a wholly different kind of complexity. The evolution of one complex organ into another can take place only because in each generation the development of individuals restarts at a simple, single-celled beginning (Dawkins, 1982, chapter 14).

Complex organisms all have a life cycle which begins with a single cell, passes through a phase of mitotic cell division in which great complexity of structure may be built up, and culminates in reproduction of new single-celled propagules of the next generation. Evolutionary change consists in genetic changes which alter the developmental process at some crucial stage in the life cycle, in such a way that the complex structure of the organism of the next generation is different. If organisms simply grew indefinitely, without returning cyclically to a single-celled zygote in a sequence of generations, the evolution of complexity at the multicellular organ level would be impossible. For lineages to evolve, individuals must develop from small beginnings in each generation. They cannot just grow from the multicellular bodies of the previous generation.

We must beware of falling into the trap of 'biotic adaptationism' here (Williams, 1966). We cannot argue that a tendency to reproduce rather than grow will evolve in order to allow evolution to happen! Rather, when we look at complex living things we are looking at the end products of an evolutionary process which could only occur because the lineages concerned showed repeated reproduction rather than just growth. A related point is that repeated cycles of reproduction are only possible if there is also death of individual vehicles, but this is not, in itself, a reason that explains why death occurs. We cannot say that the biological function of death is 'to' allow repeated reproduction and hence evolution (Medawar, 1957). But given that death and reproduction do occur in a lineage, evolution in that lineage becomes possible (Maynard Smith, 1969).

Is the distinction between growth and reproduction a rigid one? As so far defined it seems so. A life cycle which restarts with a single cell represents a new reproductive unit, a new discrete vehicle. All other apparent reproduction should be called growth. But couldn't there be a new life cycle that was initiated, not by a single-celled propagule but by a small multicellular propagule? When a new plant grows from a runner sent out by an old plant, is this reproduction or growth? If Harper's definition is rigidly applied, everything depends on an embryological detail. Are all the cells of the new 'plant' the clonal descendants of one cell at the growing tip of the runner? In this case we are dealing with reproduction. Or is the runner a broad-fronted meristem, so that some cells in the new plant are descended from one cell in the old plant, while other cells in the new plant are descended from another cell in the old plant? In this case the Harper definition forces us to classify the phenomenon as growth, not reproduction. It is, in principle, not different from the growth of a new leaf on a tree.

That is what follows from the Harper definition, but is it a sensible definition? I can think of one good reason for saying yes. It makes sense if we are regarding reproduction as the process by which a new vehicle comes into existence, and growth as the process by which an existing vehicle develops. Imagine a plant that sends out vegetative suckers which are broad-fronted meristems, and suppose that this species never reproduces sexually. How might evolutionary change occur? By mutation and selection in the usual way, but *not* by selection among multicellular organisms. A mutation would affect the cell in which it occurred, and all clonal descendants of that cell. But because the runner is broad-fronted, new 'plants' (ramets) would be heterogeneous mosaics with respect to the mutation. Some of the cells of a new plant would be mutant, others would not. As the vegetation creeps over the land, mutant cells are peppered in haphazard bunches around the 'individual' plants. The apparent individual plants, in fact, are not genetic individuals at all. Since they are genetic mosaics, the largest gene vehicle that can be discerned as having a regular life cycle is the cell. Population genetics would have to be done at the cellular level, not at the 'individual' level. And vehicle selection could give rise to adaptive modification at the cellular level, but not at the level of the whole 'plant'. The whole 'plant' would not function as a vehicle propagating the genes inside it, because different cells inside it would contain different genes. Cells would function as vehicles, and adaptations would not be for the good of the whole plant but for the good of smaller units within the plant. To qualify as a 'vehicle', an entity must come into being by reproduction, not by growth.

That is my justification for the importance of the Harper definition. But now suppose that the runner is a narrow bottleneck of mitotic cell descent, so that the life cycle consists of an alternation between a growth phase and a small, if multicellular, restarting phase. 'Individual plants' would now be statistically unlikely to be genetic mosaics. In this case vehicle selection at the level of whole plants could go on, in a statistical sense, since most, though not all, plants would be genetically uniform. Genetic variation within the cells of individual plants would be less than that between cells of different plants. A kind of 'group selection' (J. Hartung, personal communication) at the cellular level could therefore go on, leading to adaptation at the level of the multicellular vehicle, the level of the 'individual plant'. We might, therefore, tolerate a slight relaxation of Harper's criterion, using 'reproduction' whenever a life cycle is constricted into a narrow bottleneck of cells, even if that bottleneck is not always quite as narrow as a single cell.

We are now, incidentally, in a position to see a reason, additional to those normally given, why the individual organism is so much more persuasive a unit of natural selection (vehicle) than the group of organisms. Groups do not go through a regular cycle of growth (development), alternating with 'reproduction' (sending off a small 'propagule' which eventually grows into a new group). Groups grow in a vague and diffuse manner, occasionally fragmenting like pack-ice. It is significant that models of group selection which come closest to succeeding tend to incorporate some reproduction-like process. Thus Levins, and Boorman & Levitt (reviewed by Wilson, 1973) postulate a metapopulation of groups, in which populations 'reproduce' by sending out 'propagules' consisting of migrant individuals or small bands of individuals. Moreover, 'group selection' in the sense of D.S. Wilson (1980) can only work if there is some mechanism by which genetic variation between groups is kept higher than genetic variation within groups (Maynard Smith, 1976; Grafen, 1980, and in preparation). This point is analogous to the one I made in my discussion of 'cellular selection' in plants with narrow runners. In practice the most likely way for intergroup variation to be higher than intragroup variation is through genetic relatives tending to associate together. In this case we are dealing with what has been called kin-group selection. Is 'kin selection', then, an authentic case where we have a vehicle larger than the individual body, in the same way as group selection would be if it existed?

Kin selection and kin group selection

There are those who see kin selection as a special case of group selection (E.O. Wilson, 1973; D.S. Wilson, 1980; Wade, 1978). Maynard Smith (1976) disagrees, and emphatically so do I (Dawkins, 1976, 1978, 1979). Maynard Smith is too polite in suggesting that the disagreement is merely one between lumpers and splitters. Hamilton (1975) at first reading might be thought to be endorsing the lumping of kin and group selection. To avoid confusion I quote him in full

> 'If we insist that group selection is different from kin selection the term should be restricted to situations of assortation definitely not involving kin. But it seems on the whole preferable to retain a more flexible use of terms; to use group selection where groups are clearly in evidence and to qualify with mention of "kin" (as in the "kin-group" selection referred to by Brown, 1974)' (Hamilton, 1975, p. 141, citation of Brown corrected).

Hamilton is here making the distinction between kin selection and kin-group selection. Kin-group selection is the special case of group selection in which individuals tend to be closely related to other members of their own group. It is also the special case of kin selection in which the related individuals happen to go about in discrete family groups. The important point is that the theory of kin selection does not *need* to assume discrete family groups. All that is needed is that close relatives encounter one another with higher than random frequency, or have some method of recognizing each other (Maynard Smith, this volume). As Hamilton says, the term kin selection (rather than kin-group selection) 'appeals most where pedigrees are unbounded and interwoven.'

I have previously quoted Hull (1976) on mammary glands: 'mammary glands contribute to individual fitness, the individual in this case being the kinship group'. Hull is here using 'individual' in a special, philosopher's sense, as 'any spatio-temporally localized, cohesive and continuous entity'. In this sense 'organism' is not synonymous with 'individual' but is only one of the class of things that can be called individuals. Thus Ghiselin (1974) has argued that species are 'individuals'. The point I wish to make here is that the 'kinship group' is an 'individual' only if families go about in tightly concentrated bands, rigidly discriminating family members from non-members, with no half measures. There is no particular reason for expecting this kind of rigid family structure in nature, and certainly Hamilton's theory of kin selection does not demand it. As I suggested when I originally quoted Hull (Dawkins, 1978), we are not dealing with a discrete family group but with

'... an animal plus $\frac{1}{2}$ of each of its children plus $\frac{1}{2}$ of each sibling plus $\frac{1}{4}$ of each niece and grandchild plus $\frac{1}{8}$ of each first cousin plus $\frac{1}{32}$ of each second cousin : .. Far from being a tidy, discrete group, it is more like a sort of genetical octopus, a probabilistic amoeboid whose pseudopodia ramify and dissolve away into the common gene pool.

Where they exist, tightly knit family bands, or 'kin groups', may be regarded as vehicles. But the general theory of kin selection does not depend on the existence of discrete family groups. No vehicle above the organism level need be postulated.

Doing without discrete vehicles

It will have been noted that my 'vehicles' are 'individuals' in the sense of Ghiselin and Hull. They are spatiotemporally localized, cohesive and continuous entities. Much of my section on organisms was devoted to illustrating the sense in which bodies, unlike groups of bodies, are 'individuals'. My sections on vegetatively propagating plants and on kin-groups suggested that while they sometimes *may* be discrete and cohesive entities there is no reason, either in fact or in theory, for expecting that they usually will be so. Kin selection, as a logical deduction from fundamental replicator theory, still leads to interesting and intelligible adaptation, even if there are not discrete kin-group vehicles.

I now want to generalise this lesson: although selection sometimes chooses replicators by virtue of their effects on discrete vehicles, it does not have to. Let me repeat part of my quotation from Gould (1977) 'Selection simply cannot see genes and pick among them directly. It must use bodies as an intermediary.' Well, it must use *phenotypic effects* as intermediaries, but do these have to be bodies? Do they have to be discrete vehicles at all? I have suggested (Dawkins, 1982) that we should no longer think of the phenotypic expression of a gene as being limited to the particular body in which the gene sits. We are already accustomed to the idea of a snail shell as phenotypic expression of genes, even though the shell does not consist of living cells. The form and colour of the shell vary under genetic control. In principle the same is true of a caddis larva's house, though in this case building behaviour intervenes in the causal chain from genes to house. There is no reason why we should not perform a genetic study of caddis houses, and a question such as 'are round stones dominant to angular stones?' could be a perfectly sensible research question. A bird's nest and a beaver dam are also extended phenotypes. We could do a genetic study of bower bird bowers in exactly the same sense as we could do a genetic study of bird of paradise tails. I continue this conceptual progression further in the book referred to, concluding that genes in one body may have phenotypic expression in another body. For instance, I argue that genes in cuckoos have phenotypic expression in host behaviour. When we look at an animal behaving, we may have to learn to say, not 'How is it benefiting its inclusive fitness?', but rather 'Whose inclusive fitness is it benefiting?'.

Gould is right that genes are not naked to the world. They are chosen by virtue of their phenotypic consequences. But these phenotypic consequences should not be regarded as limited to the particular individual body in which the gene sits, any more than traditionally they have been seen as limited to the particular cell in which the gene sits (red blood corpuscles and sperm cells develop under the influence of genes that are not inside them). Not only is it unnecessary for us to regard the phenotypic expression of a gene as limited to the body in which it sits. It does not have to be limited to any of the discrete vehicles which it can be described as inhabiting – cell, organism, group, community, etc. The concept of the discrete vehicle may turn out to be superfluous. In this respect, if I understand him aright, I am very encouraged by Bateson (this volume, page 136) when he says 'Insistence on character selection and nothing else does not commit anyone to considering just the attributes of individual organisms. The characters could be properties of symbionts such as competing lichens or mutualistic groups such as competing bands of wolves'. However, I think Bateson could have gone further. The use of the word 'competing' in the last sentence quoted suggests that he remains somewhat wedded to the idea of discrete vehicles. An entity such as a band of wolves must be a relatively discrete vehicle if it is to be said to compete with other bands of wolves.

I see the world as populated by competing replicators in germ lines. Each replicator, when compared with its alleles, can be thought of as being attached to a suite of characters, outward and visible tokens of itself. These tokens are its phenotypic consequences, in comparison with its alleles, upon the world. They determine its success or failure in continuing to exist. To a large extent the part of the world which a gene can influence may happen to be limited to a local area which is sufficiently clearly bounded to be called a body, or some other discrete vehicle – perhaps a wolf pack. But this is not necessarily so. Some of the phenotypic consequences of a replicator, when compared with its alleles, may reach across vehicle boundaries. We may have to face the complexity of regarding the biosphere as an intricate network of overlapping fields of phenotypic power. Any particular phenotypic characteristic will have to be seen as the joint product of replicators whose influence converges from many different sources, many different bodies belonging to different species, phyla and kingdoms. This is the doctrine of the 'extended phenotype'.

Conclusion

In the present paper I have mainly tried to clear up a misunderstanding. I have tried to show that the theory of replicators, which I have previously advocated, is not incompatible with orthodox 'individual selectionism'. The confusion over 'units of selection' has arisen because we have failed to distinguish between two distinct meanings of the phrase. In one sense of the term unit, the unit that actually survives or fails to survive, nobody could seriously claim that either an individual organism or a group of organisms was a unit of selection; in this sense, the unit has to be a replicator, which will normally be a small fragment of genome. In the other sense of unit, the 'vehicle', either an individual organism or a group could be a serious contender for the title 'unit of selection'. There are reasons for coming down on the side of the individual organism rather than larger units, but it has not been a main purpose of this paper to advocate this view. My main concern has been to emphasise that, whatever the outcome of the debate about organism versus group as *vehicle*, neither the organism nor the group is a *replicator*. Controversy may exist about rival candidates for replicators and about rival candidates for vehicles, but there should be no controversy over replicators *versus* vehicles. Replicator survival and vehicle selection are two aspects of the same process. The first essential is to distinguish clearly between them. Having done so we may argue the merits of the rival candidates for each, and we may go on to ask, as I briefly did at the end, whether we really need the concept of discrete vehicles at all. If the answer to this turns out to be no, the phrase 'individual selection' may be judged to be misleading. Whatever the upshot of the latter debate about the extended phenotype, I hope here to have removed an unnecessary source of semantic confusion by exposing the difference between replicators and vehicles.

Summary

1. The question of 'units of selection' is not trivial. If we are to talk about adaptations, we need to know which entity in the hierarchy of life they are 'good' for. Adaptations for the good of the group would look quite different from adaptations for the good of the individual or the good of the gene.

2. At first sight, it appears that 'the individual' is intermediate in some nested hierarchy between the group and the gene. This paper shows, however, that the argument over 'group selection' versus 'individual selection' is a different kind of argument from that between 'individual selection' and 'gene selection'. The latter is really an argument about what we ought to *mean* by a unit of selection, a 'replicator' or a 'vehicle'.

3. A Replicator is defined as any entity in the universe of which copies are made. A DNA molecule is a good example. Replicators are classified into Active (having some 'phenotypic' effect on the world which influences the replicator's chance of being copied) and Passive. Cutting across this they are classified into Germ-line (potential ancestor of an indefinitely long line of descendant replicators) and Dead-end (e.g., a gene in a liver cell).

4. Active, germ-line replicators are important. Wherever they arise in the universe, we may expect some form of natural selection and hence evolution to follow.

5. The title of replicator should not be limited to any particular chunk of DNA such as a cistron. Any length of DNA can be treated as a replicator, but with quantitative reservations depending on its length, on recombination rates, linkage disequilibrium, selection pressures etc.

6. An individual organism is not a replicator, because alterations in it are not passed on to subsequent generations. Where reproduction is asexual, it is possible to regard an individual's whole genome as a replicator, but not the individual itself.

7. Genetic replicators are selected not directly but by proxy, via their phenotypic effects. In practice, most of these phenotypic effects are

bundled together with those of other genes in discrete 'Vehicles' – individual bodies. An individual body is not a replicator; it is a vehicle containing replicators, and it tends to work for the replicators inside it.

8. Because of its discreteness and unitariness of structure and function, we commonly phrase our discussions of adaptation at the level of the individual vehicle. We treat adaptations as though they were 'for the good of' the individual, rather than for the good of some smaller unit like a single limb, or some more inclusive vehicle such as a group or species.

9. But even the individual organism may be less unitary and discrete than is sometimes supposed. This is especially true of plants, where it seems to be necessary to define two different kinds of 'individuals', 'ramets' and 'genets'.

10. An individual may be defined as a unit of *reproduction*, as distinct from *growth*. The distinction between reproduction and growth is not an easy one, and it should not be confused with the distinction between sexual and asexual reproduction. Reproduction involves starting anew from a single-celled propagule, while growth (including vegetative 'reproduction') involves 'broad-fronted' multicellular propagation.

11. Kin selection is quite different from group selection, since it does not need to assume the existence of kin-groups as discrete vehicles. More generally, we can question the usefulness of talking about discrete vehicles at all. In some ways a more powerful way of thinking is in terms of replicators with *Extended Phenotypes* in the outside world, effects which may be confined within the borders of discrete vehicles but do not have to be.

12. The concept of the discrete vehicle is useful, however, in clarifying past discussions. The debate between 'individual selection' and 'group selection' is a debate over rival vehicles. There really should be no debate over 'gene selection' versus 'individual (or group) selection', since in the one case we are talking about replicators, in the other about vehicles. Replicator survival and vehicle selection are two views of the same process. They are not rival theories.

I have benefited from discussion with Mark Ridley, Alan Grafen, Marian Dawkins, and Pat Bateson and other members of the conference at King's College. Some of the arguments given here are incorporated, in expanded form, in chapters 5, 6 and 14 of *The Extended Phenotype* (Dawkins, 1982).

References

Alexander, R.D. (1980). *Darwinism and Human Affairs*. Pitman: London.

Alexander, R.D. & Borgia, G. (1978). Group selection, altruism, and the levels of organization of life. *Annual Review of Ecology and Systematics*, **9**, 449–74.

Benzer, S. (1957). The elementary units of heredity. In *The Chemical Basis of Heredity*, ed. W.D. McElroy & B. Glass; pp. 70–93. Johns Hopkins Press: Baltimore.

Bonner, J.T. (1974). *On Development*. Harvard University Press: Cambridge, Mass.

Bonner, J.T. (1980). *The Evolution of Culture in Animals*. Princeton University Press: Princeton, N.S.

Brown, J.L. (1974). Alternate routes to sociality in jays – with a theory for the evolution of altruism and communal breeding. *American Zoologist*, **14**, 63–80.

Clegg, M.T. (1978). Dynamics of correlated genetic systems II. Simulation studies of chromosomal segments under selection. *Theoretical Population Biology*, **13**, 1–23.

Crick, F.H.C. (1979). Split genes and RNA splicing. *Science*, **204**, 264–71.

Dawkins, R. (1976). *The Selfish Gene*. Oxford University Press: Oxford.

Dawkins, R. (1978). Replicator selection and the extended phenotype. *Zeitschrift für Tierpsychologie*, **47**, 61–76.

Dawkins, R. (1979). Twelve misunderstandings of kin selection. *Zeitschrift für Tierpsychologie*, **51**, 184–200.

Dawkins, R. (1982). *The Extended Phenotype*. Freeman: Oxford.

Dawkins, R. & Dawkins, M. (1973). Decisions and the uncertainty of behaviour. *Behaviour*, **45**, 83–103.

Doolittle, W.F. & Sapienza, C. (1980). Selfish genes, the phenotype paradigm and genome evolution. *Nature*, **284**, 601–3.

Ghiselin, M.T. (1974). A radical solution to the species problem. *Systematic Zoology*, **23**, 536–44.

Gould, S.J. (1977). Caring groups and selfish genes. *Natural History*, **86 (12)**, 20–4, (December).

Grafen, A. (1980). Models of *r* and *d*. *Nature*, **284**, 494–5.

Hamilton, W.D. (1964a). The genetical evolution of social behaviour. I. *Journal of Theoretical Biology*, **7**, 1–16.

Hamilton, W.D. (1964b). The genetical evolution of social behaviour. II. *Journal of Theoretical Biology*, **7**, 17–32.

Hamilton, W.D. (1975). Innate social aptitudes of man: an approach from evolutionary genetics. In *Biosocial Anthropology*, ed. R. Fox. Malaby Press: London.

Harper, J.L. (1977). *Population Biology of Plants*. Academic Press: London.

Hull, D.L. (1976). Are species really individuals? *Systematic Zoology*, **25**, 174–91.

Hull, D.L. (1981). The units of evolution: a metaphysical essay. In *Studies in the Concept of Evolution*, ed. U.J. Jensen & R. Harré. The Harvester Press: Hassocks.

Huxley, J.S. (1912). *The Individual in the Animal Kingdom*. Cambridge University Press: Cambridge.

Janzen, D.H. (1977). What are dandelions and aphids? *American Naturalist*, **111**, 586–9.

Leigh, E. (1977). How does selection reconcile individual advantage with the good of the group? *Proceedings of the National Academy of Sciences of the U.S.A.*, **74**, 4542–6.

Lewontin, R.C. (1970). The units of selection. *Annual Review of Ecology and Systematics*, **1**, 1–18.

Lewontin, R.C. (1974). *The Genetic Basis of Evolutionary Change*. Columbia University Press: New York and London.

Maynard Smith, J. (1969). The status of neo-Darwinism. In *Towards a Theoretical Biology* **2**: *Sketches*. Edinburgh University Press: Edinburgh.

Maynard Smith, J. (1976). Group selection. *Quarterly Review of Biology*, **51**, 277–83.

Medawar, P.B. (1957). *The Uniqueness of the Individual.* Methuen: London.

Orgel, L.E. & Crick, F.H.C. (1980). Selfish DNA: the ultimate parasite. *Nature*, **284**, 604–7.

Wade, M.J. (1978). A critical review of the models of group selection. *Quarterly Review of Biology*, **53**, 101–14.

Wallace, A.R. (1866). Letter to Charles Darwin dated July 2nd. In *More Letters of Charles Darwin*, vol. **2**, ed. F. Darwin. Murray (1903): London.

Williams, G.C. (1966). *Adaptation and Natural Selection.* Princeton University Press: New Jersey.

Williams, M.B. (1970). Deducing the consequences of evolution: a mathematical model. *Journal of Theoretical Biology*, **29**, 343–85.

Wilson, D.S. (1980). *The Natural Selection of Populations and Communities.* Benjamin Cummings: Menlo, California.

Wilson, E.O. (1973). Group selection and its significance for ecology. *Bioscience*, **23**, 631–8.

Young, R.M. (1971). Darwin's metaphor: does nature select? *The Monist*, **55**, 442–503.

4

The concept of fitness in population genetics and sociobiology

PETER O'DONALD

Introduction

'Individuals maximize their inclusive fitness' seems to have become the central dogma of sociobiology (for example, see Dawkins, 1978). Dawkins immediately corrects himself to say that what is really maximized is gene survival. But what does 'gene survival' mean? Does it maximize? In the simplest possible model of evolution, the possession of a dominant, semi-dominant or recessive character gives rise to a constant selective advantage. The allele that determines the character will then spread through a population, replacing alternative alleles. When the advantageous allele has replaced the others, its survival as a gene has certainly been maximized. The mean fitness of the population has also been maximized. But very often one allele does not completely replace another in evolution: a stable polymorphism is established in which several alleles may be maintained in a population simultaneously. Equilibrium is maintained by a balance of selective forces. If these selective forces are the result of fitnesses that are constant for each genotype, then the mean fitness is still maximized at the point of stable equilibrium. In what sense can 'gene survival' be said to be maximized unless it is a term synonymous with 'mean fitness'?

Mean fitness may be defined as the average genotypic fitness in a population. It only maximizes when alleles at one particular locus on a chromosome determine genotypes each with constant values of their fitnesses. Varying fitnesses, and interactions in fitness between alleles at different loci, do not in general lead to the maximization of mean fitness. Can we say what happens to 'inclusive fitness' in the course of evolution? 'The full effects of the individual on its own fitness and on the fitness of all its relatives, weighted by the degree of relationship to the relatives, is referred to as the "inclusive fitness"' (Wilson, 1975). In Hamilton's original formulation of a model of kin selection using the concept of inclusive fitness (Hamilton, 1964), it is implicit that inclusive fitness has a constant value for each genotype, since Hamilton inserts his inclusive fitness values into the standard equations for selection with constant fitnesses. The mean inclusive fitness will then maximize if the most fit homozygous genotype replaces the other genotypes. In kin selection, however, when formulated in population genetic terms, the genotypic fitness cannot simply be a constant. If some individuals are altruistic towards their kin, the increase in fitness derived from altruism depends on the chance of having altruistic relatives. This depends on the frequency of the gene for altruism. In altruism between sibs, for example, an individual's fitness depends partly on whether his brothers and sisters possess the altruistic genotypes. This depends on whether their parents possess these genotypes. The benefit from altruism is thus dependent on the frequencies of the altruistic and non-altruistic genotypes in the previous generation. To construct a population-genetic model, we need to know the overall fitness of each genotype. This will be a combination of the individual fitness and the average benefit received from the altruistic sibs. This fitness, which is a characteristic of the genotype in the population as a whole, is therefore different from inclusive fitness. The inclusive fitness of an *altruistic individual* combines his fitness as an individual with the benefit he gives his relatives. Until we know what proportion of altruists receive the benefits, we cannot find the *overall fitness of the altruistic genotypes*: the average effects of benefits received, combined with the effects of each genotype on the individual, determine the overall genotypic fitnesses, hence the frequencies of the genotypes and their matings after selection, and thus the relative genotypic contribution of offspring to the next generation. An explicit population genetic model can be constructed: it cannot be constructed simply by substituting inclusive fitness for fitness in population-genetic models.

Since inclusive fitness is obviously a different concept from that of fitness in population-genetic models, we are led to ask how these two concepts relate to each other and what conclusions may be drawn from a knowledge of inclusive fitnesses. In this essay, I shall first examine the concept of fitness as it is used in population-genetic models. The corresponding expressions for fitness will then be derived for several different genetic models of kin selection. We shall see how these population-genetic concepts of fitness compare with statements that have been made about inclusive fitness. Finally I shall analyse the population changes in mean fitness that occur in kin selection models. Throughout my analyses, I shall assume that the parameters measuring the fitness effects on individuals and their relatives are constants for particular genotypes. If I talk about 'individuals', this will always mean individuals with particular genotypes. Thus I interpret the statement 'individuals maximize their inclusive fitness' to mean 'the mean fitness of individuals with different genotypes is maximized in a population'. I assume that in a particular generation a particular individual is stuck with the fitness he has got: he cannot change it. This is entailed by the assumption that the fitness parameters are constant for particular genotypes. Thus I shall not consider models in which an individual might change his fitness in the course of his life by seeking some other environment or adopting some other strategy of behaviour. Such models would always be special cases. They would not be models of evolution unless genetically some individuals could alter their fitness and others could not.

The measurement of Darwinian fitness

Models of the genetical structure of populations are used to predict evolutionary changes. Evolution is caused by many factors. These include the mating system, in which sexual selection may occur; the genetic system, which produces changes by mutation and recombination and which may produce selection by unequal segregation or meiotic drive; and the environment, which may give rise to natural selection and kin selection and which also determines the intensities of natural selection, sexual selection and kin selection. Selection is not an essential factor for evolution, however: the neutral mutation theory of protein evolution is based on the premises that mutations in the amino-acid sequences of proteins are without selective effect and are fixed or lost by chance. The theory makes general predictions about the rate of accumulation of amino-acid differences and levels of heterozygosity in protein polymorphisms that are broadly in agreement with observation.

The fitness of particular genotypes or phenotypes is defined as their relative contribution of offspring to the next generation. Fitness thus depends on the chances of surviving to reproductive age, the adult survival rate and the variation in fertility during adult life. In organisms like birds and mammals with overlapping generations, we need to know the following statistics for each genotype:

(i) the age-specific survival rate, or survivorship, l_x;

(ii) the age-specific reproductive rate, b_x.

The net reproductive rate, given by

$$R_0 = \sum_x l_x b_x,$$

is often used as a measure of absolute fitness: it is the average number of offspring produced by a newly born individual of the previous generation. Since in general different genotypes will have different generation times, values of R_0 for each genotype are not completely satisfactory as measurements of fitnesses. It is better to calculate the fitnesses from the values of the intrinsic rate of increase, r, in Lotka's equation

$$\sum_x e^{-rx} l_x b_x = 1$$

The value of r can be estimated by solving the polynomial

$$\log_e R_0 = \alpha r + \beta r^2/2 + \gamma r^3/3 + \cdots$$

where

$$\alpha = R_1/R_0$$
$$\beta = \alpha^2 - R_2/R_0$$
$$\gamma = \alpha^3 - 3(R_2 R_1/R_0^2)/2 + \tfrac{1}{2} R_3/R_0$$

and

$$R_1 = \sum_x x l_x b_x$$
$$R_2 = \sum_x x^2 l_x b_x$$

etc.

O'Donald & Davis (1976) give the derivation of these expressions and apply them to the estimation of the fitnesses of the melanic and non-melanic genotypes of the arctic skua. The generation time for each genotype can be found by the formula

$$T = \alpha + \beta r/2 + \gamma r^2/3 + \cdots$$

To a first order of approximation, when terms in r^2 and higher powers of r can be considered negligible, we find immediately that

$$T = R_1/R_0$$

which is the same as the mean age of child-bearing. Then

$$r = \log_e R_0/T.$$

To a second order of approximation

$$r = \{-1 + \sqrt{[1 + 2(1 - R_2 R_0/R_1^2)\log_e R_0]}\}/(R_1/R_0 - R_2/R_1).$$

If two phenotypes or genotypes, A_1 and A_2, have intrinsic rates of increase, r_1 and r_2, then their relative fitness over the course of a generation can be estimated by the ratio

$$w = \exp(r_1 T)/\exp(r_2 T),$$

where T is the mean generation time of the population as a whole (Cavalli-Sforza & Bodmer, 1971). This is a better measure of relative fitness than the ratio of the values of R_0. But if the generation times are the same for each genotype, then

$$T_1 = T_2 = T$$

and

$$\exp(r_1 T)/\exp(r_2 T) = R_0(A_1)/R_0(A_2).$$

These measurements of fitness can be used to determine the changes in genotypic frequencies from one generation to the next. Most genetic models are described in terms of discrete, non-overlapping generations. If generations are continuous, as in humans, or overlapping from one breeding season to the next as in birds and mammals generally, the genotypic frequencies change within each generation, either continuously, or from one breeding season to the next. Unless the intrinsic rates of increase are small, the use of the values $\exp(r_1 T)$ and $\exp(r_2 T)$ as fitnesses in models with discrete generations will lead to error. In fact, in the derivation of differential equations of gene frequency change for continuous generations, it has generally been assumed that rates of change are small. Charlesworth (1974) has proposed a method of calculating the continuous changes in gene frequency based on the intrinsic rates of increase. For the purpose of calculating gene frequencies, Charlesworth's method is more satisfactory than the method using fitnesses for a complete generation; but both methods involve approximation.

The problem of how to measure fitness creates no difficulty when organisms have separate, discrete generations. Insects and annual plants are obvious examples of such organisms. Suppose we observe a population that is polymorphic for the three genotypes $A_1 A_1$, $A_1 A_2$ and $A_2 A_2$. Let their probabilities of survival to reproductive age be the viabilities l_{11}, l_{12} and l_{22}. If they survive, they then produce offspring at rates b_{11}, b_{12} and b_{22}. Therefore, their contributions to the next generation will be given by

$$R_0(A_1 A_1) = l_{11} b_{11}$$
$$R_0(A_1 A_2) = l_{12} b_{12}$$
$$R_0(A_2 A_2) = l_{22} b_{22}$$

We can allow for the relative contributions of both males and females by supposing that male fertilization rates and female egg-laying rates are each given by half of the contribution that each pair of individuals make to the next generation. By giving one of the genotypes, say the heterozygote $A_1 A_2$, an arbitrary fitness of 1.0, we can obtain the relative fitnesses of the two homozygous genotypes as follows:

$$w_{11} = (l_{11}b_{11})/(l_{12}b_{12})$$
$$w_{12} = 1.0$$
$$w_{22} = (l_{22}b_{22})/(l_{12}b_{12}).$$

A population that mates at random with respect to these three genotypes is equivalent to a population of their gametes that unite at random. If p and q are the gametic frequencies of the alleles A_1 and A_2 in generation t, and p' and q' are their gametic frequencies in generation $t + 1$, then after zygotes have formed in generation $t + 1$, the genotypic frequencies follow the Hardy – Weinberg ratios

$$\{A_1A_1\} = p^2$$
$$\{A_1A_2\} = 2pq$$
$$\{A_2A_2\} = q^2.$$

Gametes are produced in $t + 1$ at frequencies

$$p' = (p^2w_{11} + pqw_{12})/\bar{w}$$
$$q' = (q^2w_{22} + pqw_{12})/\bar{w}$$

where

$$\bar{w} = p^2w_{11} + 2pqw_{12} + q^2w_{22}.$$

The mean relative fitness is given by the expression for $\bar{w}$. It changes as the gene frequencies change until an equilibrium is reached at which

$$p' = p = p_*.$$

It is easy to show that at this point

$$p_* = (w_{12} - w_{22})/(2w_{12} - w_{11} - w_{22})$$
$$q_* = (w_{12} - w_{11})/(2w_{12} - w_{11} - w_{22}).$$

Provided that $w_{12} > w_{11}, w_{22}$, the population reaches a stable equilibrium at these gametic frequencies. The mean fitness at this equilibrium attains a maximal value given by

$$w_* = p_*^2w_{11} + 2p_*q_*w_{12} + q_*^2w_{22}.$$

Evolution has maximized the mean population fitness.

In this formulation of fitness, we have explicitly assumed that the values of w_{11}, w_{12} and w_{22} remain constant for each genotype. Although in the early days of population genetics, fitnesses were always assumed to be constant (Fisher, 1930; Haldane, 1932; Wright, 1931), this is most unlikely to be true. The fitnesses may depend on the frequency or density of the individuals with the different genotypes. There are many ecological factors that can give rise to frequency-dependent selection. It has indeed been argued that selection will almost always be frequency-dependent (Kojima,

1971). Density-dependent selection will necessarily be frequency-dependent as well.

Frequency-dependent selection is characteristic of selection for Batesian mimics of warningly coloured distasteful or harmful organisms. Predators avoid the mimics of species they have found to be distasteful. But if the mimics become common relative to their models, predators will encounter many palatable forms with warning colours and may learn to associate warning colour with palatability. Common mimics will suffer a disadvantage relative to rare ones. Predators generally tend to prefer common prey to rare prey: the common prey are the ones they have learnt and are looking for (Allen & Clarke, 1968). If genotypes utilize different environmental resources, the commoner genotypes will deplete more of the resource they need than the rare genotypes. Frequency-dependent selection of this sort has been found to maintain the stability of polymorphisms at certain allozyme loci (Kojima, 1971). In all these examples, the frequency-dependence is negative: the advantage is to the rare. Sexual selection, too, can give rise to a 'rare-male' effect as a consequence of the expression of female preference (O'Donald, 1977, 1978, 1980). Now when the values of the fitnesses are frequency-dependent, there is no reason to assume that the mean population fitness will reach a maximal value in evolution. Consider a simple model of selection dependent on genotype frequency (Clarke & O'Donald, 1964). Let r and s define a linear relationship between fitness and frequency as follows.

$$w_{11} = 1 - rp^2$$
$$w_{12} = 1 - 2spq$$
$$w_{22} = 1 - rq^2.$$

If the allele A_1 has just entered the population at a very low frequency (for example it may have just arisen by mutation), then the relative fitnesses will be given approximately by the values

$$w_{11} = 1$$
$$w_{12} = 1 - 2sp$$
$$w_{22} = 1 - r(1 - 2p).$$

The mean fitness is approximately

$$\bar{w} \simeq 1.0.$$

It can be shown that at equilibrium $p_* = q_* = \frac{1}{2}$ and the mean fitness is then

$$\bar{w} = 1 - (r + 2s)/8.$$

The value of w thus declines from its value when the allele A_1 was just starting to spread through the population. A similar result is found if the fitnesses are functions of the frequencies of dominant and recessive phenotypes. Suppose A_1 is dominant to A_2. The A_1A_1 and A_1A_2 combine to give a phenotype A_1 with frequency

$$p^2 + 2pq = 1 - q^2.$$

Thus the fitnesses will become

$$w_{11} = 1 - s(1 - q^2)$$
$$w_{12} = w_{11}$$
$$w_{22} = 1 - tq^2,$$

where s and t now define the relationship of fitness to frequency. This model might describe the selection exerted by a predator who learnt that A_1 and A_2 were palatable phenotypes and who had a tendency to pursue the commoner phenotypes he had developed a searching image for. In this model at stable equilibrium

$$p_* = 1 - \sqrt{[s/(s + t)]}$$
$$q_* = \sqrt{[s/(s + t)]}$$

and

$$\bar{w}_* = 1 - st/(s - t).$$

Therefore $\bar{w}$ is a maximum, not at equilibrium, but at the point when either A_1 or A_2 are just about to be eliminated from the population.

In general, therefore, $\bar{w}$ does not reach a maximum by natural selection. It does so only in the special case when a number of alleles at a single locus are subject to constant genotypic or phenotypic selection.

A model of kin selection

Population-genetic models of kin selection have been described by Charnov (1977), Charlesworth (1978) and Cavalli-Sforza & Feldman (1978). In Charnov's model Hardy-Weinberg frequencies were assumed, but as we shall see, this assumption is not valid for kin selection. Charlesworth obtained conditions for initial increase of an altruistic trait with partial penetrance in its genotypic expression. Cavalli-Sforza & Feldman (1978) analysed a general model of kin selection in which the allele A_1 may give rise to altruistic behaviour towards the altruist's brothers and sisters. It is a model of sib-to-sib altruism. This appears to be one example of kin selection for which an exact population genetic model can be derived. In order to formulate this model in the population-genetic terms of the models I have described in the previous section, we must consider the frequencies of the matings in generation t that will give rise to individuals with genotypes A_1A_1, A_1A_2 and A_2A_2 who may also have sibs with these genotypes. After selection has taken place, these genotypes will be present in the population at frequencies u, v and w, producing gametes with frequencies

$$p = u + \tfrac{1}{2}v$$
$$q = w + \tfrac{1}{2}v.$$

Since selection has already taken place at this stage, we cannot assume that the genotypic frequencies occur in the Hardy-Weinberg ratios, p^2, $2pq$ and q^2.

Matings take place between the genotypes with the following frequencies:

Mating	Frequency
$A_1A_1 \times A_1A_1$	u^2
$A_1A_1 \times A_1A_2$	$2uv$
$A_1A_1 \times A_2A_2$	$2uw$
$A_1A_2 \times A_1A_2$	v^2
$A_1A_2 \times A_2A_2$	$2vw$
$A_2A_2 \times A_2A_2$	w^2.

Now we can obtain the probabilities that two sibs, chosen at random, shall have specified genotypes. For example, the probability that two sibs are both genotypically A_1A_1 is given by

$$u^2 + \tfrac{1}{2} \cdot \tfrac{1}{2} \cdot 2uv + \tfrac{1}{4} \cdot \tfrac{1}{4} \cdot v^2 = (u + v/4)^2.$$

This follows because matings $A_1A_1 \times A_1A_1$ produce only A_1A_1 offspring; matings $A_1A_1 \times A_1A_2$ produce A_1A_1 offspring with probability $\tfrac{1}{2}$; and matings $A_1A_2 \times A_1A_2$ produce A_1A_1 offspring with probability $\tfrac{1}{4}$. What is the probability that an A_1A_1 individual has a sib who is also A_1A_1? In general, for two events A and B, the probability of the joint event is

$$P(A \text{ and } B) = P(A|B) \cdot P(B),$$

where $P(A|B)$ is the conditional probability of A given B. Since the probability of being A_1A_1 is simply p^2, therefore we have the conditional probability

$$P(A_1A_1|A_1A_1) = (u + v/4)^2/p^2.$$

Similarly, for sibs who are A_1A_1 and A_1A_2, we have

$$P(A_1A_1 \text{ and } A_1A_2) = \tfrac{1}{2} \cdot \tfrac{1}{2} \cdot 2uv + \tfrac{1}{2} \cdot \tfrac{1}{4} \cdot v^2 = \tfrac{1}{2}v(u + v/4).$$

Therefore

$$P(A_1 A_1 | A_1 A_2) = \tfrac{1}{2} v(u + v/4)/(2pq)$$
$$P(A_1 A_2 | A_1 A_1) = \tfrac{1}{2} v(u + v/4)/p^2.$$

Proceeding in this way for all possible pairs of genotypes of sibs, we get the conditional probability matrix of Cavalli-Sforza & Feldman (1978):

Genotype of individual	Genotypes of sibs of individual		
	$A_1 A_1$	$A_1 A_2$	$A_2 A_2$
$A_1 A_1$	$(u + v/4)^2/p^2$	$\tfrac{1}{2} v(u + v/4)/p^2$	$\tfrac{1}{16} v^2/p^2$
$A_1 A_2$	$\tfrac{1}{2} v(u + v/4)/(2pq)$	$(pq + uw)/(2pq)$	$\tfrac{1}{2} v(w + v/4)/(2pq)$
$A_2 A_2$	$\tfrac{1}{16} v^2/q^2$	$\tfrac{1}{2} v(w + v/4)/q^2$	$(w + v/4)^2/q^2.$

Since the genotypes $A_1 A_1$, $A_1 A_2$ and $A_2 A_2$ are produced with probabilities p^2, $2pq$ and q^2 after random mating, each conditional probability that they have sibs with any of these genotypes sums to unity.

Suppose individuals may perform altruistic acts for their sibs; but if they do, they reduce their own chances of survival. At the same time they may also gain in fitness if they themselves benefit from an altruistic act. Let proportions a, h and b of individuals who are $A_1 A_1$, $A_1 A_2$ and $A_2 A_2$ act as altruists. These proportions represent the 'penetrance' of the genotypes in respect of the altruistic trait. If $a = h = 1$ and $b = 0$, the allele A_1 is fully penetrant and dominant: all $A_1 A_1$ and $A_1 A_2$ individuals will be altruists. If $a = b = 0$ and $h = 1$, the heterozygotes alone will be altruists. Having determined the probabilities that an individual may have an altruist for a brother or sister, we must now consider how the components of fitness – the costs and benefits – should be combined. Prior to Cavalli-Sforza & Feldman's paper, no consideration seems to have been given to this problem, although, as we shall see, it is of crucial importance in determining the final outcome of kin selection. Consider, for example, altruistic individuals, some of whom may stand guard to warn their brothers and sisters if a predator should approach. By taking this altruistic stance, they put themselves at a greater risk from predation than their non-altruistic sibs. Will their additional risk depend on whether they themselves also benefit from the altruistic acts of others? Or will it be independent of any benefit they may gain? If it is independent, the benefit will be the same, whether or not the altruists successfully warned their sibs. This is surely the most plausible assumption: the warning may or may not have been successful, but this should not affect the chances that an altruist receives warning in his turn. On the assumption of independence, the costs and benefits to fitness must be combined multiplicatively. But if, as seems less plausible, the altruists gain a benefit only if they successfully warn their sibs, then the costs and benefits must be combined additively.

Following the logic of Cavalli-Sforza & Feldman, the individuals with genotypes $A_1 A_1$, $A_1 A_2$ and $A_2 A_2$ will benefit by having altruistic sibs with probabilities

$$f_{11} = a(u + v/4)^2/p^2 + \tfrac{1}{2}hv(u + v/4)/p^2 + \tfrac{1}{16}bv^2/p^2$$
$$f_{12} = \tfrac{1}{2}av(u + v/4)/(2pq) + h(pq + uw)/(2pq) + \tfrac{1}{2}bv(w + v/4)/(2pq)$$
$$f_{22} = \tfrac{1}{16}av^2/q^2 + \tfrac{1}{2}hv(w + v/4)/q^2 + b(w + v/4)^2/q^2.$$

The benefit, expressed as a gain in relative fitness, is then given by βf_{ij}, while the altruists lose an amount γ in fitness. Depending on whether the costs and benefits are combined multiplicatively or additively, the overall fitnesses will then be as follows.

Genotype	Multiplicative model	Additive model
$A_1 A_1$	$\phi_{11} = (1 - a\gamma)(1 + \beta f_{11})$	$\phi_{11} = 1 - a\gamma + \beta f_{11}$
$A_1 A_2$	$\phi_{12} = (1 - h\gamma)(1 + \beta f_{12})$	$\phi_{12} = 1 - h\gamma + \beta f_{12}$
$A_2 A_2$	$\phi_{22} = (1 - b\gamma)(1 + \beta f_{22})$	$\phi_{22} = 1 - b\gamma + \beta f_{22}$

As thus defined, these fitnesses have exactly the same meaning as fitnesses in any other population-genetic model: they represent the relative fitness of individuals of one genotype compared to individuals of another. They determine the relative viabilities of the individuals and hence the relative contribution of offspring to the next generation made by individuals of each genotype. They are complicated functions of the gene and genotype frequencies from the previous generation. They are obviously not what is generally understood by the concept of inclusive fitness.

Following Hamilton's original paper (1964), we should define the 'inclusive fitness effect' for an individual A by the expression

$$\delta R_A^* = \sum r(\delta a_r)_A = -\gamma + \tfrac{1}{2}\beta$$

where r is the coefficient of relationship of A and his relations, and δa_r is the effect on fitness of relatives with coefficient of relationship r. Hamilton immediately proceeds to assume that this concept can be applied without modification to genotypes and writes for the inclusive fitness of the genotypes

$$R_{ij}^* = 1 - \delta R_{ij},$$

where δR_{ij} is the inclusive fitness effect of the genotype $A_i A_j$. But while strongly asserting this, he gives no reason to show why this step is valid. To denote genotypic fitnesses, the expressions for R_{ij}^* (our ϕ_{ij}) must be complicated frequency-dependent functions. They are not simply the sums of the effects of the costs and benefits multiplied by the coefficients of relationship. Hamilton simply slots the symbols R_{ij}^* into the standard equations for constant fitnesses and concludes that the mean inclusive fitness will maximize – which it will obviously seem to do if fitnesses are taken as constants. The mean fitness, however, is really a most complicated function of the frequencies of the genes and genotypes, the behaviour of which is most unlikely to be obtained from any general analysis. This is a problem which Cavalli-Sforza & Feldman (1978) did not attempt to discuss.

I propose to discuss the evolutionary consequences of kin selection by analysing three simple models. In the first model, the altruists are assumed to be dominant, with $a = h = 1$ and $b = 0$. In the second and third models, the altruists are either heterozygotes ($a = b = 0, h = 1$) or homozygotes ($a = b = 1, h = 0$). Cavalli-Sforza & Feldman described the outcome of selection in the first of these models. The frequencies of the genotypes $A_1 A_1$, $A_1 A_2$ and $A_2 A_2$ are given by the values (u, v, w). If the point $(0, 0, 1)$ is unstable, then the altruists will be selected: the allele A_1 can enter the population and start to increase in frequency: instability of the point $(0, 0, 1)$ 'protects' the allele against loss. If the point $(1, 0, 0)$ is stable, the allele A_1 becomes fixed in the population which ultimately comes to consist only of individuals with the genotype $A_1 A_1$. If both the fixation states $(0, 0, 1)$ and $(1, 0, 0)$ are unstable, neither the allele A_1 nor A_2 can become fixed: a polymorphism is therefore maintained.

Dominance of the allele for altruism

For sib-to-sib altruism in which the allele for altruism is completely dominant, Cavalli-Sforza & Feldman obtained the following results.

Multiplicative model	Additive model
$(0, 0, 1)$ is unstable	$(0, 0, 1)$ is unstable
if $\gamma < \beta/(2 + \beta)$	if $\gamma < \frac{1}{2}\beta$
or $\beta > 2\gamma/(1 - \gamma)$	or $\beta > 2\gamma$
$(1, 0, 0)$ is stable	$(1, 0, 0)$ is stable
if $\gamma < 2\beta/(4 + 5\beta)$	if $\gamma < \frac{1}{2}\beta$
or $\beta > 4\gamma/(2 - 5\gamma)$	or $\beta > 2\gamma$

The additive model gives an outcome that is consistent with the formulation in terms of inclusive fitness. The non-altruists have an inclusive fitness of 1.0; the altruists have an inclusive fitness of $1 - \gamma + \frac{1}{2}\beta$. The altruists have the greater inclusive fitness if $\beta > 2\gamma$. This is the condition in the additive model that the gene for altruism spreads through the population ultimately reaching fixation. In the multiplicative model, the conditions for initial increase and ultimate fixation of the gene for altruism are more stringent. For example, suppose $\gamma = 0.2$. Then for 'protection' of the polymorphism, we must have

$$0.5 < \beta < 0.8$$

and for ultimate fixation

$$\beta > 0.8.$$

This is twice the value of β as given by inclusive fitness. For a smaller value of γ, say $\gamma = 0.1$, the conditions for protection are

$$0.22 < \beta < 0.27$$

and the condition for fixation

$$\beta > 0.27.$$

As the values of γ get smaller, the conditions for protection and fixation converge on those for the additive model. Cavalli-Sforza & Feldman also obtained the corresponding results for a sex-linked locus. In this case, too, the additive model gives the same conditions for protection and fixation as those based on inclusive fitness. The multiplicative model gives more stringent conditions that only converge on the inclusive fitness conditions as $\gamma \to 0$.

It should now be clear how the concept of inclusive fitness relates to the population-genetic concept of fitness. Inclusive fitness is not fitness in the population-genetic sense: it does not describe the genotypic contribution of offspring to the next generation. It relates to the conditions that an allele may enter a population and thus remain protected against loss. For the additive model of sib-to-sib altruism, inclusive fitness gives the exact conditions both for protection and for ultimate fixation. For the more realistic multiplicative model, it only gives an approximation to these conditions for small parameter values. At large parameter values, it gives conditions that may be much less stringent than the exact conditions.

In view of the frequency-dependence of kin selection, it is obvious that a general analysis of the effects of selection on mean fitness is going to be extremely difficult or impossible. However, it is easy to determine what happens to mean fitness in a particular numerical case: the changes in gene frequency and mean fitness can be calculated from one generation to the next by computer. In the model with complete dominance of the allele A_1, fitness is maximized at its fixation state. But, as we have seen, it reaches fixation only if

$$\beta > 4\gamma/(2 - 5\gamma).$$

It is eliminated if

$$\beta < 2\gamma/(1 - \gamma).$$

And it arrives at a polymorphic state if

$$2\gamma/(1 - \gamma) < \beta < 4\gamma/(2 - 5\gamma).$$

If we consider again the case when $\gamma = 0.1$, and let $\beta = 0.25$, then computer solution of the recurrence equations of the genotypic frequencies shows that a stable polymorphism is established at which A_1 has an equilibrium frequency

$$p_* = 0.6667.$$

At this frequency, the mean fitness is

$$\phi_* = 1.1126.$$

At the point at which A_1 has just entered the population, the mean fitness has its minimum value of

$$\phi_{\min} = 1.0$$

and at the point of fixation of A_1 it has its maximum value of

$$\phi_{\max} = 1.125.$$

But since the fixation states are unstable, at the point of maximum fitness, A_2 will increase in frequency until the point of stable equilibrium has been reached, the mean fitness declining from $\phi_{\max}$ to ϕ_*.

In the case when $\gamma = 0.2$, $\beta = 0.6$, we find a stable polymorphism established at the frequency

$$p_* = 0.4389$$

with

$$\phi_* = 1.2063$$
$$\phi_{\max} = 1.28$$
$$\phi_{\min} = 1.0.$$

Heterozygous altruism

Suppose the altruistic individuals are the heterozygotes, $A_1 A_2$. Then we obtain the following fitnesses in the multiplicative model:

$$\phi_{11} = 1 + \tfrac{1}{2}\beta v(u + v/4)/p^2$$
$$\phi_{12} = (1 - \gamma)[1 + \beta(pq + uw)/(2pq)]$$
$$\phi_{22} = 1 + \tfrac{1}{2}\beta v(w + v/4)/q^2.$$

As we should expect, both this and the additive model give rise to polymorphic equilibria since the fitnesses are symmetric. The genotypic frequencies from one generation to the next are given by the recurrence equations

$$\phi u' = p^2 + \tfrac{1}{2}\beta v(u + v/4)$$
$$\phi v' = 2pq(1 - \gamma) + \beta(1 - \gamma)(pq + uw)$$
$$\phi w' = q^2 + \tfrac{1}{2}\beta v(w + v/4)$$

where the mean fitness is

$$\phi = 1 - 2\gamma pq + 2\beta pq - \beta\gamma(pq + uw).$$

This gives the result

$$u' - w' = (u - w)(1 + \tfrac{1}{2}\beta v)/\phi$$

so that at equilibrium

$$u_* = w_*$$
$$p_* = q_* = \tfrac{1}{2}.$$

Although this is a point of equilibrium, it may not be stable: if it is not stable, the less common allele will be lost. Stability is determined by the condition

$$(1 + \tfrac{1}{2}\beta v)/\phi < 1$$

since if this condition holds, the values of $u - w$ in successive generations must converge to zero. It is not easy to evaluate the constraints on the parameters that this condition imposes. Suppose, however, that the values of β and γ are small, so that terms like $\beta^2, \gamma^2, \beta\gamma$ can all be considered to be negligible. We may then assume that approximately the genotypic frequencies will follow the Hardy-Weinberg Law, giving equilibrium frequencies

$$u_* = w_* = \tfrac{1}{4}$$
$$v_* = \tfrac{1}{2}.$$

The condition for stability thus becomes

$$\beta > 2\gamma/(1 + 5\gamma/4).$$

Since by expansion of the right hand side we obtain

$$2\gamma/(1 + 5\gamma/4) = 2\gamma[1 - 5\gamma/4 + (5\gamma/4)^2 - \cdots]$$
$$\simeq 2\gamma$$

then approximately

$$\beta > 2\gamma.$$

This approximate condition for stability is the same as saying that the altruists must have a greater inclusive fitness than the non-altruists. This is also the condition for stability in the corresponding additive model.

When squares and higher powers of the parameters are no longer thought to be negligible, the condition based on the inclusive fitness no longer holds. For example, if $\gamma = 0.2$, then the central equilibrium at $p_* = \frac{1}{2}$ is stable if $\beta > 0.5$. This condition is more stringent than that given by inclusive fitness. It is nevertheless remarkable that even in the case of heterozygous altruism, use of inclusive fitness gives the most important result – the conditions for protection of a polymorphism – to close approximation for small parameter values.

In this model of heterozygous altruism, mean fitness is maximized if the polymorphism is stable. The value of ϕ obviously takes its maximal value when $p = q$ and $u = w$, which are the values at equilibrium. If the equilibrium is not stable, then the point $p = \frac{1}{2}$ defines the domains of convergence to the fixation states: if $p > \frac{1}{2}$, A_1 is fixed; if $p < \frac{1}{2}$, A_2 is fixed.

Homozygous altruism

If homozygous individuals are the altruists towards their sibs, a monomorphic population will necessarily consist entirely of altruists who may be genotypically either $A_1 A_1$ or $A_2 A_2$. This case is the opposite of heterozygous altruism and is obviously unrealistic. Nevertheless, as I shall show, inclusive fitness still provides the approximate conditions for the maintenance of the altruist population, even in this extreme and unlikely genetical model. We should expect that the allele A_2 could only invade an $A_1 A_1$ population (and similarly, A_1 could only invade an $A_2 A_2$ population) if the selfish heterozygotes that were introduced had an inclusive fitness greater than that of the altruists. For sib-to-sib altruism, this would entail the condition

$$\beta < 2\gamma.$$

As before, β is the benefit received as a result of the altruism and γ the cost of being altruistic. Then for the multiplicative model, we obtain the following recurrence equations from Cavalli-Sforza & Feldman's conditional probability matrix

$$\phi u' = p^2(1 - \gamma) + \tfrac{1}{2}\beta(1 - \gamma)(p^2 + u^2)$$
$$\phi v' = 2pq + \tfrac{1}{2}\beta v(1 - \tfrac{1}{2}v)$$
$$\phi w' = q^2(1 - \gamma) + \tfrac{1}{2}\beta(1 - \gamma)(q^2 + w^2).$$

Therefore

$$\phi(u' - w') = (u - w)(1 - \gamma)(1 + \beta - \tfrac{1}{2}\beta v)$$

where

$$\phi = 1 + (\beta - \gamma)(p^2 + q^2) - \tfrac{1}{2}\beta\gamma(p^2 + q^2 + u^2 + w^2).$$

At equilibrium

$$u_* = w_*$$
$$p_* = \tfrac{1}{2}.$$

Assuming that β and γ are only small quantities and the Hardy-Weinberg Law holds approximately after selection, then

$$\phi \approx 1 - \tfrac{1}{2}\gamma + \tfrac{1}{2}\beta$$
$$u' - w' = (u - w)(1 - \gamma + \tfrac{3}{4}\beta)/(1 - \tfrac{1}{2}\gamma + \tfrac{1}{2}\beta).$$

Therefore

$$u' - w' \to 0$$

provided that

$$(1 - \gamma + \tfrac{3}{4}\beta)/(1 - \tfrac{1}{2}\gamma + \tfrac{1}{2}\beta) < 1$$

or $\quad \beta < 2\gamma,$

which is exactly the condition suggested by the values of inclusive fitness. The additive model gives the same result. In fact, the values of β can be much greater than this: the condition for maintaining an altruist population is always more stringent than the condition based on inclusive fitness. The deviations from the Hardy-Weinberg Law are always considerable unless the parameter values are very small. These deviations from Hardy-Weinberg seem to make an exact analysis impossible.

The recurrence equations are easy to analyse numerically, however. As expected, the multiplicative and additive models give different results, the conditions for the maintenance of a monomorphic population being more stringent in the multiplicative model.

Multiplicative model. (i) $\gamma = 0.1$ A stable polymorphic equilibrium is attained at the frequency $p_* = \tfrac{1}{2}$ provided that $\beta \leq 0.25$.
(ii) $\gamma = 0.2$ The polymorphic equilibrium is stable provided that $\beta \leq 0.667$.

Additive model. (i) $\gamma = 0.1$ The polymorphic equilibrium is stable provided that $\beta \leq 0.204$. The value $\beta = 0.204$ gives rise to only local stability of the equilibrium point at $p_* = \tfrac{1}{2}$; the value $\beta \leq 0.2$ gives rise to global stability. When $\beta = 0.204$, the conditions

$$0.287 \leq p \leq 0.713$$

define the domain of convergence to $p_* = \tfrac{1}{2}$.
(ii) $\gamma = 0.2$ The polymorphic equilibrium is stable provided that

$\beta \le 0.419$. When $\beta = 0.419$, the equilibrium $p_* = \frac{1}{2}$ is locally stable with domain of convergence given by the conditions

$$0.409 \le p \le 0.591,$$

but when $\beta \le 0.4$ the equilibrium is globally stable.

In each of these four numerical examples, an allele giving rise to a selfish heterozygote may invade an homozygous altruist population and establish a stable polymorphism of both altruistic and selfish individuals. The conditions for initial invasion and final stability are always at least somewhat more stringent than the conditions obtained from the inclusive fitnesses. In the multiplicative model, they are much more stringent. With very small parameter values, however, the Hardy-Weinberg Law gives a good approximation to the genotypic frequencies after selection and the argument from inclusive fitness becomes exact.

Conclusions

In sociobiology, the concept of inclusive fitness has been used very widely in order to determine the evolutionary consequences of altruistic behaviour that raises the fitness of the relatives of the altruist. In this paper, I have analysed the simplest example of kin selection to which the concept of inclusive fitness has been applied – that of sib-to-sib altruism. Cavalli-Sforza & Feldman (1978) derived a general and explicit population-genetic model for sib-to-sib altruism. On the basis that an altruist reduces his own chances of survival by the fraction γ, but increases his sibs' chances by β, his inclusive fitness would be given by

$$R_A = 1 - \gamma + \tfrac{1}{2}\beta.$$

This quantity is different from the fitness of individuals possessing particular genes or genotypes. Genotypic fitnesses, which are required to formulate a population-genetic model of the selection of the altruists, are found to be complicated functions of the genotypic frequencies in the previous generation. These functions bear no simple relationship to inclusive fitness. Inclusive fitness is therefore a different concept from that of fitness as used in population genetics. Inclusive fitness relates to the conditions for initial increase and ultimate fixation of a gene for altruism.

The values of the parameters β and γ determine the possible outcomes of the process of kin selection: (i) the gene for altruism may be lost from the population; (ii) it may be protected from loss and ultimately reach some stable polymorphic state; or (iii) it may become fixed. In the limiting case when the parameter values tend to zero, the condition $\beta > 2\gamma$ ensures that the gene for altruism will be protected against loss and may therefore increase in frequency either to fixation or to a polymorphic equilibrium; if the population consists of homozygous altruists, this condition ensures that selfish individuals cannot invade the altruist population. This result is exactly what we obtain from inclusive fitness by requiring that the benefit given to relatives, when multiplied by the coefficient of relationship r ($r = \frac{1}{2}$ for sibs), must exceed the cost of being altruistic, or that $- \gamma + \frac{1}{2}\beta > 0$. This condition holds for three completely different genetical models: altruism which is dominant; altruism which is heterozygous; and altruism which is homozygous.

If the parameter values are not extremely small, then the conditions for the protection of an altruistic gene may become much more stringent than the condition given by inclusive fitness. Particularly, this depends on the formulation of the model: a model in which the costs and benefits are combined multiplicatively can easily give rise to a value for the benefit that may be twice the value given by inclusive fitness; in such a case altruism would only evolve if the benefit to the sibs were more than four times the cost suffered by the altruist. The probable magnitudes of the parameters as well as the nature of the process of giving and receiving benefits must therefore be considered as factors in determining whether altruism may evolve.

Summary

1. In population-genetic models, the fitness of particular genotypes or phenotypes is defined as their relative contribution of offspring to the next generation. Demographic data on survival and reproductive rates of each genotype can be used to estimate their relative fitnesses. If the fitnesses are constant from one generation to the next, the mean fitness of the population is eventually maximized. In many examples of selection, however, a genotype's fitness depends on its frequency: mean fitness does not then reach a maximum; it often declines in the course of evolution.

2. In a model of kin selection in which individuals may act altruistically towards their brothers and sisters, the genotypic fitnesses are shown to be complicated functions of the genotypic frequencies in the previous generation. As a result of this frequency-dependence, the mean fitness does not necessarily maximize. Inclusive fitness is defined as an individual's own fitness plus his effect on his relatives' fitness weighted by his degree of relationship to them. This is not frequency-dependent and shows that inclusive fitness is a different concept from that of genotypic fitness in population genetic

models. Inclusive fitness relates to the conditions that a gene for altruism may enter a population and remain protected against loss.

3. In models of selection for altruism, an altruist's own fitness may be combined either additively or multiplicatively with the benefit gained from sibs' altruism. In the additive model, inclusive fitness gives the conditions for the protection of the gene for altruism. In the multiplicative model, inclusive fitness gives the conditions for protection only if the effects of selection are small, tending to zero. If altruism has large effects on an individual and his relatives, the conditions for protection become much more stringent than those obtained from the inclusive fitness: relatives must receive much greater benefits before the gene for altruism can start to increase in frequency in the population. These conclusions are only slightly affected by the genetics of the altruistic character: dominant, heterozygous and homozygous characters for altruism are each maintained in a population under approximately the same conditions. In every case, inclusive fitness gives the conditions for the maintenance of altruism when parameters of selection are small.

References

Allen, J.A. & Clarke, B.C. (1968). Evidence for apostatic selection on the part of wild passerines. *Nature*, **220**, 501–2.

Cavalli-Sforza, L.L. & Bodmer, W.F. (1971). *The Genetics of Human Populations*. W.H. Freeman: San Francisco.

Cavalli-Sforza, L.L. & Feldman, M.W. (1978). Darwinian selection and "altruism". *Theoretical Population Biology*, **14**, 268–80.

Charlesworth, B. (1974). Selection in populations with overlapping generations VI. Rates of change of gene frequency and population growth rate. *Theoretical Population Biology*, **6**, 108–33.

Charlesworth, B. (1978). Some models of the evolution of altruistic behaviour between siblings. *Journal of Theoretical Biology*, **72**, 297–317.

Charnov, E.L. (1977). An elementary treatment of the genetical theory of kin-selection. *Journal of Theoretical Biology*, **66**, 541–50.

Clarke, B.C. & O'Donald, P. (1964). Frequency-dependent selection. *Heredity*, **19**, 201–6.

Dawkins, R. (1978). Replicator selection and the extended phenotype. *Zeitschrift für Tierpsychologie*, **47**, 61–76.

Fisher, R.A. (1930). *The Genetical Theory of Natural Selection*. Clarendon Press: Oxford.

Haldane, J.B.S. (1932). *The Causes of Evolution*. Longmans, Green: London.

Hamilton, W.D. (1964). The genetical evolution of social behaviour. I. II. *Journal of Theoretical Biology*, **7**, 1–52.

Kojima, K. (1971). Is there a constant fitness value for a given genotype? No! *Evolution*, **25**, 281–5.

O'Donald, P. (1977). The mating advantage of rare males in models of sexual selection. *Nature*, **267**, 151–4.

O'Donald, P. (1978). Rare male mating advantage. *Nature*, **272**, 189.
O'Donald, P. (1980). *Genetic Models of Sexual Selection*. Cambridge University Press: Cambridge.
O'Donald, P. & Davis, J.W.F. (1976). A demographic analysis of the components of selection in a population of Arctic Skuas. *Heredity*, **36**, 343–50.
Wilson, E.O. (1975). *Sociobiology*. Belknap Press: Massachusetts.
Wright, S. (1931). Evolution in Mendelian populations. *Genetics*, **16**, 97–159.

....

II

Complexity in evolutionary processes

Edited by
D.I. RUBENSTEIN

Natural selection may be the most potent agent of evolutionary change, but it is not the only one. As every first-year biology student knows other factors such as genetic drift and allometry can lead to the modification of species. This obvious fact is often forgotten, however, when biologists construct arguments to account for the evolution of various adaptations. Today reliance on selection is virtually complete, even if the selection being envisaged is somewhat simplistic. Criticism of this pan-selectionist approach to evolution began when Darwin first proposed his theory, and it has not diminished in intensity as sociobiology has gained prominence. By critically examining the role that natural selection plays in evolution, and the complexities involved in this interaction, the essays in Section II attempt to provide insights into why some of the objections to sociobiology are fair, whereas others are not.

First, Rubenstein examines conceptual limitations arising from a too narrow view of the selection process. By focusing on how natural selection operates in environments that change, he shows that natural selection does not always favour behaviour that on average yields the highest payoffs or produces the most offspring. At least for behaviour associated with foraging, reproduction and sociality, alternatives having lower average success as well as lower variance in success may often be favoured by natural selection. The consequences of expanding the traditional view of how selection operates will undoubtably affect not only the ways in which evolutionary hypotheses are formulated or the ways in which experiments are designed to test them, but also the means by which field workers evaluate the success of alternative patterns of behaviour.

In the next essay Thompson examines how evolution proceeds in the absence of selection. She shows how the structure of a population – its size, rate of change, family size and mating patterns – affect a gene's probability of survival. In diploid organisms reproducing sexually the survival of one gene reduces the survival prospect of a rival gene. As Thompson shows, bottlenecks or decreases in family size both significantly increase such negative correlations in gene survival. Perhaps her most intriguing finding that illustrates how effective population structure can be in causing evolutionary change pertains to explaining the presence of incest taboos. Selectionists suggest that the avoidance of mating with close relations is favoured because it decreases the likelihood of lethal homozygous recessives appearing in offspring. Thompson's structuralist interpretation, however, proposes that since the correlation of gene extinctions between any two individuals in a population is highest among mates, the avoidance of inbreeding simply represents the avoidance of competition by descendants of a common ancestor trying to propagate replicates of the same gene. Because she shows that the effects of structure are significant, the magnitude of the change they bring about in a population's composition must be assessed as a baseline against which to compare the change associated with a selectionist, or 'adaptationist' argument.

Selectionists often fail to appreciate that there are limits to the effectiveness of natural selection. In the third essay, Bateson shows that developmental processes will often serve as such constraints. By preventing many genetic changes from being expressed in the phenotype, plasticity in an individual's development may hide genetic changes from the action of natural selection. But if development can prevent selection from producing the best of all possible worlds, Bateson explores the idea that development can create some new worlds as well. By amplifying the effects of small mutations, developmental plasticity may create the hopeful monsters envisaged by Goldschmidt. It is clear that developmental biology is taking on a more prominent role in deciphering the complexities of natural selection. But as Bateson also emphasises, evolutionary theory is unravelling some tangled developmental problems as more and more aspects of an individual's ontogeny are scrutinised in terms of their adaptive value.

Just as developmental biology is benefitting from an association with evolutionary theory, so is ecology as Łomnicki reveals in the last essay of Section II. A principle so central to evolution – that individuals are different – has largely been omitted from ecological theory. When Łomnicki allows competitors to vary in their ability to acquire resources, he finds that the dynamics and stability of populations change dramatically. By examining patterns of animal dispersal he shows how these two bodies of theory can be married to produce the ecological patterns that biologists encounter in nature. This analysis shows the value of making ecological models more realistic by making them consistent with evolutionary principles, even if accomplishing the task will not be easy.

5

Risk, uncertainty and evolutionary strategies

DANIEL I. RUBENSTEIN

Introduction

Biologists have long appreciated that animals live in habitats that are spatially heterogeneous and that change over time. That most biologists subscribe to the view of natural selection favouring individuals that obtain the highest *expected* lifetime reproductive success, or genotypes which leave, *on average*, the most mature offspring, shows they also believe this variation plays an important role in evolution. Yet this belief is not echoed in most models of the evolutionary process. Apart from some models of life history evolution (Cohen, 1966, 1968; MacArthur, 1972; and Schaffer, 1974), the role of environmental variation has largely been ignored by implicitly assuming that strategies always manifest their expected fitness. In effect, the certainty of obtaining an average reward has been substituted for the uncertainty of obtaining any one of a variety of rewards.

Such a change raises the question of whether it is possible to de-emphasise the role of environmental variation in the evolutionary process without distorting our understanding of the process. An elegant analysis by Gillespie (1977) suggests that the answer is likely to be no. When he compared genotypes with the same expected reproductive success he found that natural selection favoured those with the smallest variances in reproductive success. The implication is clear: behaviour maximising average fitness may not always be the best strategy that an animal can choose. Much will depend on how environmental variation affects the likelihood of a strategy actually manifesting its expected fitness.

The purpose of this chapter is to investigate how risk and uncertainty affect behavioural decision-making and optimal patterns of resource allocation. I begin by examining the relationship between expected payoffs and their variances, and develop a fitness measure based on this relationship.

Then I use these concepts to investigate how environmentally induced uncertainty affects strategies of reproduction, foraging and social interaction.

From determinism to uncertainty: a general model

The model is based on the assumption that at any point in time an animal will have a limited amount of resources (R_0) that can be invested in a variety of activities. If the activity adopted is unaffected by the vagaries of nature this investment will result in $\phi(R_0)$ units of fitness. Otherwise, if the strategy is sensitive to environmental fluctuations then the amount actually converted to fitness may be more or less than R_0. As a consequence the fitness of such a strategy would be $E[\phi(R_0)]$, the expected value of the various fitness possibilities.

For the purpose of the general model it does not really matter whether the individual's investment is used to increase fitness by increasing its own survival prospects, by increasing those of its existing offspring or other relatives, or even by producing offspring now or in the future. What does matter, however, is the form of the relationship between the appropriate fitness measure and the level of resource investment. The most realistic form of this relationship will be S-shaped (Fig. 5.1). This means that although increased investment always increases fitness ($\phi'(R_0) > 0$) the rate at which fitness changes with additional investment varies. What begins as a gradual increase in fitness accelerates as investment is further increased, but eventually declines as investment levels become extremely high. Such sigmoid curves have mathematical properties such that to the left of the inflexion point each additional unit of investment brings increasing returns ($\phi''(R_0) > 0$), whereas to the right of the inflexion point each additional unit brings diminishing returns ($\phi''(R_0) < 0$). It appears that most animals are operating in the range of diminishing returns (Smith & Fretwell, 1974; Wilbur, 1977), but exceptions do occur and will be particularly illuminating.

Given this fitness characterisation we are now in a position to examine how environmental uncertainty affects animals confronted with only two strategies: one in which the payoff is certain and the other in which the payoff is not. In one of the simplest situations an animal has the option of investing its R_0 resources in a strategy which will yield exactly R_1 resources at the end of the time period, or in another strategy which will yield, with equal probability, either $R_1 + \gamma$ or $R_1 - \gamma$ resources at the end of the time period. On average, the 'risky' strategy will yield R_1 resources, the same payoff as the 'certain' strategy. The fitnesses of the certain and risky strategies are $\phi(R_1)$ and $\frac{1}{2}\phi(R_1 + \gamma) + \frac{1}{2}\phi(R_1 - \gamma)$ respectively. According to Jensen's inequality (Breimen, 1968) when the fitness function is concave ($\phi''(R_1) < 0$), which will occur to the right of the inflexion point, $\phi[E(R_1)] > E[\phi(R_1)]$. Hence,

$$\phi(R_1) > \tfrac{1}{2}\phi(R_1 + \gamma) + \tfrac{1}{2}\phi(R_1 - \gamma). \tag{1}$$

Thus when animals face the prospects that increasing investments will increase fitness but at an ever-declining rate, they should select among strategies offering the same expected fitness, the one with the lowest variance. However, when the function is convex, which will occur to the left of the inflexion point, the converse should occur as the riskier strategy will have the higher expected fitness.

These relationships can be clearly demonstrated by graphical means (Fig. 5.1). For convenience a symmetric sigmoid fitness function was chosen; its inflexion point is located on the ordinate halfway between the origin and the asymptote, and thus on the abscissa halfway between the origin and $2R$, the point at which the asymptote is reached. For the first

Fig. 5.1. Example of how a sigmoid fitness function affects the fitness of strategies producing payoffs with certainty and uncertainty. In situations of diminishing returns the fitness of the conservative strategy [$\phi_c(Y)$] is greater than that of the risky strategy [$\phi_R(Y)$]. In situations of increasing returns the risky strategy [$\phi_R(X)$] is superior to the conservative one [$\phi_c(X)$].

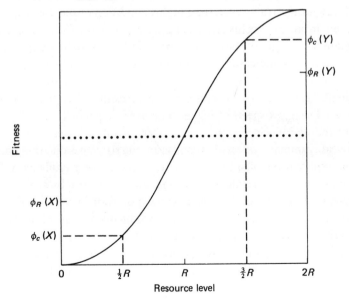

case let us consider a situation to the right of the inflexion point where the expected payoff of both strategies is $Y = 3R/2$, but where the risky strategy offers the prospects of obtaining payoffs of $2R$ and R with equal probabilities. From Fig. 5.1 it is clear that in this case the fitness of the certain strategy is $\phi_c(Y)$ and is greater than $\phi_r(Y)$, which is the average of $\phi(R)$ and $\phi(2R)$. For the second case let us consider a situation to the left of the inflexion point in which the expected payoffs of both strategies are $X = R/2$, but where the payoffs of the risky strategy are either 0 or R and occur with equal frequency. Here Fig. 5.1 shows that the situation is reversed as the fitness of the certain strategy is $\phi_c(X)$ which is less than $\phi_r(X)$, the average of $\phi(0)$ and $\phi(R)$. Thus in one case the risky strategy has a higher fitness than the certain strategy, but in the other it does not. Apparently much depends on the relationship between the initial level of investment and expected payoff, and the position of the latter with respect to the inflexion point of the fitness function.

These results suggest a variety of consequences for the ways in which animals should behave in the face of environmental uncertainty. In one sense the model predicts that animals in good bodily condition, or in favourable environments (both conditions generating returns on investments that augment fitness but at an ever-decreasing rate) should not adopt risky strategies – those offering high losses as well as high gains – if they only provide the same average payoffs as a certain strategy. In another sense the model predicts that animals should switch from risk-averting to risk-favouring strategies as their bodily condition or the favourableness of the environment declines. As long as initial resource levels or payoffs remain to the right of the inflexion point animals should attempt to reduce their decline or increase their reserves by shunning risky strategies. But as soon as initial resource levels or payoffs drop below this critical point animals should abandon conservative investment strategies and adopt those offering prospects of higher than average payoffs.

In the real world few strategies offer payoffs with certainty. In most situations animals will have to choose among strategies differing not only in their expected payoffs, but in their distribution of payoffs as well. How animals make such strategic decisions can best be seen by characterising a strategy's fitness in terms of its payoff expectation as well as its variance.

In effect, the fitness of any strategy producing a range of unpredictably occurring outcomes is simply the sum of the products of the fitness of each payoff and its weighting factor as measured by its likelihood of occurrence. Thus where the payoff of a strategy is a random variable whose expectation can be represented by $E(X)$ the fitness of the strategy is

$$w(X) = \int_{-\infty}^{\infty} \phi(x)f(x)\mathrm{d}x = E[\phi(X)].\tag{2}$$

Here $f(x)$ is a normal probability density function of X with expectation μ and variance σ^2. If the sigmoid fitness function $\phi(x)$ is represented as a normal cumulative distribution $G(x)$, the analysis is greatly simplified. When this is done the fitness of the strategy becomes

$$w(X) = \int_{-\infty}^{\infty} G(x)f(x)\mathrm{d}x.\tag{3}$$

After expanding $G(x)$ about the mean ($x = \mu$) (see Appendix I for details), the fitness of the risky strategy simplifies to

$$w(X) = \phi(\mu) + \tfrac{1}{2}\sigma^2\phi''(\mu).\tag{4}$$

This fitness characterisation shows exactly how variance affects a strategy's fitness. If we assume that most animals operate in the range of investment levels where diminishing returns occur ($\phi''(\mu) < 0$), then any change of strategy that leaves the expected payoff unchanged but increases the variance will reduce the fitness of that strategy. The most important point to note about (4) is that both mean and variance considerations are often likely to be of the same order of magnitude. Hence selection for minimising the uncertainty surrounding a strategy's expected payoff should be no less strong than that for maximising a strategy's expected payoff.

Few data have been collected that demonstrate that animals adopt behavioural strategies specifically to minimise the effects of uncertainty. But much circumstantial evidence suggests that one of the main effects of natural selection has been the evolution of adaptations, such as behavioural diversification, storage of resources, increases in body size, and increases in mobility, that buffer animals against the effects of fluctuating environments. In times of uncertainty animals often diversify their behaviour to reduce risk. Some foraging animals become generalists sampling from a wider range of food types than they otherwise would (Oster & Heinrich, 1976) and some reproducing plants set a greater proportion of seeds that will lie dormant than they otherwise would (Cohen, 1966). Presumably diversifying investment greatly reduces the variance about a strategy's expectation. Whether such diversification yields lower expected payoffs than non-diversification is presently unknown but worth investigating.

Other animals reduce risk by adopting strategies that involve resource storage. One of the most compelling examples involves marine zooplankton (Bevison, Lee & Nevenzel, 1972; Lee, 1975). In seasonal environments some species invest a significant proportion of their energy acquired during periods of resource abundance in the production of wax esters. Later, during periods of resource shortage, these are utilized for energy. In less seasonal environments, zooplankton are rarely seen accumulating wax esters. Again this increased homeostasis reduces the impact of environmental variability, and it may also be achieved with a reduction in the expected payoff.

The evolution of larger body sizes may also represent a long-term response to changes in the magnitude of seasonally induced environmental uncertainty. Although an animal's absolute energy requirements increase with increases in size, the weight-specific, or relative energy requirements, show the opposite trend. Jarman (1974) and Bell (1971) argue that these relationships enable large animals to subsist on lower quality vegetation than smaller animals, as long as they can consume and process it in large quantities. One consequence of being able to utilise abundant sources of low-quality vegetation is that the pressure for animals to forage selectively is relaxed. As a result even in changing environments the probability is high that alternative low-quality food types will be available. Even if they are not available locally, increases in body size reduce the energetic constraints on travelling long distances to obtain these alternative foods (Pennycuick, 1979). Large size then may have evolved in part because it enabled diversification of behaviour in response to fluctuating environments. Boyce (1979) has even suggested that Bergman's rule – the average increase in mammalian body size with increasing latitude – is a consequence of the increasing seasonality that also increases with increasing latitude.

The fitness function (4) also suggests that when two strategies differ both in their expected payoff and their variances, situations are likely to occur in which the strategy with the higher fitness will have the lower expected payoff. That is,

$$\phi(\mu_1) + \tfrac{1}{2}\sigma_1^2\phi''(\mu_1) > \phi(\mu_2) + \tfrac{1}{2}\sigma_2^2\phi''(\mu_2) \tag{5}$$

but where $\phi(\mu_2) > \phi(\mu_1)$. Obviously for this situation to arise reductions in the mean payoff must be offset by reductions in the variance. To determine how extensive the changes in expectations must be to offset changes in variance, and vice versa, we can examine the slope and curvature of the line connecting strategies exhibiting equivalent fitnesses but having different means and variances. After some manipulation (see Appendix II for details), we can show that the slope of this line is

$$\left(\frac{\partial \mu}{\partial \sigma}\right)_{w(\mu)} = \frac{-\phi''(\mu)\sigma}{\phi'(\mu)}, \tag{6}$$

and that its curvature is

$$\left(\frac{\partial^2 \mu}{\partial \sigma^2}\right)_{w(\mu)} = \frac{-\phi'''(\mu)}{\phi''(\mu)} \tag{7}$$

In most biological circumstances $\phi''(\mu) < 0$ and $\phi'''(\mu) > 0$ (see Appendix I for the case in which $\phi(X)$ is represented by a normal cumulative frequency distribution). Therefore $(\partial \mu / \partial \sigma)_{w(\mu)} > 0$ and $(\partial^2 \mu / \partial \sigma^2)_{w(\mu)} > 0$. This means that for strategies manifesting identical fitnesses, those with larger variances must also have disproportionately larger means. It also means that strategies which significantly reduce variation can tolerate even larger reductions in their expectations and still be equally successful alternatives. That equally successful alternative strategies can have different expected payoffs is an important consequence of this analysis. For the most part, behavioural ecologists evaluate the adaptive value of alternative patterns of behaviour that so often appear within populations (Maynard Smith, 1976; Rubenstein, 1980; Dunbar, 1981) solely in terms of expected payoffs. Because differences in variance can have significant effects on a strategy's adaptive value, the previous criteria are no longer sufficient. Doubtless, accounting for variance will make the field worker's task more difficult. Fortunately, equation (7) specifies quantitatively exactly how large these compensatory shifts must be in order to maintain equality among strategies. This should prevent all compensatory changes in expectations and their variances being automatically considered as offsetting.

The purpose of developing this general model was to show how uncertainty affects fitness by unravelling the relationship between a strategy's expected payoff and the variation about this expectation. Now we will use the model to investigate how variation affects decision-making in a few specific situations.

Reproductive strategies

Reproduction often involves the allocation of limited resources among a variety of competing processes. In this section we consider how environmental variation affects the optimal (a) allocation of resources among current versus future reproduction, (b) distribution of investment among good and bad years, and (c) dispersion of young among a few or many nests.

Dispersal in time

We begin by considering the reproductive behaviour of an individual having R_0 resources that it can mobilise and either invest in current reproduction or store and invest in reproduction the following year. We will assume that the 'stored' reserves can in fact be used in the period between reproductive episodes in ways which increase, on average, the resources the individual will have available for reproduction the following year. As long as the animal inhabits an environment that is unpredictable there will be variation in the rate of return on the stored resources. During harsh periods the reserves will actually decline, while during mild periods they will dramatically increase.

For such an animal, in which the rate of return on the risky investment can be represented by a random variable X with $E[X] > 0$, its fitness for the two years would be

$$w(s) = \phi(P) + E[\phi(F)]. \tag{8}$$

Here P and F are the amounts invested in present and future reproduction respectively. Note that we are assuming that the fitness of investment in current reproduction is without uncertainty. If s represents the proportion of the R_0 resources allocated for storage, then $P = (1 - s)R_0$ and $F = sR_0X$. The optimal level of storage, s^*, obtains when

$$w'(s) = E[\phi'(F)X] - \phi'(P) = 0. \tag{9}$$

Given that we can find this optimal level we can ask how s^* is affected by changes in (a) the expected rate of return, (b) the dispersion about this expectation, and (c) the initial amounts of resources, R_0.

Shifting the expectation of the distribution can be accomplished simply by adding a constant to X, $X(c) = X + c$. Changing the dispersion, however, is more complex but can be accomplished by adjusting X as follows, $X(c) = X + Xc - c^2$, where $c = E(X)$. (In effect, this adjustment first moves the centre of the distribution to the origin, expands the dispersion and then moves the centre back to its original position.)

Upon rewriting, (9) becomes

$$w'(s) = E[\phi'[F(c)]X(c)] - \phi'(P) = 0 \tag{10}$$

where $F(c) = sR_0X(c)$. Since $dP/dc = 0$ and $dF/dc = s[dX/dc] + X(c)[dr/dc]$, differentiating (10) with respect to c yields

$$E[\phi''(F)\{sR_0[dX/dc] + X(c)[ds/dc]R_0\}X(c) + \phi'(F)[dX/dc]] = 0. \tag{11}$$

When this is solved for ds/dc we get

$$\frac{\mathrm{d}s}{\mathrm{d}c} = \frac{-E[\{sR_0\phi''(F)X(c) + \phi'(F)\}\mathrm{d}X/\mathrm{d}c]}{R_0E\{\phi''(F)[X(c)]^2\}}. \tag{12}$$

In the case of shifts in the expectation $\mathrm{d}X/\mathrm{d}c = 1$. And when $\phi''(\cdot) < 0$, the biologically important range of the fitness function, it can be shown that the denominator is negative and that the numerator is positive. Hence $\mathrm{d}s/\mathrm{d}c > 0$. For changes in dispersion, however, $\mathrm{d}X/\mathrm{d}c < 0$, and therefore $\mathrm{d}s/\mathrm{d}c < 0$. Thus whereas increases in the expected rate of return for storage increase the proportion invested in delayed reproduction, increases in the dispersion about the mean increase the proportion invested in current reproduction. So far these results parallel those of Schaffer (1974).

To see how changing the amount of resources available for investment affects the investment strategy we differentiate (10) with respect to R_0. This yields

$$\frac{\mathrm{d}s}{\mathrm{d}R_0} = \frac{\phi''(P)(1 - s) - E[\phi''(F)X^2]s}{R_0\{E[\phi''(F)X^2] + \phi''(P)\}}. \tag{13}$$

Clearly as R_0 increases the proportion invested in the risky strategy of delayed reproduction can increase, decrease, or remain unchanged. When $\phi''(\cdot) < 0$ the denominator is negative, and at least for fitness functions represented by exponential functions the numerator is positive because $E[\phi''(F)X^2]s > \phi''(P)(1 - s)$. Hence $\mathrm{d}s/\mathrm{d}R_0 < 0$.

This conclusion is particularly striking. It suggests that individuals in good bodily condition or with large amounts of resources to invest in reproduction should avoid investing in the risky strategy and devote a greater proportion of their resources to immediate reproduction than individuals in poorer condition. This prediction might explain why young animals and those in moderate bodily condition delay reproduction, adopt alternative mating tactics that are less costly and less risky, or even become helpers, assisting other adults in their reproduction. All three strategies enable individuals to invest greater proportion of their meagre resources in activities that will increase their chances of success in the future.

Reproductive timing

If the environment changes in a regular and predictable manner then selection should favour animals that track the environment. But under such conditions should animals invest heavily in reproduction during the good years, and abstain from reproduction in bad years, or should they invest the same amount in all years? In terms of the general model should animals invest R_0 in all years, or should they invest $R_0 + y$ in good years and $R_0 - y$ in bad years? Intuition, as well as an analysis by MacArthur (1968), suggests that selection should favour animals that adopt the boom-bust strategy of investing all their resources in the good year, and none in the bad year. The answer, however, is not so simple, and depends on the magnitude of the yearly fluctuations.

If we assume (a) that the fitness functions for good years (ϕ_G) and bad years (ϕ_B) are the same shape, only differing in their slopes and asymptotes, (b) that the level of resource investment is sufficiently high so that $\phi''_{G\,or\,B}(\cdot) < 0$, and most importantly (c) that the difference between good and bad years is not too large (see Fig. 5.2), then

$$E[\phi_G(R_0) + \phi_B(R_0)] > E[\phi_G(R_0 + y) + \phi_B(R_0 - y)]. \tag{14}$$

Under such conditions animals should minimise the variance about their mean yearly investment by investing equally in good and bad years. However, if the fluctuations between good and bad years are catastrophic, then the inequality in (14) is reversed and animals should increase the variance about their mean yearly investment by adopting the boom-bust strategy. This can be shown graphically by an example in which a good year follows

Fig. 5.2. Relationships between fitness of a strategy involving constant investment in good and bad years (E), and one involving no investment in bad years and twice the normal investment in good years (BB). $\phi_G(R) = R^{0.3}; \phi_B(R) = 0.5R^{0.3}; \phi_{VB}(R) = 0.1R^{0.3}; \phi_{CB}(R) = 0.23R^{0.3}$. The critical fitness function has the property that $\phi_B(R_0) - \phi_B(R_0 - y) > \phi_G(R_0 + y) - \phi_G(R_0)$. After rearranging, (14) results.

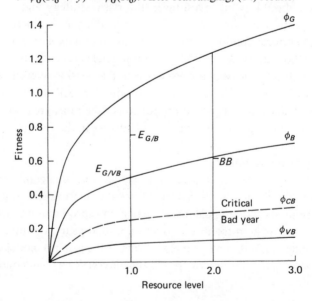

a bad year (Fig. 5.2). In the first case, for every unit invested, the fitness of the bad year is 50% of that of a good year. Over the two-year period the average fitness of the less variable strategy, which involves 1 unit of investment in each year, is 0.75. Over the same period, that of the more variable boom-bust strategy, which involves no investment in the bad year but 2 units in the good year, is 0.62. In the second case, the fluctuations between years is more severe and the fitness function of the very bad year is only 10% of that of a good year. Under such conditions the fitness of the boom-bust strategy is still 0.62, whereas that of the equal strategy is only 0.55.

Inspection of Fig. 5.2 shows that inequality (14) is robust and will be true for fairly severe yearly fluctuations. That the predictions of the model diverge from those of our intuition raises questions about the assumptions underlying the problem, particularly those concerning how the lack of investment in one year affects the level of investment in the following year. If, for example, an animal will be able to add on to next year's amount more than it could have invested in the bad year, then it is possible that the boom-bust strategy could be more profitable even when the difference between good and bad years is small. But because of diminishing returns much will still depend on how large this 'surplus' is. Data are therefore needed to determine exactly how environmental variation affects the accumulation of resources by 'missing out' a season.

Dispersal in space

The last question I want to consider in which variation will affect reproduction concerns strategies of nest laying – should a female lay all her eggs in one nest, or should she scatter them in a variety of nests? If her decision depends simply on each strategy's expected reproductive success, then both would yield the same fitness and she should be indifferent as to which strategy to adopt. But what if females are not attempting to maximise their average reproductive success? Suppose females are attempting to maximise the likelihood that at least one offspring survives to independence. Here the two strategies produce very different results.

If the probability of a nest escaping being preyed upon is s_0 then the probability that none of a female's n nests survive is $(1 - s_0)^n$. This means that the probability of at least one nest surviving is $P_s = 1 - (1 - s_0)^n$ and this increases as n increases. Clearly, animals increase their chances of being represented in the next generation by distributing their young among a variety of nests. One interesting aspect of this prediction is that this 'insurance' against extinction is acquired without diminishing average reproductive success. Another is that this principle of minimising the likelihood of extinction is achieved by a reduction in the variance of nestling survival. As Wilbur (1977) has shown, the variance about the expected reproductive success is $ne^2 s_0(1 - s_0)$ where e is the number of eggs per nest. Thus given the fact that a female lays a fixed number of eggs, by reducing the number of eggs per nest she reduces the variance to such an extent that it offsets the increase in variance that occurs by her distributing the eggs in more nests.

To determine if a nesting strategy with the same average nestling success as another but with a smaller variance is an evolutionary stable strategy (ESS), I ran some computer simulations. According to Maynard Smith (1976), an ESS is a strategy that when rare can successfully invade a population and spread to fixation, and when fixed can resist invasion by any alternative, 'mutant' strategy. In the simulation, a female adopting the normal strategy laid 40 eggs in one nest, whereas a female adopting the mutant strategy laid 10 eggs in each of four nests. The habitat contained 100 nest sites, and the initial population consisted of one mutant and 96 normal females. Then 20 nests were chosen at random. From these all the nestlings survived to become adults. But because of nest limitations, they too were subjected to random mortality. Individuals were chosen at random and assigned one or four nests depending on their nesting strategy. When all 100 nests were occupied the cycle was completed and random nest predation began again. A total of 100 simulations were run, each beginning with a different random sequence. Both nesting strategies served as rare mutants in half the simulations, and within each series half involved moderate ($s_0 = 0.5$) or high ($s_0 = 0.2$) predation levels.

The results are in Table 5.1 and clearly show that the nest dispersing strategy was able to invade in about 75% of the simulations and was only displaced in about 5% of the simulations when it was common. In addition

Table 5.1. *Effects of nest predation on the fixation success of dispersed and clumped nesting strategies*

		Predation intensity			
		low		high	
		Dispersed fixates	Clumped fixates	Dispersed fixates	Clumped fixates
Clumped strategy	common	17	8	20	5
	rare	23	2	25	0

the advantage of nest dispersion seemed to increase as the intensity of predation increased. Thus it appears that reducing variance in nestling survival is an important factor that selection can operate on. The extent to which females will be able to reduce the variance in nestling mortality by increasing the number of nests they make, will depend on many other factors. The costs of making, provisioning, or frequenting more than one nest, in terms of reduced parental survival or diminished overall clutch size, and whether this behaviour increases or decreases the likelihood of each nest being taken by the predator, may be particularly relevant.

Foraging strategies

Because foraging involves the expenditure of energy in the pursuit of even larger amounts of energy, it is a risky venture. Few animals will always succeed in acquiring more than they expend, and the likelihood of their doing so is affected by changes in the environment. The link between foraging success and fitness is indirect, but its existence means that environmentally induced variation in a strategy's rewards will affect fitness.

In fact, the general model can be applied directly to evaluate how uncertainty affects the choice of foraging strategies. Imagine animals having two foraging options: one in which the average yield over the period is fairly small, but whose distribution of gains is spread closely about the average, and another in which the average gain is slightly larger, but whose distribution of gains is spread widely about the average. In particular $\mu_2 > \mu_1$, and $\sigma_2^2 > \sigma_1^2$. According to (4), animals should choose the second more risky strategy when they are in good bodily condition ($\phi''(\mu) < 0$) and $\phi(\mu_1) - \phi(\mu_2) < \frac{1}{2}\sigma_2^2\phi''(\mu_2) - \frac{1}{2}\sigma_1^2\phi''(\mu_1)$. But as (6) and (7) have shown, the relative advantage of the more risky strategy diminishes as the difference between the variances increases. When animals are in poor bodily condition ($\phi''(\mu) > 0$) the risky strategy will always be preferable. Thus as an animal's condition changes, due either to random or consistent small events, the general model predicts that major shifts from risk-favouring to risk-averting strategies, or vice versa, are likely. It is interesting to note that in computer simulations of bird foraging behaviour Thompson, Vertinsky & Krebs (1974) showed that the formation of flocks had a stronger effect on reducing the risk of feeding failure than it did on increasing average success.

Sociality

One of the cornerstones of sociobiology was Hamilton's (1964) development of the concept of inclusive fitness because it helped explain the evolution of altruistic behaviour. According to Hamilton, altruism would spread as long as the ratio of the costs to the altruist divided by the benefits to the recipient were exceeded by r, the coefficient of relatedness among the two individuals. Describing relatedness has taken two forms. In one, r measures the probability that a particular gene will appear in a relative. In the other, it measures the proportion of an individual's genome represented in a relative. These two interpretations are very different, and, in fact, only the former formulation has been demonstrated to be consistent with population-genetic models of the spread of altruism in populations (Charlesworth, 1979).

Recently Barash, Holmes & Green (1977) have shown that associated with the proportionate interpretation is the fact that relationships among relatives consisting of identical values of r may differ in the variances in the proportion of genome held in common. They cite the example that for any parent and its offspring *exactly* 50% of the genome will be shared, whereas for any two siblings only *on average* will they share 50% of their genome. This variation occurs because there is a 25% chance that two siblings will not share any genes, a 50% chance that they will share one, and a 25% chance that they will share two. Barash *et al.* suggest that one consequence of this variation is that it should significantly alter the types of altruistic behaviour shown among parents and offspring, and among siblings. They suggest that siblings should become more discriminatory, bestowing their favours on those most similar to them, and that no such discrimination should develop among parents towards their different offspring. If such discrimination could indeed happen, then there should be greater conflict among siblings than among parents and offspring.

But, as Dawkins (1979) has pointed out, even if it is unreasonable to assume that there is any linkage between genes that control recognition and the genes that predispose an individual to behave altruistically to relatives, then parents should also discriminate among those siblings possessing the altruistic gene and those that do not. An individual either does or does not possess the particular gene, and it does not matter whether the relation in question involves siblings or parents and offspring. The probability of sharing a particular piece of DNA is exactly $\frac{1}{2}$. Thus the variance considerations described by Barash *et al.* should not have a significant influence on the quality of social relationships among relatives.

This does not mean, however, that variance considerations do not influence the likelihood of an animal behaving altruistically to a relative, or for that matter, a non-relative. As stressed throughout this chapter investments in most activities produce uncertain returns. Assisting other individuals is no exception.

Consider a hypothetical pedigree as shown in Fig. 5.3. Given that the probability is $\frac{1}{2}$ that Ego's prospective full sibling and prospective daughter will share with Ego a common altruistic gene, we can ask whether Ego should sacrifice its own reproduction in order to help its mother produce a sibling. Obviously, ecological factors affecting the likelihood of Ego obtaining the necessary resources to breed successfully will affect her decision. If Ego's likelihood of breeding is low then it should assist its mother who has the resources and experience to reproduce successfully (West-Eberhart 1975). As Ego's chances of success improve she should, at some point, reproduce by herself. Although this is an important consideration we will assume that Ego and her mother both have the same expectation of success. In either case, there will be uncertainty associated with the success of Ego's investment and this might lead to differences in the variance about the expected success of each strategy. If we assume that more investment increases the survival or reproductive capabilities of the newborn, but that each additional unit does so at an ever decreasing rate, then from (4) and as in Fig. 5.1, Ego should invest her resources in the strategy with the smaller variance in reproductive success. To a large extent, the strategy Ego chooses will depend on her ability to influence the effectiveness of her investment. It seems most likely that by relinquishing control over the investment to her mother a larger variance about the expected return will be produced, than by maintaining control herself. In one sense, any investment in the sibling or its mother could be manipulated by the mother and

Fig. 5.3. Hypothetical pedigree showing the relationship between Ego and its offspring and its mother's offspring.

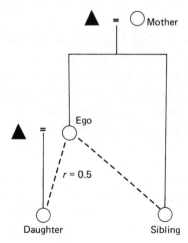

might reduce its effectiveness from Ego's perspective. In another sense, the mother's age or experience might enable her to invest the resources more efficiently than Ego. Unless Ego can ascertain the outcome of her investment before parting with it, the variance associated with caring for her own offspring will be less than that associated with assisting her sibling. As a consequence parental care should be favoured by natural selection.

Social relationships need not occur only when relatives assist each other. Natural selection will favour cooperation and the development of sociality when all parties benefit by the interaction. It will also favour sociality that develops among strangers based on altruistic interactions as long as the altruistic act is repaid in the future either to one's self or to one's kin (Trivers, 1971). Obviously, this investment carries with it an expectation and variance about both the probability of repayment and the value of the repayment. As in (4), and the example of kin-directed altruism, when investment in strangers brings diminishing returns, individuals should assist strangers only if the altruist can reduce the variance about these two expectations. Therefore it would seem likely that such altruism would occur in closely knit groups where contact is frequent or where conflicts of interest are few, or among kin where the risk is automatically reduced to some extent simply by the increased survival or reproductive prospects of the recipient relative.

In a few circumstances, however, we might expect to see individuals increasing their fitness by behaving altruistically in situations where the uncertainties attached to the probability of repayment and the value of the repayment are high. Since the fitness function is convex for animals with few resources to invest, or those in poor bodily condition, then according to (4) their fitnesses can be increased by adopting risky strategies. It is precisely these individuals that might be favoured by adopting extreme reciprocally altruistic behaviour. If subordinate group members corresponded to this class of individuals, then we might expect them to be more altruistic than the dominants. This offers the interesting prospect that despite their very different investment strategies and their apparent conflicts of interests in many areas, on at least this issue of investment in others, their relationship is symbiotic and mutually advantageous.

Concluding remarks

The aim of this chapter was to investigate whether we could ignore the role of environmental variation in the evolutionary process without distorting our understanding of the process. As the fitness characterisation (4) shows, the answer is no. For most animals in most circumstances, increases in the variance of a strategy's outcomes will lower the fitness of that strategy. If this increased variation is accompanied by an increase in the strategy's average success, then it is possible for the strategy's fitness to remain unchanged or even increase. But, as expressions (6) and (7) show, the average increases will have to be large indeed.

In general then, animals should adopt strategies yielding small variances in their outcomes. But if animals are unable to do so by switching strategies, then they should use their resources to reduce the variance about the present strategy's expected outcome, or divert greater proportions of their resources away from the risky aspects of the strategy and invest them in those aspects with more certain outcomes, even if they have lower expected success. Exceptions to this pattern should occur, but only occasionally. Whenever animals find themselves in situations where further investments yield higher and higher returns they should choose risky strategies. Here the fitnesses of the few high-gain outcomes more than compensate for the low fitnesses associated with the rare disasters. But such conditions can only occur to the left of the inflexion point on the fitness curve, and it seems likely that selection will push this point near the origin. As a result, few animals will find themselves in this range. Nevertheless, the model indicates that some individuals, especially the disadvantaged ones, should exhibit this 'aberrant' behaviour.

At least in theory, variance considerations will have about the same impact on fitness as considerations of average success. Now it is up to field workers and experimentalists to determine whether animals behave in accordance with both considerations.

Summary

1. The purpose of this chapter is to show that environmental variability can have a major impact on shaping animal investment patterns.

2. A general model is developed based on the idea that animals invest their limited resources in activities yielding payoffs that are then converted into units of fitness. In a constant environment, the payoff is certain. In a variable environment, a range of payoffs and thus fitness prospects are possible.

3. If higher payoffs produce higher fitnesses, but each payoff increment increases fitness somewhat less than the previous increment (diminishing returns), then, of strategies yielding equivalent payoff expectations, the one with the smallest variance will have the highest fitness. Conversely, if each additional payoff increment

increases fitness somewhat more than the previous increment (increasing returns), then the situation is reversed and the strategy with the largest payoff variance will have the highest fitness.

4. Often strategies differ in both their expected payoffs and their distribution of payoffs. If two such strategies manifest equivalent fitnesses, then the one with the larger variance must have a disproportionately larger expectation. As an example, animals in good bodily condition should choose riskier foraging strategies (large payoff variances) only if the expected payoffs are very high.

5. When animals reproduce they are faced with many investment choices. One involves animals investing some or all of their resources in current reproduction that yields a payoff with certainty, or waiting and investing their resources in future reproduction. Such a delay may increase the expected payoff, but because of the intervening period and environmental uncertainty investment in future reproduction will yield a wide range of payoffs. In such situations, increases in the dispersion of payoffs about the mean, or in the amount of resources available for investment, select for increases in the proportion of resources devoted to current as opposed to future reproduction.

6. When environments change predictably, animals can either invest more of their resources in reproduction during the good year and less during the bad year, or they can divide the resources equally between the two. As long as the fluctuations between years are not too severe selection favours investing equally in both years. When the fluctuations are catastrophic, however, a boom-bust strategy is favoured.

7. When nest predation is common and destroys all the eggs or nestlings present, laying all one's eggs in one nest results in the same expected reproductive success as scattering one's eggs in a variety of nests. Making multiple nests, however, lowers the variance in reproductive success and increases the likelihood that at least one offspring will survive to independence. All else being equal, making many nests is an evolutionary stable strategy.

8. Social relationships involve investing resources in others. As a consequence, the types of social relationships that evolve will be influenced by uncertainty attached to expected payoffs. Because the variance in the effectiveness of investment in offspring is less than that in close kin, parental care will be more common than sibling care. Similarly, reciprocity should evolve most readily in

closely knit or kin groups where the variance in the probability and value of repayment is small.

I thank the Fellows of King's College for their continuous support during the project. I also thank H.E. Daniels, R.I.M. Dunbar, A. Grafen, and R.W. Wrangham for their comments on an earlier draft of the manuscript.

Appendix I

(A) Given an environment in which the outcomes of a strategy are variable, and a function $\phi(x)$ which converts a strategy's payoff x into fitness we can represent such a strategy's fitness as the expectation

$$w(X) = \int_{-\infty}^{\infty} \phi(x)f(x)\mathrm{d}x \tag{A1}$$

Here we assume that $f(x)$ is a density function with mean μ, and variance σ^2. Since we want $\phi(x)$ to be sigmoid in shape, we can represent it as a cumulative distribution function $\phi(x) = \int_{-\infty}^{x} g(u)\mathrm{d}u$ with mean $m = \int_{-\infty}^{\infty} xg(x)\mathrm{d}x$ and variance $\sigma^2 = \int_{-\infty}^{\infty} (x - m)^2 g(x)\mathrm{d}x$. By expanding $\phi(x)$ about $x = \mu$, we get

$$w(X) = \int_{-\infty}^{\infty} \left[\phi(\mu) + (x - \mu)\phi'(\mu) + \frac{1}{2}(x - \mu)^2\phi''(\mu) \right. $$
$$\left. + \frac{1}{6}(x - \mu)^3\phi'''(\mu) + \frac{1}{24}(x - \mu)^4\phi^{\mathrm{iv}}(x_1) \right] f(x)\mathrm{d}x \tag{A2}$$

where x_1 lies between x and μ. If $\phi(x)$ is symmetric then the odd terms in (A2) drop out, leaving

$$w(X) = \phi(\mu) + \frac{1}{2}\phi''(\mu)\sigma^2 + R \tag{A7}$$

where $R \leq \frac{1}{24}\mu_4 \cdot \max|\phi^{\mathrm{iv}}(X)|$.

To find out the magnitude of R we can suppose that $\phi(x)$ is a normal distribution function. Then $\phi(x) = \Phi((x - m)/s) = \Phi(z)$. Since $\phi^{(r)}\mu = r\Phi^{(r)}((\mu - m)/s)/s$

and $\quad \Phi^{(r)}(z) = \dfrac{\mathrm{d}^{r-1}}{\mathrm{d}z^{r-1}} \cdot \dfrac{\exp[-z^2/2]}{(2\pi)^{\frac{1}{2}}}$

then $\Phi^{(\mathrm{iv})}(z) = (3z - z^3) \cdot \exp[-z^2/2]/(2\pi)^{\frac{1}{2}}$. As a result $\Phi^{(\mathrm{iv})}(z)$ takes on its maximum value 0.5506 at $z = 0.72$. The maximum error is therefore $\frac{1}{24}\mu_4(0.5506/54) = 0.023\mu_4/s^4$. If we assume that $f(x)$ is normal with mean μ, and standard deviation σ, then $\mu_4 = 3\sigma^4$ and the maximum error is $0.0688\left(\dfrac{\sigma}{s}\right)^4$. If $\sigma/s = \frac{1}{3}$ then $R < 0.0076$, which is small.

(B) Now we substitute normal density functions for $\phi'(x)$ and $f(x)$ to get an explicit expression for $w(X)$. The first three derivatives of $\phi(x)$ are:

$$\phi'(\mu) = \frac{\exp[-(\mu - m)^2/2s^2]}{s(2\pi)^{\frac{1}{2}}};$$

$$\phi''(\mu) = \frac{-(\mu - m)\exp[-(\mu - m)^2/2s^2]}{s^3(2\pi)^{\frac{1}{2}}}$$

and $\quad \phi'''(\mu) = \left[\dfrac{-1}{s^3(2\pi)^{\frac{1}{2}}} + \dfrac{(\mu - m)^2}{s^5(2\pi)^{\frac{1}{2}}}\right]\exp[-(\mu - m)^2/2s^2]$

Thus where $\mu > m$, $\phi'(\mu) > 0$, $\phi''(\mu) < 0$, and $\phi'''(\mu) > 0$. This means that when the centre of $f(x)$, the payoff distribution, is to the right of the inflexion point of the fitness function (s), increases in the dispersion of $f(x)$ will lower $w(X)$.

The mathematics of this Appendix are the work of Professor H.E. Daniels and are greatly appreciated.

Appendix II

If $w(X) = \phi(\mu) + \frac{1}{2}\sigma^2\phi'''(\mu)$ then

$\partial w/\partial\mu = \phi'(\mu) + \frac{1}{2}\sigma^2{}'''(\mu)$, $\partial^2 w/\partial\mu^2 = \phi''(\mu) + \frac{1}{2}\sigma^2\phi^{iv}(\mu)$,
$\partial w/\partial\sigma = \sigma\phi''(\mu)$ and $\partial^2 w/\partial\sigma^2 = \phi'''(\mu)$.

By assuming that terms of order higher than 2 will not add to fitness we can simplify and combine these partial derivatives to yield the slope

$$\frac{\partial\mu}{\partial\sigma} \approx \frac{-\phi''(\mu)\sigma}{\phi'(\mu)}$$

and curvature

$$\frac{\partial^2\mu}{\partial\sigma^2} = \frac{-\phi'''(\mu)}{\phi''(\mu)}$$

for the line containing all strategies manifesting the same fitness, $w(X)$.

References

Barash, D.P., Holmes, W.G. & Greene, P.J. (1978). Exact versus probabilistic coefficients of relationship: some implications for sociobiology. *American Naturalist*, **112**, 355–63.

Bell, R.H.V. (1971). A grazing ecosystem in the Serengeti. *Scientific American*, **225**, 86–93.

Bevison, A.A., Lee, R.F. & Nevenzel, J.C. (1972). Wax esters: major marine metabolic energy sources. *Biochemistry Society Symposium*, **35**, 175–87.

Boyce, M.S. (1979). Seasonality and patterns of natural selection for life histories. *American Naturalist*, **114**, 569–83.

Breimen, L. (1968). *Probability*. Addison-Wesley: Reading, Mass.

Charlesworth, B. (1979). A note on the evolution of altruism in structured demes. *American Naturalist*, **113**, 601–5.

Cohen, D. (1966). Optimising reproduction in a randomly varying environment. *Journal of Theoretical Biology*, **12**, 119–29.

Cohen, D. (1968). A general model of optimal reproduction in a randomly varying environment. *Journal of Ecology*, **56**, 219–28.

Dawkins, R. (1979). Twelve misunderstandings of kin selection. *Zeitschrift für Tierpsychologie*, **51**, 184–200.

Dunbar, R.I.M. (1981). Determinants and evolutionary consequences of dominance among female gelada baboons. *Behavioural Ecology and Sociobiology* (in press).

Gillespie, J.H. (1977). Natural selection for variances in offspring numbers: a new evolutionary principle. *American Naturalist*, **111**, 1010–14.

Jarman, P.J. (1974). The social organisation of antelope in relation to their ecology. *Behaviour*, **48**, 215–69.

Lee, R.F. (1975). Lipids in the mesopelagic copepod, *Gaussia princeps*. Wax ester utilization during starvation. *Comparative Biochemistry and Physiology*, B, **50**, 1–4.

MacArthur, R.H. (1968). Selection for life tables in periodic environments. *American Naturalist*, **102**, 381–3.

MacArthur, R.H. (1972). *Geographical Ecology. Patterns in the Distribution of Species*. Harper and Row: New York.

Maynard Smith, J. (1976). Evolution and the theory of games. *American Scientist*, **64**, 41–5.

Oster, G. & B. Heinrich (1976). Why do bumble bees major? A mathematical model. *Ecological Monographs*, **46**, 129–33.

Pennycuick, C.J. (1979). Energy costs of locomotion and the concept of "Foraging Radius". In *Serengeti: Dynamics of an Ecosystem*, ed. A.E.R. Sinclair & M. Norton-Griffiths, pp. 164–84. Chicago University Press: Chicago.

Rubenstein, D.I. (1980). On the evolution of alternative mating strategies. In *Limits to Action. The Allocation of Individual Behaviour*, ed. J.E.R. Staffon, pp. 65–100. Academic Press, New York.

Schaffer, W.M. (1974). Optimal reproductive effort in fluctuating environments. *American Naturalist*, **108**, 783–91.

Smith, C.C. & Fretwell, S.D. (1974). The optimal balance between size and number of offspring. *American Naturalist*, **108**, 499–506.

Thompson, W.A., Vertinsky, I. & Krebs, J.R. (1974). The survival value of flocking in birds: a simulation model. *Journal of Animal Ecology*, **43**, 785–820.

Trivers, R.L. (1971). The evolution of reciprocal altruism. *Quarterly Review of Biology*, **46**, 35–57.

Wilbur, H.M. (1977). Propagule size, number, and dispersion pattern in *Ambystoma* and *Asclepias*. *American Naturalist*, **111**, 43–68.

West-Eberhard, M.J. (1975). The evolution of social behaviour by kin selection. *Quarterly Review of Biology*, **50**, 1–34.

6

Gene competition without selection

E.A. THOMPSON

Evolution and gene extinction

The evolution of a population is the differential survival of its genes, through their replication in offspring. This obvious comment is implicit in every discussion of evolution, whether genetic, anthropological or sociobiological, but it too often becomes submerged beneath concepts of inclusive fitness and discussions of intraspecific competition. The aim of this chapter is therefore to present some basic results on possibilities and probabilities of gene survival, unencumbered even by any assumed effects on individual phenotype. Selection on phenotype, although of central importance in any evolutionary superstructure, can obscure the underlying framework of gene survival within which, and through which, it must operate.

Also of central importance in any analysis of evolution, whether a theoretical analysis of potential evolution or a statistical analysis of population data, is the variability within and between populations. Variability between populations, whether of behavioural characteristics or simple genetic traits, is often a reflection of differing environmental histories, and hence a consequence of selective forces. Yet again, this selection operates on, and in parallel with, genetic variability arising as a result of chance events. Only when the limits of this underlying variability are understood, is there any possibility of justifiably ascribing population differences to differential selection.

Equally important is an understanding of the processes which maintain variability within a population. Mutation provides the basic elements of variability and selection acts upon them, but the establishment of a new mutation, and the maintenance of within-population variability, are primarily functions of population structure. Different structures provide different patterns of gene survival, and different levels of variability. These, in turn, affect the potential for future evolution and adaptability under changing environments. Thus an understanding of processes determining the short-term survival patterns of genes, is an important element in assessing the possibilities of long-term survival of populations.

Although data necessarily consist of observations on individuals that have survived, causes of survival are sometimes not easy to assess. On the other hand, whether considering behavioural, physiological or biochemical traits, it is often straightforward to specify some requirements for survival, and hence conversely causes of extinction. Similarly, in our analysis of effects of population structure on patterns of gene survival, it is mathematically easier to consider patterns of gene extinction. This should not, however, obscure the underlying motivation (an understanding of the observable results of evolution), any more than in a discussion of Darwinian selection. However, the transfer of a discussion of selection from the fitness of the survivors to the extinction of the failures also relates to the problem of selection of individuals versus extinction of groups (Łomnicki, 1978). As selection operates only on the phenotype of an individual, so in the first instance can population structure be viewed via its effect on survival of individual genes. But as the traits of individuals may control the survival of their population, so structure may be considered as a group feature determining the variety of genes. We are not here referring to functional interactions between genes, nor to genetic linkage between traits, although these may offer an explanation for some observed phenomena (Stern, 1960; Wagener & Cavalli-Sforza, 1973). Our interest will be restricted to the fundamental framework of genes at a single (autosomal) locus.

The behavioural characteristics of individuals which determine population structure may also be viewed as evolving in response to evolutionary pressures. The structure's 'evolutionary advantage' to an individual may be considered, both with respect to ensuring survival of replicates of his genes, and with respect to ensuring stability of the population group (Chagnon, 1979). Yet such an evolutionary pressure cannot be quantified, or its importance assessed, without an understanding of the effects of a given structure on individual gene survival and on the variety of genes in a population. Structure maintains genetic variation without which it could not itself evolve. Thus here we shall take the structure as given, and discuss its genetic effects.

Components of structure

To investigate evolutionary consequences of population structure, this must first itself be characterised. There are two basic levels, which we shall call macro- and microstructure. Macrostructure relates to the population as a whole, and its relation with others. Thus it includes such elements as population size, rates of increase or decrease, and rates and sources of migration. We shall consider the effects of changing population size, and in particular the effect of bottlenecks – sudden and severe but shortlived restrictions of the population size. Migration, although also an important factor, raises theoretical difficulties as a problem of several interdependent populations. It is more easily considered in the context of subdivision of a single population, which we shall discuss briefly. From this viewpoint it is rather an aspect of microstructure – the mating patterns and sibship distributions within a population. Thompson (1979*b*) has proposed that microstructure be quantified via its effects on patterns of gene extinction, but this presupposes an understanding of these effects. Here we discuss only the necessary preliminary: an investigation of the consequences of the well specified structural features of family-size distributions and regular mating systems.

There are two aspects of an analysis of gene survival. One is the more classical approach of studies of gene identity and loss of heterozygosity (Wright, 1921); the other is our current analysis of gene extinction. The two aspects are of course related, but they are not equivalent. In an analysis of gene identity the emphasis is upon common ancestry, and the descent of single ancestral genes to a variety of current individuals. In an analysis of gene extinction we consider the variety of ancestors, and descent of their genes to common descendants who can carry only a limited number of these genes. Both aspects are important, but the theoretical problems are different, and the results illuminate different aspects of the problem.

Where individuals have common ancestors, they may carry identical replicates of genes in such an ancestor. Knowledge that an individual carries a certain allele increases the probability that a relative does so, and hence the probability that the allele exists elsewhere in the population. This is an aspect of gene identity from common ancestry. An individual passes on one of his two genes at an autosomal locus independently to each child. If he has only one child, he cannot pass on both. Even if he has more, knowledge that a particular one of his genes survives in the current population decreases the probability that the homologous one does so also. Conversely, knowledge of the extinction of a given gene decreases the probability of extinction of the other. This is an aspect of interactions in gene extinction, induced by passage of different ancestral genes via the same common descendants. The offspring of a couple in turn pass to each of their offspring either their maternal or their paternal gene. Thus the survival of a given gene decreases the survival probability of a gene of a spouse. At the next generation, genes segregate in the grandchildren of original founders, inducing dependence between the survival of genes in co-grandparents, and so on. A specified genealogy may be regarded as a framework within which genes are competing for survival; competing not in any selectionist sense, but simply by virtue of the limited paths of descent from ancestors. Some genes must survive, if the population does so, but it is unlikely that all can do so, even for a few generations.

The interactions between two genes, or more generally two disjoint sets of genes, can be measured via the correlation between the zero-one random variables indexing the events of their extinction (Thompson, 1979b). That is, if the two sets of genes have extinction probabilities p_1 and p_2, and the probability that both sets are extinct is q, we have that the correlation

$$\rho = (q - p_1 p_2)/\{p_1(1 - p_1)p_2(1 - p_2)\}^{\frac{1}{2}}.$$

In our case we have always $\rho < 0$, and for zero-one variables it can further be shown that

$$|\rho| \leq \min\left\{\left(\frac{p_1 p_2}{(1 - p_1)(1 - p_2)}\right)^{\frac{1}{2}}, \left(\frac{(1 - p_1)(1 - p_2)}{p_1 p_2}\right)^{\frac{1}{2}}\right\}.$$

Thus correlations do not directly illuminate the structural features of a genealogy, since they are dominated by the macrostructure – the population size, and number of generations elapsed, which determine the order of magnitude of p_1 and p_2. Thus it is more useful to consider a normalised correlation which can take values throughout the range 0 to 1. In particular, we define the *index of extinction association*

$$\alpha_E = |\rho|\{(1 - p_1)(1 - p_2)/p_1 p_2\}^{\frac{1}{2}}.$$

This is 1 if extinction of one set of genes precludes that of the other, and is zero if the extinctions are independent. The latter can be the case only if relevant ancestors have no common descendants.

It is mathematically convenient to define survival as the negative of extinction; thus survival of a set of genes is taken to mean survival of any gene in the set. Since we can consider arbitrary sets of genes, there is no loss of generality in this definition. We may therefore define also an *index of survival association*

$$\alpha_S = |\rho|\{p_1 p_2/(1 - p_1)(1 - p_2)\}^{\frac{1}{2}}.$$

This index also lies between 0 and 1, and measures the extent to which survival of one set of genes precludes that of the other. It is 1 if the survival events are mutually exclusive, and 0 if they are independent. The indices α_E and α_S are alternative normalisations of the same correlation, but are appropriate to different situations. In an increasing population, survival of a gene will rarely preclude that of another, and α_E is the index of interest.

Conversely, in a decreasing population, $\alpha_E \approx 0$ and α_S is more illuminating. Over long periods of time, individual gene survival probabilities are small and again α_S is the relevant index, whereas over a few generations α_E is more useful.

The above discussion applies to a specified genealogical structure. Where we consider a class of structures generated by a given process, correlations need not be negative and the association indices may not lie between 0 and 1. Consider, for example, outbreeding genealogies generated by an offspring distribution which has a high probability of zero offspring. Here knowledge of the extinction of a founder gene increases the conditional probability that the founder had no offspring, and hence *increases* the probability of extinction of the homologous gene of the same founder.

Effects of population and family size

We consider now the effect on gene extinction of the distribution of offspring number and of bottlenecks in the population size. Both these features have been previously considered, with reference to the problem of *effective population size*. This is a measure of rate of increasing gene identity, and the ratio of effective to actual population size is thus a measure of structure. Where a population's size is changing, effective size is approximately the harmonic mean of actual sizes, and where a dioecious population has, at a given generation, n_m males and n_f females, the effective size resulting from immediate segregations is $4(n_m^{-1} + n_f^{-1})^{-1}$ (Wright, 1931). Thus population-size restrictions (bottlenecks) are the dominating features. Crow (1954) considered the case of an offspring distribution with mean m and coefficient of variation c, in a population size n, giving an effective size of $2(n - 2)/(m(1 + c^2) - 1)$. When the variance of the off-spring distribution is large, many individuals will have no offspring. Even if the remainder compensate ($m = 2$), the effect is again as of a bottleneck, destroying the survival chances of many genes. Nei (1972) has considered more fully the effects of bottlenecks in population size on within-population gene identity.

To analyse the effects of bottlenecks on gene extinction, consider first the simplest case. A population of N genes is assumed to lose all except a randomly chosen r, and we quantify the effect of this disaster alone. Consider disjoint sets of k and l homologous autosomal genes existing before the bottleneck; these are genes of one or several individuals. The probability of extinction of any set of s genes in the bottleneck is

$$\binom{N - s}{r} \Big/ \binom{N}{r}$$

and hence the association in extinction, between the two disjoint sets, is

$$\alpha_E = \left\{ \binom{N-k}{r}\binom{N-l}{r} - \binom{N-k-l}{r}\binom{N}{r} \right\} \Bigg/ \left\{ \binom{N-k}{r}\binom{N-l}{r} \right\}^{\frac{1}{2}}$$

with a similar expression for α_S. For a single pair of genes ($k = l = 1$), we have

$$\alpha_E = r/(N-1)(N-r) \quad \text{and} \quad \alpha_S = (N-r)/r(N-1).$$

The interdependence in survival is greatest when r is small, when $\alpha_S \approx 1/r$. The interdependence in extinction is greatest when $r \approx N$, when $\alpha_E \approx 1/(N-r)$. For a severe bottleneck, α_E is of little interest; most genes become extinct, and extinction of one has little effect on that of others. However, survival of one has a large effect on survival of others, since few can survive, and we see that this effect is inversely proportional to the size immediately following the bottleneck, regardless of previous size.

The effect of family-size distribution may be assessed by considering extinction of genes over only a two-generation transition from a couple to their grandchildren, assuming absence of sib mating. For convenience we shall consider a general probability generating function (p.g.f.), $h(z)$, for offspring number, although where a genealogy specifies k offspring we have the particular form z^k. We shall also denote by $g^{(t)}(z)$ the p.g.f. of the number of replicates of a given gene after t generations. Then, for an outbreeding genealogy,

$$g^{(t+1)}(z) = h(\tfrac{1}{2} + \tfrac{1}{2}g^{(t)}(z)); \ g^{(0)}(z) = z,$$

since at every segregation a specified gene is passed to an offspring with probability of $\frac{1}{2}$ (Thompson, 1979b). Since the probability of no replicates after t generations is $g^{(t)}(0)$. We have

p(gene not passed to any offspring) $= g^{(1)}(0) = h(\tfrac{1}{2})$
p(gene not passed to any grandchild) $= g^{(2)}(0) = h(\tfrac{1}{2}(1 + h(\tfrac{1}{2})))$.

Further we have, for passage of genes to offspring,

p (neither gene of individual survives) $= p$ (no offspring) $= h(0)$,

and, for passage of genes to grandchildren,

p (neither gene of individual survives) $= h(h(\tfrac{1}{2}))$
p (neither of two specified genes, one in each member of a couple, survives) $= h((1 + 2h(\tfrac{1}{2}) + h(0))/4)$.

Thus the association in extinction between the two genes of an individual, by virtue of segregations to his offspring, is $\alpha_E^{(1)} =$

$1 - h(0)/(h(\frac{1}{2}))^2$. However, given the existence of offspring, $h(0) = 0$ and $\alpha_E^{(1)} = 1$. This is of little interest. Over two generations we have

$$\alpha_E^{(2:W)} = 1 - h(h(\tfrac{1}{2}))/\{h(\tfrac{1}{2} + \tfrac{1}{2}h(\tfrac{1}{2}))\}^2$$

and $\quad \alpha_E^{(2:B)} = 1 - h(\tfrac{1}{4} + \tfrac{1}{2}h(\tfrac{1}{2}) + \tfrac{1}{4}h(0))/\{h(\tfrac{1}{2} + \tfrac{1}{2}h(\tfrac{1}{2}))\})^2$

for extinction association between two genes within and between a grand-parental couple, respectively. The function h, a p.g.f., is convex, increasing with $h(1) = 1$. Thus

$$\tfrac{1}{4} + \tfrac{1}{2}h(\tfrac{1}{2}) + \tfrac{1}{4}h(0) > h(\tfrac{1}{2})$$

and association between genes between individuals is always less than between genes within individuals. This is the major conclusion, and can be extended to individuals with more distant common descendants (Thompson, 1979b).

Even from this simplest case, we see that associations in extinction depend on the complete distribution of offspring number, and not simply mean and variance (c.f. Crow, 1954). For a specified k offspring ($h(z) = z^k$), associations in survival decrease exponentially with k, while associations in extinction converge exponentially to one. All unnormalised correlations converge to zero; for large families, passages of parental genes become largely independent. As measured by our normalised index, however, extinction of some parental genes precludes extinction of others to a high degree, the normalisation removing the effect of overall small probabilities of extinction.

Random mating populations

A random-mating population provides a base-point for assessment of within-population structure, and a simple framework for analysis of effects of changing population size and of subdivision. Although gene identity has been extensively considered, even for the case of subdivision (Wright, 1951), the problem of gene extinction is more complex. The simplest cases have been analysed (Felsenstein, 1971; Karlin, 1966), and the results applied to correlations in gene extinction (Thompson, 1979b), but the effects of population subdivision remain to be studied.

Another aspect of gene survival probability is its dependence on changing population size. This is indirectly an aspect of gene competition, since this is lessened in an expanding population and heightened in a contracting one. The fate of a new mutation is heavily dependent on its performance in its first few generations (Fisher, 1930), and its probability of survival is greatly increased if it arises in an expanding population (Ewens, 1967). Many small populations undergo marked fluctuations in size; periods of gradual increase can be reversed by epidemics or famine. The effect of such fluctuations on mutant survival probabilities have been considered by Thompson & Neel (1978). These survival probabilities affect in turn the number of observable polymorphic variants in a population (Neel & Thompson, 1978).

Any analysis of population data is an analysis of the survivors. For a selectionist interpretation, survivors are inferred to be selectively advantaged. The interpretation of data on the basis of population structure infers that surviving mutants arose at periods of population increase. The differential survival probability of new mutations arising throughout a cycle of population size provide relative likelihoods of times of occurrence of surviving variants. Whereas selectively advantageous variants may be regarded as active survivors, their own traits contributing to that survival, the structurally advantageous mutant survives by the chance of its position, and at the expense of genes to which it may even be selectively inferior.

To quantify the discussion, we consider a branching process model for the replication of a variant gene, with the standard two-parameter negative exponential offspring distribution at generation t;

$$p^{(t)}(k \text{ offspring}) = \begin{cases} r_t & (k = 0) \\ (1 - r_t)(1 - c_t)c_t^{k-1} & (k = 1, 2, \ldots). \end{cases}$$

As well as providing a good fit to naturally occurring distributions, this form has the mathematical convenience of compounding to the same form over any number of generations, even when the parameters vary with t (Keiding & Nielson, 1975). Over T generations the expected number of replicates is $M_T = \prod_{t=1}^{T}(1 - r_t)/(1 - c_t)$ and the probability of extinction is

$$R_T = 1 - \left\{1 + \sum_{t=1}^{T} \{r_t/(1 - r_t)M_{t-1}\}\right\}^{-1}$$

The probability of more than k replicates is

$$Q_T(k) = (1 - R_T)G_T^k \text{ where } G_T = (M_T + R_T - 1)/M_T$$

(Thompson & Neel, 1978).

Using these formulae, the effect of cycles, gradual increase and abrupt declines in population size may be considered. The major conclusion is that long-term survival probability is proportional to expected number of replicates immediately preceding the first decline the variant undergoes. The effect of changing the length of cycles, and rates of gradual increase, may also be considered. These two factors determine the factor of population decline required to restore long-term equilibrium, and in fact this last single factor is the major determinant of results. If the extent of decline is catastrophic (for example, 10-fold or more), there will be very few variants to be seen in a population, but those that do survive will be present in large numbers. If falls in population size are slight more variants will survive, but none will achieve large numbers (Neel & Thompson, 1978). One advantage of the above model is that selection can be easily incorporated, simply by assuming that the mean number of replicate offspring $((1 - r_i)/(1 - c_i))$ for the variant is different from that for the general population. Where the means are of the same order of magnitude, effects of time of origin in the population cycle outweigh those of selective advantage, although the precise relative importance depends of course on the exact patterns of the population cycle.

The above discussion has assumed random mating over the whole population. Subdivision affects population variability, and levels of migration between subdivisions determine the degree of structurally induced competition between mutants arising in different components. Subdivision has been extensively analysed via its effect on gene identity by descent, and rate of loss of variability. Wright (1943) considers F-statistics and isolation by distance models, while Kimura & Weiss (1964) have analysed the stepping-stone models of migration between disjoint colonies. Maruyama (1970a) shows that mutant fixation probability is unaffected by partial subdivision of a population, even where, subject to certain conditions, mutations are not selectively neutral. If migration rates are very small, however, times between fixations may become so prolonged that this is no longer a relevant criterion. Maruyama (1970b) considers the effect of partial subdivision on the asymptotic rate of decrease of variability in a linear stepping-stone model. If the migration rate to neighbours is m, and there are k colonies each of N diploid individuals, this rate is approximately min. $\{1/2Nk, m\pi^2/2k^2\}$ when k is large. Thus if m is very small, subdivision dominates the process, and variability is lost at a rate proportional to the migration rate. If migration is more than a certain level (viz. $k/N\pi^2$) the population acts, in this respect, as a panmictic unit. The transition between the two behaviours seems to be sharply determined.

In assessing genetic evidence from natural populations, an analysis based only on equilibria and asymptotic rates is not sufficient. There are large variances inherent in the processes of loss of genetic variability and of increasing gene identity by descent. Further the covariances between the processes are slight (Thompson, 1976), levels of coancestry do not precisely determine levels of variability, and cannot be inferred from them. Nei & Chakravarti (1977) and Nei, Chakravarti & Tateno (1977) consider more directly the process of decreasing heterozygosity both in the case of isolated populations, and in the case of partial subdivision. Again they conclude that variances are large; standard deviations of changes are larger than mean changes. Thus, although structure has a major effect on the survival of mutants and hence on genetic variability within a population, there is a wide scope for 'chance effects' within any structural framework. General structural parameters (e.g. coancestry) cannot be inferred from general genetic parameters (e.g. population heterozygosity); it is thus difficult to delimit the effects of structure. In the next section we shall find that, in some cases, there are parameters which characterise structure more precisely, and that in these cases the effects of structure can be more precisely quantified.

There is a further aspect of subdivision relevant to the present discussion. Thompson (1979c) has superposed a fission model of population subdivision on the branching-process model of mutant replication, and considered the effect of mean offspring number on the variation in mutant replicate numbers between subdivisions. Conversely, observed variation may be used to estimate rate of mutant increase, and estimated rates for different mutants may be compared. Again there are large variances inherent in the process; the subdividing structure may, by chance, have very different effects on different rare mutants. Differing rates of mutant increase may be simply an effect of differing rates of population increase in the sections of the population where different mutants are located. Nonetheless, comparison of rates of increase quantifies the outcome of a 'selection' process, even if the effects of genetic and structural selection are difficult to disentangle. Genetic selection is a long-term process for biochemical mutant variants, and even for behavioural traits of large selective effect the time-scale is much greater than for the consequences of chance events of demographic history. But the short-term effects of structural events can have long-term genetic consequences, and only by first considering these can we infer where genetic selection has also been operative.

Structure and mating systems

The structures of natural populations have been characterised mainly in terms of their rates of inbreeding. The random mating population discussed above may be used as a base level for comparison, but it is useful also to compare natural populations with those of simple structure which may be analysed theoretically. We therefore consider the regular mating systems, which have themselves long been characterised by their asymptotic inbreeding rates (Wright, 1921). However, it has also been recognised that this alone is an insufficient characterisation (Kimura &

Crow, 1963; Robertson, 1964). In a small population, the genetic contributions of different ancestors can alter markedly, even over a few generations. The detailed structure of such a population is thus better characterised by its short-term effects than by asymptotic properties. Structures do not remain constant for long periods, and asymptotic properties will seldom have immediate practical consequences, although this is not to deny their use as general descriptive parameters. Although we may consider short-term coancestry and gene identity, it is more illuminating to characterise structures of populations by their effect on gene extinction. In particular, since it is the *joint* survival pattern of genes that is the feature of structure relevant to the evolution of a population, we consider interactions in extinction between disjoint sets of genes.

Consider first the case of a pair of genes. In a completely random-mating population, correlations in extinction are the same for every pair. In a random-mating population of diploids there are two values: that between genes initially in the same individual, and that between genes in different individuals. As more structure is imposed, we obtain sets of individuals between whom there are different degrees of relationship, and hence more possible values. Further, the larger a population the more different levels of structure it is possible to impose. Yet even in populations of the same size, and the same number of degrees of relationship there are different levels of structure. For example, consider groups of size four and the regular systems of half-sib and double-first cousin mating (Fig. 6.1*a*, *b*). In both cases there are pairs of genes within individuals, between spouses, and between cograndparents. The cousin system has the greater structure, consisting of full sibships, and provides the more extreme extinction correlations. These values span those for half-sib mating which in turn span those for the less-structured systems of diploid random mating and random union of gametes (Table 6.1). In addition to the two well known regular systems, there is an intermediate mixed system (Fig. 1*c*). Although it is not regular in the sense of equivalence of individuals, and is therefore a first step towards natural populations, it remains well characterised by the correlations it generates (Table 6.1), these designating it as intermediate in structure. Further results and discussion are given by Thompson (1979*b*).

Thus associations or correlations in extinction do provide a useful characterisation of the level of internal structure of a system, in terms of its short-term effects, even when only gene pairs are considered. Of more practical importance are the survival possibilities and probabilities for larger sets. In this connection, note that avoidance of mating with close relatives not only decreases homozygosity of offspring, but also the degree of competition of genes with those of close relatives. We have already seen that the most intense structurally imposed competition is that between spouses, through segregation in their offspring. The survival of one's genes makes that of a spouse's less likely. Thus incest avoidance may be selected for not as an avoidance of selectively disadvantaged offspring, but as an avoidance of competition in descendants between genes which are in fact replicates of the same. Both explanations arise by virtue of coancestry between members of the mating, but whereas one requires the genetic explanation of heterozygote advantage the other is a purely structural phenomenon.

There is no difficulty in considering the extinction probabilities of specified sets of genes of arbitrary size, using the methods of Cannings, Thompson & Skolnick (1978) for computing probabilities on pedigrees. However an overall analysis raises difficulties, because there are too many

Fig. 6.1. Mating systems in bisexual populations of size 4. Males, A, C; females, B, D.

(a) Half-sib mating

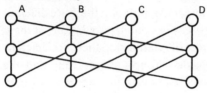

(b) Double-first cousin mating

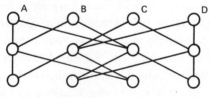

(c) Mixed system

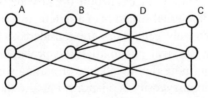

possible sets to compare. In the case of regular mating systems (Thompson, 1979*b*) we have concentrated on the sets of immediate practical interest; both genes in a given individual, all genes in cograndparents, all genes in individuals of a given sex etc. In this way we can begin to build up a picture of the intensity of competition between different segments of the population. Again analysis of these systems shows that associations in gene extinction provide a consistent measure of degree of internal structure.

At this stage comparisons have been made only between parallel sets of genes in different structures – for example cograndparents in half-sib and in cousin mating. However a more extended analysis, which would for example, compare spouses in cousin mating with cograndparents in half-sib mating, has not been attempted. The full interrelationship of structures in their effect on the survival of a variety of genes in small populations cannot therefore yet be assessed. This is a massive task, but also important. Natural populations are a mixture of many different mating types, and cannot be fully characterised without a comparative analysis of all levels of structurally imposed gene competition. However there is one aspect of competition between larger sets of genes that can be considered; namely, an analysis of any specified genealogy. This is a much smaller problem than

Table 6.1 *Extinction correlations in systems of size 4*

	Generation			
	5	10	20	∞
Random union of gametes				
Any gene pair	−0.094	−0.103	−0.123	−0.143
Random mating of individuals				
Gene pair in same founder	−0.138	−0.124	−0.127	−0.143
Gene pair in different founders	−0.085	−0.096	−0.117	−0.143
Half sib mating (Fig. 6.1*a*)				
Gene pair in same founder	−0.290	−0.215	−0.162	−0.143
Gene pair in (A, B)	−0.072	−0.092	−0.104	−0.143
Gene pair in (A, C)	−0.023	−0.054	−0.084	−0.143
Double first cousin (Fig. 6.1*b*)				
Gene pair in same founder	−0.262	−0.192	−0.130	−0.143
Gene pair in (A, B)[a]	−0.097	−0.106	−0.113	−0.143
Gene pair in (A, C)	−0.036	−0.066	−0.094	−0.143
Mixed system (Fig. 6.1*c*)				
Gene pair in (A, B)	−0.071	−0.088	−0.104	−0.143
Gene pair in (A, C)	−0.068	−0.088	−0.104	−0.143
Gene pair in (A, D)	−0.025	−0.036	−0.087	−0.143

[a]See Fig. 6.1

the general characterisation of an arbitrary genealogy, or over the distribution of genealogies and corresponding effects that arise under a population model, yet it provides a complete solution with respect to the particular genealogy of interest. Our final section thus discusses this analysis for the complex genealogy of the population of Tristan da Cunha.

Structure of an island population

The population of the small and isolated South-Atlantic island of Tristan da Cunha descends almost entirely from thirteen original founders of diverse ethnic origin (Roberts, 1971). Following temporary evacuation of the island in 1961 a detailed study was made of the genealogical history, and of the genetic and medical characteristics of current members. The complex nature of the genealogy, the existence of two bottlenecks arising at periods when the survival of the population was in doubt, the small number of founders, and our detailed knowledge of all of these things, makes it an ideal structure on which to analyse genetic effects of genealogy (Thompson, 1979a). Further, the current genetic observations can be analysed in the light of conclusions regarding the consequences of genealogical history. Each illuminates the other.

Our present interest is in the effect of the genealogy on the joint survival of genes. We wish to obtain an overall view of the complete set of interactions in gene survival or extinction, and this requires an overall analysis of the extinction probabilities of all possible subsets of original founder genes. Even for this small population, a complete analysis with respect to all twenty-six homologous autosomal genes of thirteen original founders is not feasible. Two of the thirteen are not of great interest with respect to gene survival, however; they arrived on the island as recently as 1892, and had still-living offspring in the population sample in 1961. Further, the remaining eleven are found to fall conveniently into two groups, with respect to their intermarriages, and those of their immediate descendants (Fig. 6.2). There are six individuals in each group, one founder being in both. The descent of genes from each group is largely independent of that from the other, and a complete analysis of the interactions *within* each group is possible (Thompson, 1979a).

For each set of 6 founders (12 genes) there are 2^{12} distinct subsets of genes whose extinction probabilities must be computed and analysed. Symmetry between the two genes of each founder reduces this figure to $3^6 = 729$, but although computation is readily achieved (Cannings *et al.*, 1978; Thompson, 1979a), overall analysis of a set of 729 probabilities is not simple. Our major interest is in interactions in the extinction of genes, and these correlations are a multiplicative component in probabilities of extinction. An additive log-linear model therefore facilitates a precise quantification of these interactions. The full model, and the analysis based upon it, are given by Thompson (1979*a*); we discuss here only the results.

The aim in fitting a standard log-linear model is to partition variability in extinction probabilities, and hence to assess interactions. Each log-probability is partitioned first into a term attributable to the effect of each founder in the set under consideration. Having taken out these 'main effects' the residual is partitioned into terms attributable to the interaction between each founder pair. The further residual is partitioned into terms attributable to interactions between triples, over and above the pairwise correlations; and so on. This hierarchic structure has several attractive features. Where descents of genes from sets of founders are independent, fitted interaction terms are zero. If a given interaction is found to be zero, so also is any higher-order interaction involving these individuals. For example

$$\langle A \cdot B \rangle = 0 \Rightarrow \langle A \cdot B \cdot C \rangle = 0 \text{ for any other founder C.}$$

The two groups of founders give very different results. In the first, 83% of the variation is attributable to effects of single founders, a further 13% to

Fig. 6.2. Intermarriages between the founders of the Tristan da Cunha population.

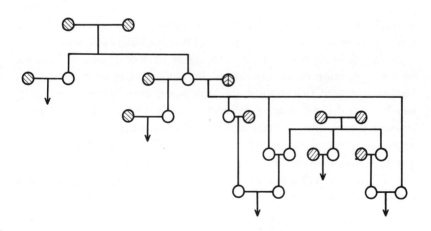

pairwise interactions, 3.5% to three-founder interactions, leaving 0.5% to higher-order terms. In the other group the figures are 18, 34, 30.5 and 17.5%, respectively. Thus the extinctions of genes of the first group are largely independent, the only significant restrictions on descent being amongst offspring of original founders. The second group is characterised by intense competition in gene survival over several generations, the descent from the whole group passing mainly through a very limited number of marriages between descendants of several members of the group. The interactions within each group of founders may be analysed further; unusually large components of interaction may be traced to key marriages, which are constrictions through which genes must pass to survive to the current population. A full discussion of features of the genealogy thereby illuminated is given by Thompson (1979a).

Joint survival of genes is closely related to observable distributions of allelic types. The extent to which genealogical structure has influenced gene descent can be investigated via an analysis of the extent to which founder genotypes can be inferred from current genetic data. Where descents of genes are largely independent, separate inferences about founder types can be made. Where there are significant interactions, acceptance of any hypothesis about the allelic type of one founder gene completely changes inferences about others. An inference about a founder allele, from current genetic data, is an assessment about the descent of that founder gene to certain segments of the current population and not to others. Due to interactions between genes, this is equally an assessment regarding the fates of other founder genes. Thus the effects of structure on genetic composition can be quantified via the connecting consideration of joint survival of genes. Structure implies a joint survival pattern which determines genotypic distributions. Conversely, an observed genotype distribution, through an analysis of implied genotypes of ancestors, provides information on interactions in gene survival that have actually occurred.

In the above discussion we have assumed absence of selection; we are now in a position to incorporate it. In analysis of genetic data it may become apparent that certain ancestral genes have spread particularly widely, or perhaps that genes of several founders have done so, and that amongst these certain alleles are highly represented. By analysing the ancestral genealogy we may delimit the distorting effect of structure on genotype distributions, and hence ultimately have concrete evidence for selection, and an estimate of its magnitude. There are, of course, problems. For biochemical traits selection effects may be slight, and very large amounts of data required to detect them. For behavioural traits, selection effects are probably much larger and detectable over a few generations, but these are not determined by single loci. Nonetheless, only when structural effects are fully understood will it be possible to trace or infer the genetic evolution of an adaptive trait in a natural population.

Summary

1. The long-term evolution of a species depends primarily on the provision of new mutations, and selection acting upon them. However, the distribution of alleles within a small population is primarily a function of short-term structure.

2. This structure is an important aspect of reproductive strategy, having, through its effect on gene survival, long-term consequences in population survival and evolution. Structure may be divided into macrostructure and microstructure.

3. The important effect of macrostructure is the major part it can play in establishing a new mutation, and in enhancing the number of replicates of a variant. Under assumptions of equilibrium and stable populations, a high-frequency private variant may be explainable only by selective advantage. But varying population size can produce the same effects. It is thus important, in interpreting data, first to delimit the potential evolutionary consequences of structure.

4. The important effect of microstructure is in the dependence it induces in the survival of different genes, and hence its effect on within-population diversity. Again, whereas analysis on the basis of large-population equilibria may lead to inferences of selection, the within-population distribution of a polymorphism may be a consequence of infrastructure.

5. Although associations in gene survival provide clear characterisations of simple models and mating systems, a general model for a complete population provides too much complexity. We can, however, consider any particular population with a completely specified genealogy, and we have done so for the Tristan da Cunha population.

6. By an adoption of a standard statistical procedure, we can obtain an overall view of the patterns of gene competition induced by the genealogy. By analysis of the observable genetic data we may quantify the effects of this competition.

7. To do so in general remains a major problem, but only in this way shall we obtain a rigorous framework within which to assess the evolution of adaptive traits in natural populations.

References

Cannings, C., Thompson, E.A. & Skolnick, M.H. (1978). Probability functions on complex pedigrees. *Advances in Applied Probability*, **10**, 26–61.

Chagnon, N.A (1979). Mate competition, favouring close kin, and village fissioning among the Yanomama. In *Evolutionary Biology and Human Social Behaviour: An Anthropological Perspective*, ed. N. Chagnon & W. Irons, pp. 86–132. Duxbury Press: North Scituate, Mass.

Crow, J.F. (1954). Breeding structure of population; effective population number. In *Statistics and Mathematics in Biology*, pp. 543–56. Iowa University Press: Ames, Iowa.

Ewens, W.J. (1967) The probability of survival of a new mutant in a fluctuating environment *Heredity*, **22**, 438–43.

Felsenstein, J. (1971). The rate of loss of multiple alleles in finite haploid populations. *Theoretical Population Biology*, **2**, 391–403.

Fisher, R.A. (1930) *The Genetical Theory of Natural Selection*, Clarendon Press: Oxford.

Karlin, S. (1966). *A First Course in Stochastic Processes*. Academic Press: New York.

Keiding, N. & Nielson, J.E. (1975). Branching processes with varying and random geometric offspring distributions. *Journal of Applied Probability*, **12**, 135–41.

Kimura, M. & Crow, J.F. (1963). On the maximum avoidance of inbreeding. *Genetical Research*, **4**, 399–415.

Kimura, M. & Weiss, G.H. (1964). The stepping-stone model of population structure, and of genetic correlation with distance. *Genetics*, **49**, 561–76.

Łomnicki, A. (1978) Individual differences between animals and natural regulation of their numbers. *Journal of Animal Ecology*, **47**, 461–75.

Maruyama, T. (1970a). On the fixation probability of mutant genes in a subdivided population. *Genetical Research*, **15**, 221–5.

Maruyama, T. (1970b). Rate of decrease of genetic variability in a subdivided population. *Biometrika*, **57**, 299–311.

Neel, J.V. & Thompson, E.A. (1978). Founder effect and number of private polymorphisms observed in Amerindian tribes. *Proceedings of the National Academy of Sciences of the USA.*, **75**, 1904–8.

Nei, M. (1972). Genetic distance between populations. *American Naturalist*, **106**, 283–92.

Nei, M., Chakravarti, A. & Tateno, Y. (1977). Mean and variance of F_{ST} in a finite number of incompletely isolated populations. *Theoretical Population Biology*, **11**, 291–306.

Nei, M. & Chakravarti, A. (1977). Drift variances of F_{ST} and G_{ST} statistics, obtained from a finite number of isolated populations. *Theoretical Population Biology*, **11**, 307–25.

Roberts, D.F. (1971). The demography of Tristan da Cunha. *Population Studies*, **25**, 465–79.

Robertson, A. (1964). The effect of non-random mating within inbred lines on the rate of inbreeding. *Genetical Research*, **5**, 164–7.

Stern, C. (1960). *Principles of Human Genetics*. W.H. Freeman and Co.: San Francisco.

Thompson, E.A. (1976). Population correlation and population kinship, *Theoretical Population Biology*, **10**, 203–26.

Thompson, E.A. (1979a). Ancestral inference. III. The ancestral structure of the population of Tristan da Cunha. *Annals of Human Genetics*, **43**, 167–76.

Thompson, E.A. (1979*b*). Genealogical structure and correlations in gene extinction. *Theoretical Population Biology*, **16**, 191–222.

Thompson, E.A. (1979*c*). Fission models of population variability. *Genetics*, **93**, 479–95.

Thompson, E.A. & Neel, J.V. (1978). The probability of founder effect in a tribal population. *Proceedings of the National Academy of Sciences of the USA*, **75**, 1442–5.

Wagener, D.K. & Cavalli-Sforza, L.L. (1973). Ethnic variation in genetic disease: possible roles of hitchhiking and epistasis. *American Journal of Human Genetics*, **27**, 348–64.

Wright, S. (1921). Systems of mating. *Genetics*, **6**, 111–78.

Wright, S. (1931). Evolution in Mendelian populations. *Genetics*, **16**, 97–159.

Wright, S. (1943). Isolation by distance. *Genetics*, **28**, 114–38.

Wright, S. (1951). The genetical structure of populations. *Annals of Eugenics*, **15**, 323–54.

7

Behavioural development and evolutionary processes

PATRICK BATESON

Introduction

In this chapter I want to forge some links between studies of evolution and development. It might be thought unwise to do this, since if anything got sociobiology a bad name it was the way in which evolutionary theories were used to justify a naive form of genetic determinism in the development of individuals. The pity of it was that the whole subject of sociobiology was tainted by an apparent assumption that some simple correspondence would be found between genes and behaviour. This made a lot of people very angry and for some years a useful dialogue between sociobiologists and developmentalists seemed impossible. Anyway, the time has come to take a calmer look at both the shortcomings and the possibilities of a legal marriage between ontogeny and phylogeny in studies of behaviour. The process has already been started by, for instance, Burghardt & Bekoff (1978), Richard (1979) and Plotkin & Odling-Smee (1979) and given a valuable spur by the thinking of Gould (1977). Nevertheless, a lot still needs to be said.

On the face of it, the chances of a marriage seem remote since phylogeny and ontogeny relate to logically distinct issues. We could take any piece of machinery, animate or inanimate, and be told in detail what it was for and how the design had gradually evolved. Armed with all this knowledge we should still be completely in the dark about how that particular machine had been assembled. It is not immediately obvious, then, how a functional approach to ontogeny is going to help anybody to understand the nature of developmental processes. Equally, knowledge of development does not help us straightforwardly to understand past and present selection pressures. If that was all that could be said, however, I could stop my chapter here. It is not, and I shall go on to argue that the two distinct styles of thought can actively nourish each other.

The functional approach to biological problems encourages us to think teleologically and, since human beings are inveterate planners of their own lives, thinking of outcomes as goals can help us to get our minds round complex processes. Everybody agrees that the development of behaviour is complicated so why should we deny ourselves such aid? The dangers of muddling a tool with a solution should make us cautious. Even so, I for one am quite content to use teleological explanations as tools (or crutches as an irreverent friend calls them). The view, which I shall attempt to justify later in this chapter, is that functional arguments can help us to focus on evidence which simply would be ignored in the all too common absence of satisfactory causal theories of development.

Looking the other way from ontogeny to phylogeny, the argument is rather different. Theories about evolution require knowledge of the constraints on an animal at all stages of its life cycle, as well as its propensity to behave in particular kinds of ways. Knowledge of what happens in development should, therefore, be as much a part of the stock-in-trade of an evolutionary thinker as the knowledge of how an adult lives and behaves. Equally important, the ontogenetic processes of self-regulation and plasticity strongly suggest that random genetic mutation will rarely mean random variation in phenotypes. This conclusion has a number of implications for evolutionary theory and requires a good deal more thought than has been given to it in the past. I deal with these issues in the final part of the chapter.

The two-way flow of nourishment between studies of ontogeny and phylogeny poses problems of real scientific interest. Before dealing with them, though, it is necessary to consider the miscommunication that commonly arises when evolutionary theorists talk to people like me who are primarily interested in the development of behaviour. These are the current problems *with* sociobiology when seen from a developmental perspective at least.

Problems with language
Genes for characters

When sociobiologists in general are attacked for their genetic determinism, the criticism is undoubtedly indiscriminate. It is not fair to tar everybody with the same brush. Indeed, nobody contributing to this book disagreed with the following statements about the famous (though still hypothetical) 'gene for altruism'. (a) The mutant gene makes the difference between an animal behaving altruistically and not doing so if other things are equal. (b) The mutant gene is not sufficient for the expression of the behavioural character because it works with a great many other necessary conditions to produce the behaviour pattern. (c) The developmental process generating the behaviour must be influenced by many facets of the environment and may involve learning; change the environment or opportunities for learning and the nature of the behaviour may be dramatically altered.

Evolutionary theories that consider the costs and benefits of possessing a gene which exerts a specific influence in a particular context, must necessarily be silent on how the developmental process works. But it is not enough to gain acceptance on this point because much of the language used by contemporary sociobiology is preformationist in character and implies that a behavioural trait spreading through a population in the course of evolution is somehow represented in miniature form in the relevant gene. The effect is that critics and naive disciples alike believe that the developmental process has been dismissed as being altogether trivial and uninteresting. I accept that the majority of those who are playing an important role in forming opinion about sociobiology do not believe that. Nevertheless, confusions will persist until the language is cleared up.

I believe, then, that the 'gene for a character' language should not be used even as a shorthand. The long-winded 'gene that makes the difference between one character and another' admittedly uses more type but at least it is unambiguous. Only those who are incurably convinced that a source of a difference is a sufficient condition for obtaining that difference would then remain muddled about what sociobiologists are trying to say.

What is selected?

'We now know that selection acts primarily at the level of the individual, or to be more precise, at the level of the gene ...' (Krebs & Davies, 1978, p. 8). Confident statements like this abound in modern text books and are, I shall argue, a major cause of muddle. Two separate processes are run together. The competition between characters (if that indeed is what is involved in evolutionary change) and the way in which the characters are replicated are quite distinct. Let me illustrate this point with an analogy. Having told the public for many years that there was no demand for crusty bread, a few supermarkets cautiously offered such bread along with the flabby stuff which was supposed to be so popular. Many people immediately started to select the crusty bread. The presumed effect of the selection pressure was that recipes used for making crusty bread proliferated at the expense of those used for making the other kind. The notion of selfish recipes manipulating consumers is entertaining. Nevertheless, normal usage of language does not imply that when you buy your bread what you are really doing is selecting the recipes.

Returning now to biology, a behaviour pattern such as licking offspring may be favoured by natural selection in the sense that offspring are more likely to survive if they are licked. Now, at one stage in evolution the difference between those parents that licked and those that did not may have been one gene (defined as a unit of mutation). But does it follow that the gene is where natural selection has acted, as Williams (1966) and Dawkins (1976, 1978) have argued? For me, at least, Darwin's metaphor does not have that connotation. Darwin contrasted natural selection with the artificial selection of plant and animal breeders. He was specifically thinking of analogies with the way a breeder might, for instance, select pigeons with more tail feathers than was usual and he was concerned with the natural selection of *characters* – not selection of recipes for making those characters.

The importance of separating the set of processes by which one character competes with another in a natural environment from the set of processes by which characters are transmitted from one generation to the next, is that these sets are so different and involve such dissimilar issues (Bateson, 1978*a*). Richard Dawkins (this volume) now makes a distinction – between 'vehicle' and 'replicator' – a change in his thinking which is all the more welcome since he refers to 'replicator survival' rather than 'replicator selection'.

I should perhaps emphasise that my insistence on character selection does not commit me to considering just the attributes of individual organisms. The characters could be properties of symbionts such as competing lichens or mutualistic groups such as competing bands of wolves. Of course, if characters are transmitted genetically from one generation to the next, character selection must necessarily involve changes in gene frequency, but these changes are *consequences* of selection. I accept that the gene's-eye-view approach to evolution, of which Dawkins is the most brilliant exponent, has brought a sharp new light to bear on old problems, one of them being animal communication (see Dawkins & Krebs, 1978). However, a subtle difficulty arises at the point where the operational character-selection language appears to intersect with the teleological selfish-gene language. A winning character is defined in *relation* to another one while genetic replicators are thought about in *absolute* and atomistic terms. The difficulty is brought home if you ask yourself, what exactly is Dawkins' replicator. You might answer: 'That bit of genetic material making the difference between the winning and losing characters'. You would have stated that a replicator must be defined in relation to something else. Alternatively, your reply might be: 'A replicator consists of all the genes required for the expression of the surviving character'. In that case you are saddled with a complex and unwieldy concept. Either way your answer would show how misleading it is to think of replicators as the atoms of evolution.

To return to the main point, varieties of competition raise questions that are central to a particular set of theories about evolution. Varieties of methods of replication and transmission raise questions that are mainly to do with the way critical information passes from one generation to the next but also touch on how that information is expressed in an individual's development. That is why it is so important to keep the different kinds of process apart in our minds. The distinction ravages the fatal allure of the idea that the character is the gene. If the conceptual membrane separating studies of phylogeny and ontogeny is to be made more permeable to thought, the selection metaphor should be used, as Darwin originally intended, for the differential survival of characters.

The question of innateness

Anybody interested in natural selection is bound to become involved sooner or later with the issue of inheritance. So it was perhaps inevitable that the resurgence of interest in evolutionary theory should have revived terms like 'innate behaviour', 'genetically programmed behaviour', and so forth. However, in resurrecting the old innate/learned dichotomy, a crucial technical discussion about behavioural development has simply been ignored. The practical problems of how to recognise 'innate behaviour' are not trivial (see for instance, Hinde, 1968; Lehrman, 1970; Bateson, 1976a). And the difficulties are compounded if we wish to recognise higher order 'innate rules' for development.

I must emphasise that this difficulty of using 'innate behaviour' as one part of a field of possibilities is not one of principle. It is easy to conceive of adaptive behaviour that does not require learning processes for its development and which owes its qualitatively distinct character to genes specifically affecting it and nothing else. That having been said, the occurrence of the behaviour may be facultatively dependent on environmental conditions. In locusts, many generations may go by without migratory behaviour being expressed (e.g. Dempster, 1963). Furthermore, the form of the behaviour may depend on external conditions that are normally constant from one generation to the next. This becomes especially obvious when animals are brought into the laboratory. For instance, in an environment of ad libitum food, constant temperature, constant humidity and so forth, rat mothers do not care for their pups as much as they would in natural conditions. The deprivation has a major effect on their offspring's behavioural development (see Thoman & Levine, 1970). The long-term effects can be prevented if the pups are handled by humans while they are still with the mother. The presumption is that the handled pups emit ultrasonic distress calls which stimulate the mother to behave more as she would have done in the natural environment. (The irony of this particular example is that for many years the unhandled rats were regarded as the 'control group'.) Buffering mechanisms required to cope with the ill-effects of having non-maternal mothers presumably never evolved because such mothers do not exist outside laboratories.

When 'innate behaviour' is used in the sense of 'behaviour that is not learned' it seems to invite a dichotomy. A moment's thought, though, makes it obvious that the degree to which a given pattern of behaviour had been influenced by external events could vary from a little to a lot. However, I do not think it is enough to emphasise this point by breaking up the continuum of possibilities into a larger number of arbitrary categories. Alcock (1979), for instance, has used four categories ranging from 'closed instincts' to 'flexible learning'. While this is an improvement over the old dichotomies it ignores the variety of ways in which environmental conditions can influence development (see Bateson, 1976a; Gottlieb, 1976a). In my view any classification of behaviour in terms of its origins that does not take account of the multidimensional character of developmental determination is doomed to immediate failure. The major *practical* difficulty with the category of 'innate behaviour' in a multidimensional field of possibilities is the problem of interpretation that arises when dealing with experiments that purport to have excluded learning. Ambiguities arise for a number of quite separate reasons.

(a) *The specific–general continuum.* Konrad Lorenz (1965) proposed the metaphor of a blueprint for the origin of behaviour patterns which he thought were 'coded in the genome'. The metaphor was helpful in the sense that nobody would suppose that blueprints were sufficient for a building. Clearly, to raise a building, a workforce is required along with bricks, mortar, and so forth. However, a sharp distinction had been made by Lorenz between the 'information' on which the detailed characteristics of the finished building depend, and the conditions necessary for translating that blueprint into a building. The distinction is between an influence with a specific and qualitatively distinct effect on behaviour and an influence which has a general effect on all behaviour. In practice, this distinction does create problems. It is extremely difficult to know what to do when considering a spectrum of environmental conditions ranging from those that exert a highly specific effect on behaviour, such as those required for learning, through to those that produce general effects on behaviour such as a low protein diet. Where do we draw the line and say from here on the experiences are no longer providing relevant information? For instance, simple exposure to patterned light can speed up the processes by which chicks peck accurately at seed, approach potential foster-parents, and learn about visual targets (see Bateson, 1976*a*; Cherfas, 1977, 1978). In Lorenz's sense, are these environmental supplements to the blueprint, or are they part of the workforce? It really does not matter, and if we insist on an answer we have been trapped by the metaphor. Nature is not necessarily going to package herself conveniently to match our distinctions.

(b) *Equivalence.* Even when considering experiences that have a specific effect on behaviour it may be very difficult to know in advance when an animal is likely to generalise the effects from one kind of training to a novel situation. Can we really be so certain that we know what are equivalent types of experience for an animal? We might, for example, be inclined to treat tactile input as being so different from visual information that experiences of an object in one modality would not help recognition of that object when using the other modality. In rhesus monkeys, opportunities to discriminate between potential pieces of food in the dark, using tactile cues, make it easier for them to discriminate between the same objects in the light when they have to choose on the basis of visual cues (Cowey & Weiskrantz, 1975; Weiskrantz & Cowey, 1975). It is difficult to have useful intuitions about these kinds of equivalences in animals living in different perceptual worlds from ourselves.

(c) *Equifinality.* It is possible for a given pattern of behaviour to develop by several different routes (Bateson, 1976*b*). The term 'equifinality' is used for cases in which the given end point can be reached in more than one way (von Bertalanffy, 1971). An isolation experiment that deprives an animal of a particular kind of experience may force it to develop a pattern of behaviour that normally depends on such experience in another way. While this result would be very interesting, it would not show that the excluded environmental factor had no influence on development when it was normally available. To argue like that would be similar to arguing that travellers who are forced to use bicycles because of a fuel shortage do not need petrol to run their cars.

(d) *Self stimulation.* Even though an animal is isolated from relevant experience in its environment, it may do things to itself which enable it to perform an adaptive response later on. Normally treated Mallard ducklings are able to respond preferentially to the maternal call of their own species (Gottlieb, 1971). However, if they are devocalised in the egg so that they do not make sounds and thereby stimulate themselves, they do not show the same ability to recognise the calls of their own species (Gottlieb, 1976b). In other words, feedback from their own activity is an integral part of normal development. In many cases it may be difficult to cut such feedback.

It is because of all these difficulties that people who study the development of behaviour generally regard the concept of innateness as giving more trouble than it is worth. I mention all this as a warning. Sociobiologists have a hard enough time translating principle into practice because of problems of determining paternity, measuring fitness, and so forth. The introduction of 'innate behaviour' or 'innate rules' into the vocabulary simply compounds the difficulties of doing decent empirical research. In any event, 'innateness' is unnecessary to an evolutionary argument. If we accept that natural selection acts on phenotypic characters the precise way in which a character develops is irrelevant. It does not matter to the evolutionary argument that normal development may depend on instruction from a stable or reliable feature of the environment.

Functional approaches to development

When Konrad Lorenz (1935) first put the process of imprinting in birds on the map he set it in a functional context. He argued that the process is concerned with learning the characteristics of the species. Although Lorenz saw imprinting as a single process, a distinction was increasingly made between filial imprinting which has a short term influence on social preferences early in life, and sexual imprinting which influences mate choice. By degrees evidence accumulated that sexual imprinting takes place later in development than filial imprinting (e.g. Schutz, 1965; Gallagher, 1977; Vidal, 1980). In addition, it has become increasingly apparent over the years that neither process need play an essential role in species recognition, because a bird that can be imprinted can also show a predisposition to respond to members of its own species, even when it has had no direct previous experience with any of them except itself (Schutz, 1965; Immelmann, 1969; Gottlieb, 1971). A possible explanation is, then, that both filial and sexual imprinting have evolved to enable birds to recognise their close kin, but that the necessity for kin recognition is different in young and adult (Bateson, 1979).

The young bird needs to discriminate between the parent that cares for it and other members of its species because parents discriminate between their own offspring and other young in the same species, and may actually attack young that are not their own. Adult behaviour of this kind is well known in many mammals and birds (e.g. Burtt, 1977). In most cases the parent that cares exclusively for its own young will be more likely to rear them to independence than a parent that accepts and cares for all the stray young that come up to it. The suggestion is then, that filial imprinting is required for individual recognition of parents and is a secondary consequence of the selective pressures on parents to discriminate between their own and other young. In each generation individuals may differ in the stage of development when their filial responsiveness to parent-like objects first increases. Those that do it too early obtain inappropriate or insufficient information about their parents. They might, for instance, have inadequate opportunities to explore all facets of their parent and so fail to recognise it quickly enough later on when quick recognition is important. Those that do it too late respond in a friendly way to hostile members of their own species and consequently suffer. In these different ways the optimal timing for the increase in intrinsic responsiveness could have evolved. It would be critically affected by how rapidly the parents learn to discriminate between their own young and other young.

The evolutionary pressures that gave rise to sexual imprinting are likely to have been quite different. The suggestion is that sexual imprinting enables an animal to learn the characteristics of its close kin and subsequently it can choose a mate that appears slightly different (but not too different) from its parents and siblings. The advantage of behaving in this way arises because of the evolutionary pressures to avoid inbreeding on the one hand, and excessive outbreeding on the other (Mather, 1943). Just what constitutes excessive outbreeding is a matter of debate at the moment (Maynard Smith, 1978; Bateson, 1980). But assuming that some balance has to be struck between inbreeding and outbreeding the solution is for each individual, using the sexual imprinting process, to learn the characteristics of its parents and siblings and, when adult, to choose a mate that looks a bit different from its immediate kin. The underlying assumption is, of course, that there is a correlation between relatedness and similarity of external appearance – an assumption which is backed by some evidence (e.g. Bateson, Lotwick & Scott, 1980).

If these speculations about the functions of filial and sexual imprinting are correct, some sense can be made of why sexual imprinting occurs later in development than filial imprinting. In order for a bird to maximise its chances of recognising close kin when selecting a mate, it should delay learning about them until its siblings are old enough for their juvenile characteristics to provide a strong indication of their adult appearance.

What, then, has been gained by these functional considerations? How does it help the study of developmental mechanism? I think the major benefit is that it gives us a way of thinking about the differences between filial and sexual imprinting and, more importantly, about the differences in the underlying timing mechanisms. If filial and sexual imprinting continue to be treated in the classical way as though they were part of the same general process, then the difference in timing has no significance and is quickly forgotten about. With a shift in functional perspective, difference in timing becomes crucially important. So with our attention focussed on the problem, we can now look for mechanisms responsible for the timing.

Functional explanations draw attention to particular kinds of evidence and, what is particularly important to the experimentalist, can also suggest factors that may be important sources of variation. For instance, any one species of mammal can show astonishing variability in the age at which the young are weaned. In the cat a number of striking behavioural changes can occur after weaning and can be linked functionally with the changing ecology of the young (Bateson, 1981). This possibility suggested an experiment which showed that age of separation from the mother had a marked influence on the development of play in cats. The kittens that had been separated early played significantly more with each other and with objects than those in the control group (Bateson & Young, 1981). It was as though they were responding facultatively to conditions that would normally lead to a curtailed period of development in which to acquire necessary skills by playing. They pack in the experience while they have a chance.

Developmental approaches to evolution
The influence of evidence
One promising point of contact between developmental evidence and evolutionary theories is in the realm of life-history strategies (e.g. Gadgil & Bossert, 1970; Gould, 1977; Horn, 1978; Stearns, 1977). Up to now the theorising has been principally concerned with trade-offs between growth and reproductive rate and how these will be related to such forms of behaviour as parental care and dispersal. Fagen (1977, 1981) has begun to explore the utility of life-history models in relation to the timing of play in development. In the present context the interesting point is that Fagen is working a two-way street. It is not difficult to see how knowledge of what happens in development could influence life-history models. For instance, one benefit of slow development is that it provides time for acquiring skills

and for becoming familiar with the environment. The selection pressure deriving from those benefits would be expected to oppose subsequent pressures pushing towards a reduction in generation time. A longer discussion of this issue is provided by Mason (1979).

A second example of how developmental evidence can influence evolutionary thought is provided by the phenomenon of sexual imprinting and the role it might play in speciation. Following a suggestion of Huxley's (1955), many theoreticians have explored the possibility that, by being imprinted with parents and preferring to mate with an individual looking like the parents, two morphs of the same species could become reproductively isolated from each other (reviewed by Immelmann, 1975). All this work has taken as axiomatic the classical view of imprinting that the preferred mate closely resembles the individual to which the bird was exposed early in life. However, the ideas about optimal outbreeding and, of more relevance, the *evidence* that birds choose mates that differ somewhat from the familiar individuals (e.g. Bateson, 1978*b*, 1980) suggests that the assumption may have been wrong. Furthermore, in Cooke's (1978) field studies of the polymorphic snow goose, a certain proportion mated with a morph different from the one to which they had been exposed in early life – contrary to his expectations. These birds could represent the tail of the distribution of preferences which had its peak markedly displaced from the kind of plumage with which the geese were imprinted when young. Scudo (1976) foresaw some of the complications that would be introduced by assortative mating that was neither wholly positive nor wholly negative. However, the precise implications cannot be fully worked out until the genetic relatedness of maximally preferred mates is known in any one case. The point is that detailed knowledge of what development does to adult mating preferences can have an effect on the character of the evolutionary models.

Intellectually more interesting than empirical provisioning is the possibility that developmental studies will provide some theoretical insights into evolutionary changes. I shall next consider some of the implications of two concepts that have dominated much of the thinking about the processes involved in the ontogeny of behaviour. These are the notions of plasticity and developmental homeostasis.

Developmental plasticity

Plasticity in development describes not only learning in all its multifarious forms but also conditional strategies (see Davies, this volume). In the most obvious forms of learning the effects on behaviour are highly specific and correspond to the external conditions that gave rise to them. The male chaffinch, for instance, produces a song like the one he was exposed to when he was young. In the most obvious conditional strategies such as caste determination in social insects, the effects on behaviour are general and bear no correspondence to the determining events. In many cases, though, it is exceedingly hard to decide whether some environmental conditions have acted as a set of instructions or have selected patterns of development that were already latent within the animal. For the purposes of the present discussion these practical difficulties are unimportant. The relevant point is that environmental variation can generate adaptive variability in the phenotype.

The obvious implication of ontogenetic plasticity is that the phenotype changes adaptively with the nature of the environment. A less obvious implication is that ontogenetic adaptation to some environments may be costly for animals equipped with particular kinds of genotype. They can do it but there is a more efficient way. Furthermore, when pushed by an environment that changes steadily in one direction most members of a species will eventually use up their capacity for adaptive ontogenetic change (G. Bateson, 1963). The sudden appearance on the East African plains of very fast cheetah may not mean that antelope are doomed. The majority of antelope may be able to produce an extra burst of speed and so elude even the super cheetah. However, the strains and energy costs of doing so could provide an additional selection pressure favouring antelope that can run very fast at lower cost than others.

In such cases the environmental change producing a quick response by individuals also exposes the population to a new selection pressure. The short-term plasticity gives the selection pressure time to work. This is one of the few ways in which the so-called Baldwin effect could work, if as was implied by Baldwin (1896), the adaptive short-term response was necessary for the subsequent phylogenetic change.

The Baldwin hypothesis has often been treated as though it were identical with Waddington's notion of genetic assimilation. However, the classic evidence produced by Waddington (1953) in favour of his ideas suggests an alternative, though equally interesting interpretation. It is worth summarising his experiment. Fruitfly pupae were exposed to a heat shock (40°C for four hours). When adult some 40% of the flies lacked cross-veins in their wings. These were selected, bred and the process continued for many generations. A proportion of the pupae in each generation was not exposed to heat shock and after 14 generations a few untreated flies developed cross-veinless wings spontaneously. The proportion rose as selection continued. On the face of it, the experiment seemed to have provided good evidence for the inheritance of acquired characters. However, as Waddington himself argued, the heat shock may have revealed to the world a part of the population that carried particular genes. These were the genes making the flies more likely to develop cross-veinless wings. Waddington elaborated an explanation in terms of his concept of canalisation but precisely what he had in mind was not made really clear. I think it is possible to explain his results in a way which is more explicit and therefore easier to understand (see also Futuyma, 1979; Maynard Smith, 1975; Rendel, 1967).

Suppose that the difference between normal and cross-veinless wings depends crucially on a pair of alleles. *VV* gives rise to normal wings, *vv* to cross-veinless wings and *Vv* in a normal environment to normal wings. (In view of my strictures about 'genes for characters' let me emphasise that the *V* allele is not meant to be sufficient for the development of a normal wing. It is the difference between *VV* and *vv* that makes the difference between normal and cross-veinless wings.) Now, suppose that when subjected to heat shock early in development the heterozygotes *Vv* develop cross-veinless wings. In other words, dominance depends on environmental conditions. If, as was the case, the experimenters selected for cross-veinless wings, subjecting the whole population to heat shock would have meant that all the selected flies carried the *v* allele even though most of them would have been heterozygotes. As the selection process continued, the frequency of the *vv* homozygotes, which spontaneously developed cross-veinless wings, would inevitably have increased. In fact this simple explanation for Waddington's result is too simple because he showed that the spontaneous development of the cross-veinless wings was dependent on genes at a number of different loci. However, it is not difficult to elaborate the explanation a little by postulating several allelic pairs all of which respond to heat shock as does the *Vv* pair in the simple model.

If an environmental event that triggered the evolutionary change was also one that involved learning processes, could a similar explanation operate? I believe so. Consider the classic case of cultural transmission in birds, namely the opening of milk bottles by blue tits (Hinde & Fisher, 1951). In an environment of milk bottles but with no culture for opening milk bottles *MM* and *Mm* blue tits cannot open milk bottles, but *mm* blue tits can. (Again, these are genes that make the difference between behaving one way and another.) In an environment of milk bottles and with a milk bottle-opening culture already developed, *Mm* blue tits can now open bottles and *MM* still cannot or are much poorer at it. Given that the cream at the top of milk bottles is an important resource, particularly in cold winters, birds that can get it are strongly favoured by natural selection and the *m* allele should spread at a greater rate in the presence of the culture than in its absence. The prediction is that the incidence of spontaneous opening of milk bottles by blue tits that have never seen another bird do it should rise more rapidly in areas where the culture exists. Once again, it would almost certainly be a crashing over-simplification to represent birds that can spontaneously open milk bottles and those that cannot as differing in only one allele. However, the general form of the argument could still be right, and the spread of culture might have the interesting effect of increasing the frequency of spontaneous bottle opening in blue tits that had never seen others do it. Whether or not that particular idea should prove fruitful, the general point remains. When the environment changes on a long-term basis, selection pressures that result in genotypic change may well operate on those animals that are capable of plasticity, but the genotypic change lags a long way behind the prompt phenotypic response.

Developmental homeostasis

While plasticity generates variability in the phenotype, other processes gobble up variation. This kind of *elasticity* relates to all the buffering mechanisms that are variously labelled developmental homeostasis, homeorhesis, canalisation and catch-up. It is particularly obvious in growth curves. Growing animals that have been starved or have fallen ill, fall behind other members of their own species of the same age, in size and weight. However, if the discrepancy does not exceed a certain critical value they rapidly catch up as soon as they obtain adequate supplies of food or recover from their illness (see Bateson, 1976b). Such elasticity in developmental processes has some important implications for evolutionary thinking as Mayr (1963, p. 230) clearly perceived. If the homeostatic mechanisms can cope with deviations from the norm initiated from inside as well as from without, genetic mutations may well have no observable phenotypic effect (Waddington, 1957). In the short term at least, the mutations will be neutralised. This would restrain certain kinds of evolutionary change.

If mutations are neutral in outcome and the cost of operating homeostatic machinery is trivial they may spread through a population. For instance, the mutant gene might possibly have pleiotropic effects one of which was expressed and carried selective advantages while the others were neutralised. The gene could spread quickly. Now consider the possibility that in two different areas two different mutant genes are silently spreading and then, as the result of migration between the two areas, the populations mix. What if the self-regulating process in development cannot cope with the presence of both mutant genes, and a new phenotype is generated by their interactions? Clearly in certain circumstances, the new phenotype could have a competitive edge over the old one and rapidly replace it. Moreover, consideration of the involvement of developmental homeo-stasis in the early stages of the evolutionary process opens up some interest-ing possibilities. The phenotypes arising from the interaction of the mutant genes could be radically different from the phenotypes of animals contain-ing no more than one of the mutant genes. But these new creatures would not necessarily suffer the fate normally attributed to Goldschmidt's (1940) hopeful monsters because, in the right conditions, they would not be out there on their own. Indeed, monsters might be thrown together because they were not chosen or accepted as mates by normal-looking members of the population. In brief, the involvement of ontogenetic buffering might provide the first step of the take-off condition for occasional saltations in evolution (cf. Gould & Eldredge, 1977). It suggests a way by which some members of a new generation could find themselves, in Sewall Wright's (1932) terms, on a different adaptive peak from their parents.

Conclusion

This chapter has a critical part and a part that invites criticism. I am critical of the untidy linguistic habits that continue to give sociobiology a bad name. It is not enough to claim that you know how to clean up the house if you go on living in a mess. The time has come to get the broom out. As is doubtless evident, I am not arguing for order in all the conceptual rooms – only those where we really do know where things belong.

In the speculative part of this chapter I have tried to explore some rooms of the sociobiological mansion where my own research interests in behavioural development impinge most strongly. In doing so I am very much aware of the dangers. The disorder generated by these new problems may spread back into the other bits of the house where some of the junk has been cleared off the floor. Maybe the tension between creative mess and rigorous tidiness can never be adequately resolved. Anyway, the functional approach seems to me an exceptionally promising way of opening up new questions in behavioural development and, looking the other way, the two key develop-mental concepts of plasticity and homeostasis should, at the very least, provoke some fresh thinking about the nature of evolutionary processes.

Summary

1. The purpose of this chapter is to forge some links between studies of behavioural development and evolutionary theory. The first part is critical of some sociobiological language which seems

particularly misleading when seen from a developmental perspective. The second part explores how valuable nourishment might flow both ways between the separate kinds of study.

2. The 'gene for a character' shorthand is liable to encourage preformationist thinking as is the view that natural selection acts on genes. Character differences should, where appropriate, be related to genetic differences. The metaphor of selection should be confined to differential survival of characters which need not necessarily be the property of individuals alone.

3. The concept of innateness encourages dichotomous classifications of behaviour which are misleading. This is partly because external events having specific and qualitatively distinct effects on behaviour can vary from few to many. Also the influences of experience cannot be arranged on a single dimension. Since the practical difficulties of operationally defining 'innate behaviour' are many and serious, the term causes more trouble than it is worth.

4. Functional explanations for behavioural development are helpful because they draw attention to evidence that might otherwise be ignored and suggest factors that can prove to be important as sources of variation. This point is exemplified by a functional discussion of the timing of filial and sexual imprinting in birds.

5. The importance of plasticity in development as an influence on evolutionary processes is discussed in relation to models of life-history strategies and the notion of genetic assimilation. If dominance within an allelic pair is influenced by external conditions and these in turn are affected by behaviour, it is possible to see how, for instance, culturally transmitted behaviour could change gene frequencies.

6. The existence of homeostatic processes in development implies that random genetic mutation cannot bring with it random phenotypic variation. This means that some kind of evolutionary change may not occur easily. More interestingly, homeostatic mechanisms permit the silent spread of mutant genes through a population. When two previously separated populations meet, different genes, whose effects were neutralised on their own, could interact and break through the homeostatic machinery to generate radically new phenotypes.

I should like to thank the following for their helpful comments on earlier drafts of the chapter: Tim Caro, Richard Dawkins, Gabriel Dover, Paul Martin and Dan Rubenstein.

References

Alcock, J. (1979). *Animal Behavior: An Evolutionary Approach*, 2nd edn. Sinauer: Sunderland, Mass.

Baldwin, J.M. (1896). A new factor in evolution. *American Naturalist*, **30**, 441–51, 536–53.

Bateson, G. (1963). The role of somatic change in evolution. *Evolution*, **17**, 529–39.

Bateson, P.P.G. (1976a). Specificity and the origins of behavior. In *Advances in the Study of Behaviour*, vol. 6, ed. J. Rosenblatt, R.A. Hinde & C. Beer, pp. 1–20. Academic Press: New York.

Bateson, P.P.G. (1976b). Rules and reciprocity in behavioural development. In *Growing Points in Ethology*, ed. P.P.G. Bateson & R.A. Hinde, pp. 401–21. Cambridge University Press: Cambridge.

Bateson, P. (1978a). Review of Richard Dawkins' 'The Selfish Gene'. *Animal Behaviour*, **26**, 316–18.

Bateson, P. (1978b). Sexual imprinting and optimal outbreeding. *Nature*, **273**, 659–60.

Bateson, P. (1979). How do sensitive periods arise and what are they for? *Animal Behaviour*, **27**, 470–86.

Bateson, P. (1980). Optimal outbreeding and the development of sexual preferences in Japanese quail. *Zeitschrift für Tierpsychologie*, **53**, 231–44.

Bateson, P. (1981). Discontinuities in development and changes in the organisation of play in cats. In *Behavioral Development*, ed. K. Immelmann, G. Barlow, M. Main & L. Petrinovich. Cambridge University Press: Cambridge, New York. (In press.)

Bateson, P., Lotwick, W. & Scott, D.K. (1980). Similarities between the faces of parents and offspring in Bewick's swan and the differences between mates. *Journal of Zoology*, **191**, 61–74.

Bateson, P. & Young, M. (1981). Separation from the mother and the development of play in cats. *Animal Behaviour*, **29**, 173–80.

Bertalanffy, L. von (1971). *General System Theory*. Penguin: London.

Burghardt, G.M. & Bekoff, M. (1978). *The Development of Behavior: Comparative and Evolutionary Aspects*. Garland STPM Press: New York.

Burtt, E.H. (1977). Some factors in the timing of parent–chick recognitions in swallows. *Animal Behaviour*, **25**, 231–9.

Cherfas, J.J. (1977). Visual system activation in the chick: one-trial avoidance learning affected by duration and patterning of light exposure. *Behavioural Biology*, **21**, 52–65.

Cherfas, J.J. (1978). Simultaneous colour discrimination in chicks is improved by brief exposure to light. *Animal Behaviour*, **26**, 1–5.

Cooke, F. (1978). Early learning and its effect on population structure. Studies of a wild population of snow geese. *Zeitschrift für Tierpsychologie*, **46**, 344–58.

Cowey, A. & Weiskrantz, L. (1975). Demonstration of cross-modal matching in rhesus monkeys, *Macaca mulatta*. *Neuropsychologia*, **13**, 117–20.

Dawkins, R. (1976). *The Selfish Gene*. Oxford University Press: Oxford.

Dawkins, R. (1978). Replicator selection and the extended phenotype. *Zeitschrift für Tierpsychologie*, **47**, 61–76.

Dawkins, R. & Krebs, J.R. (1978). Animal signals: information or manipulation. In *Behavioural Ecology*, ed. J.R. Krebs & N.B. Davies, pp. 1–18. Blackwell: Oxford.

Dempster, J.P. (1963). The population dynamics of grasshopper and locusts. Biological Reviews, **38**, 490–529.

Fagen, R.M. (1977). Selection for optimal age-dependent schedules of play behavior. *American Naturalist*, **111**, 395–414.

Fagen, R.M. (1981). *Animal Play Behavior*. Oxford University Press: Oxford, New York.

Futuyma, D.J. (1979). *Evolutionary Biology*. Sinauer: Sunderland, Mass.

Gadgil, M. & Bossert, W.H. (1970). Life history consequences of natural selection. *American Naturalist*, **104**, 1–24.

Gallagher, J.E. (1977). Sexual imprinting: a sensitive period in Japanese quail (*Corturnix coturnix japonica*). *Journal of Comparative and Physiological Psychology*, **91**, 72–8.

Goldschmidt, R. (1940). *The Material Basis of Evolution*. Yale University Press: New Haven, Conn.

Gottlieb, G. (1971). *Development of Species Identification in Birds*. University of Chicago Press: Chicago.

Gottlieb, G. (1976*a*). The roles of experience in the development of behavior and the nervous system. In *Neural and Behavioral Specificity. Studies on the Development of Behavior and the Nervous System*, vol. **3**, ed. G. Gottlieb, pp. 25–54. Academic Press: New York.

Gottlieb, G. (1976*b*). Early development of species-specific auditory perception in birds. In *Neural and Behavioral Specificity. Studies on the Development of Behavior and the Nervous System*, vol. **3**, ed. G. Gottlieb, pp. 237–80. Academic Press: New York.

Gould, S.J. (1977). *Ontogeny and Phylogeny*. Belknap Press: Cambridge, Mass.

Gould, S.J. & Eldredge, N. (1977). Punctuated equilibria: the tempo and mode of evolution reconsidered. *Paleobiology*, **3**, 115–51.

Hinde, R.A. (1968). Dichotomies in the study of development. In *Genetic and Environmental Influences on Behaviour*, ed. J.M. Thoday & A.S. Parkes, pp. 3–14. Oliver & Boyd: Edinburgh.

Hinde, R.A. & Fisher, J. (1951). Further observations on the opening of milk bottles by birds. *British Birds*, **44**, 393–6.

Horn, H.S. (1978). Optimal tactics of reproduction and life-history. In *Behavioural Ecology*, ed. J.R. Krebs & N.B. Davies, pp. 411–29. Blackwell: Oxford.

Huxley, J. (1955). Morphism in birds. *Acta XI Congressus Internationalis Ornithologica. Experientia Suppl. III*, 309–28.

Immelmann, K. (1969). Über den Einfluss frühkindlicher Erfahrungen auf die geschlechtliche Objektfixierung bei Estrildiden. *Zeitschrift für Tierpsychologie*, **26**, 677–81.

Immelmann, K. (1975). Ecological significance of imprinting and early learning. *Annual Review of Ecology and Systematics*, **6**, 15–37.

Krebs, J.R. & Davies, N.B. (1978). *Behavioural Ecology: An Evolutionary Approach.* Blackwell: Oxford.

Lehrman, D.S. (1970). Semantic and conceptual issues in the nature–nurture problem. In *Development and Evolution of Behavior*, ed. L.R. Aronson, E. Tobach, D.S. Lehrman & J.S. Rosenblatt, pp. 17–52. Freeman: San Francisco.

Lorenz, K. (1935) Der Kumpan in der Umvelt des Vögels. *Journal of Ornithology*, **83**, 137–213, 289–413.

Lorenz, K. (1965). *Evolution and Modification of Behavior*. University of Chicago Press: Chicago.

Mason, W. (1979). Ontogeny of social behavior. In *Handbook of Behavioral Neurobiology*, vol. **3**, *Social Behavior and Communication*. Plenum Press: New York.

Mather, K. (1943). Polygenic inheritance and natural selection. *Biological Reviews*, **18**, 32–64.

Maynard Smith, J. (1975). *The Theory of Evolution*. Penguin: London.

Maynard Smith, J. (1978). *The Evolution of Sex*. Cambridge University Press: Cambridge.

Mayr, E. (1963). *Animal Species and Evolution*. Harvard University Press: Cambridge, Mass.

Plotkin, H.C. & Odling-Smee, F.J. (1979). Learning, change and evolution. An enquiry into the teleonomy of learning. In *Advances in the Study of Behavior*, vol. **10**, ed. J.S. Rosenblatt, R.A. Hinde, C. Beer & M.C. Busnel, pp. 1–41. Academic Press: New York.

Rendel, J.M. (1967). *Canalisation and Gene Control*. Logos Press: London.

Richard, G. (1979). Ontogenesis and phylogenesis: Mutual constraints. In *Advances in the Study of Behavior*, vol. **9**, ed. J.B. Rosenblatt, R.A. Hinde, C. Beer & M.C. Busnel, pp. 229–78. Academic Press: New York.

Schutz, F. (1965). Sexuelle Prägung bei Anatiden. *Zeitschrift für Tierpsychologie*, **22**, 50–103.

Scudo, F.M. (1976). "Imprinting", speciation and avoidance of inbreeding. *Evolutionary Biology, Prague*, 375–92.

Stearns, S.C. (1977). The evolution of life history traits: A critique of the theory and a review of the data. *Annual Review of Ecology and Systematics*, **8**, 145–71.

Thoman, E.B. & Levine, S. (1970). Hormonal and behavioral changes in the rat mother as a function of early experience treatments of the offspring. *Physiology and Behavior*, **5**, 1417–21.

Vidal, J.M. (1980). Filial and sexual imprinting in chickens. *Animal Behaviour*, **28**, 880–91.

Waddington, C.H. (1953). Genetic assimilation of an acquired character. *Evolution*, **7**, 118–26.

Waddington, C.H. (1957). *The Strategy of the Genes*. Allen & Unwin: London.

Weiskrantz, L. & Cowey, A. (1975). Cross-modal matching in the rhesus monkey using a single pair of stimuli. *Neuropsychologia*, **13**, 257–61.

Williams, G.C. (1966). *Adaptation and Natural Selection: A Critique of Some Current Evolutionary Thought*. Princeton University Press: Princeton, New Jersey.

Wright, S. (1932). The roles of mutation, inbreeding, cross-breeding, and selection in evolution. *Proceedings XI International Congress Genetics*, **1**, 356–66.

8

Individual heterogeneity and population regulation

ADAM ŁOMNICKI

Introduction

Since ecology developed as a part of biology, it is not too surprising that the first attempts to describe and understand ecological phenomena were based on concepts and analogies derived from the morphology and physiology of a single organism. A forest, a meadow or a lake ecosystem were approached as a type of supraorganism, and there seemed to be good reasons for this. First, they are obviously not random collections of plants and animals; rather, they appear to be integrated units. Second, breeding of plants or animals outside their ecosystems can be as difficult as keeping a tissue culture outside the organism. And third, a detailed analysis of all interrelations between the components of an ecosystem would be a monumental task.

The impact of this holistic approach on ecological theory can hardly be overestimated. While other biologists were analysing the elements of a single organism to find out how it worked, ecologists attempted to describe the features and behaviour of entire ecological systems, very often without taking into account the properties of their elements. Although not explicitly stated, there was a widespread belief among ecologists that epiphenomenal descriptions of an entire population or an entire ecosystem would allow us to manipulate and manage those ecological units in the way we manipulate and manage single organisms. This approach was especially well pronounced in the study of plant and animal communities, but it was also applied to single-species populations (Allee *et al.*, 1949). I think that the very well known and popular ecological models, like the logistic equation or competition equations, were designed to describe an entire population, not to derive the properties of this population from the properties of its members. A reduction of per capita population with increasing population density is not a property of an individual but of the entire population, even though it has sometimes been reinterpreted as the 'average' individual's reproductive contribution (Rubenstein, 1981).

The theory of population self-regulation as proposed by Wynne-Edwards (1962) was a further logical step in this holistic approach: if a population were a supraorganism, it should be able to regulate its size, and consequently one can expect intrapopulation selection to bring about such a self-regulation. Due to this important contribution, biologists have become aware of the problem on which level natural selection operates. During the eighteen years since the publication of *Animal Dispersion in Relation to Social Behaviour*, we witnessed this well known progress in evolutionary ecology and ethology as marked by papers on group selection (Maynard Smith, 1964; Matessi & Jayakar, 1976), kin selection (Hamilton, 1964) and the evolutionarily stable strategies (Maynard Smith & Price, 1973). The impact of this development on ethology and behavioural ecology is discussed in other contributions to this book. In this chapter I would like to discuss some of the consequences of this progress on population ecology and especially on the theory of population dynamics and natural regulation of animal density in the field.

If natural selection operates on the individual or gene level, not on the level of entire populations, then it seems reasonable to consider population members more as independent entities and entire populations less like integrated systems than was previously assumed. If these conditions prevail, the properties of entire populations should be derived from the properties of their members, which implies a reductionist instead of holistic approach to ecological theory. In spite of recent progress in evolutionary ecology, ecological theory still carries the heritage of its traditional holistic approach, even in such concepts as the r- and K-selection. The proposition presented here is to overcome this holistic bias by proposing an alternative to the logistic equation and related models, and inspecting the consequences of this alternative.

Population-limited growth: two simple models and their consequences

Consider a population of N individuals supplied with V units of resources per unit of time. To avoid unnecessary complications, these models assume non-overlapping generations and discrete time periods equal to generation time. The most general property of all living creatures is the requirement of energy and other resources. Assume an upper limit a of the amount of resources an individual can take per unit of time, and a lower limit m required for its growth and survival to the time of reproduction. If $N_t < V/a$, then each individual can take a units of resources from which m units are used to maintain itself, while $(a - m)$ units are used to produce its progeny. Therefore, the population size in the next generation is given by

$$N_{t+1} = N_t(a - m)h, \tag{1}$$

where h denotes the efficiency of converting resources into progeny. By setting $R = (a - m)h$, equation (1) changes into the familiar equation of unlimited population growth.

Unlimited population growth brings about a population increase to the point when $N_t > V/a$. Let us assume that in the beginning the resources are evenly partitioned among the population members, so that each individual gets V/N units of resources. This implies that

$$N_{t+1} = (V - mN_t)h. \tag{2}$$

A complete analysis of the system described by equations (1) and (2) is presented in Fig. 8.1b which is developed elsewhere (Łomnicki, 1980). The most important result of this analysis is that the system is locally and globally stable only if

$$m < 1/h. \tag{3}$$

This inequality is a biologically important one. It shows that no stable population with equal resource partitioning is possible if the cost of growth and maintenance of a single individual (m) is higher than the cost of producing a single offspring ($1/h$). Since $m > 1/h$ for the majority of plants and animals, we have to reject the concept that population members are

Fig. 8.1. N_{t+1} as functions of N_t for three different models: (a) the logistic equation in discrete time units; (b) extremely equal resource partitioning as defined by equations (1) and (2); and (c) extremely unequal resource partitioning as defined by equations (1) and (4). The equilibrium points are given by the intersection of N_{t+1} (solid) and N_t (dashed) lines.

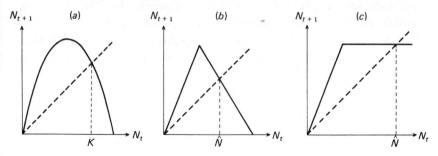

like molecules indistinguishable one from another which evenly divide among themselves the available resources.

Consider another extreme case, that of a population comprised of organisms partitioning resources unequally among themselves, such that some members get as many resources as they can, while others get none. If $N_t < V/a$, each individual gets a units of resources, and the population dynamics are described by equation (1). If $N_t > V/a$, then $L = V/a$ individuals get a units of resources, while $(N_t - L)$ get nothing. Therefore

$$N_{t+1} = hV(1 - m/a). \qquad (4)$$

The system described by equations (1) and (4) and presented in Fig. 8.1c is globally and locally stable, because N_{t+1} is independent of N_t.

These two simple models show how important resource partitioning within a population is for the stability of a single species population, and consequently for the stability of the entire ecosystem. This is not to imply that unequal resource partitioning is an adaptation to assure population stability. To the contrary, it is a by-product of physiological and behavioural processes, which implies that these physiological and behavioural processes should be studied in order to understand ecological phenomena.

At present, there is obviously a great gap between progress in behavioural ecology and traditional ecological theory. The basic ecological model, the logistic equation, ignores any individual variation in resource intake. A comparison of this equation to the models presented herein (Fig. 8.1) shows that the logistic assumption has effects similar to those of the assumption of equal resource partitioning. The models presented here are mathematically much less elegant than the logistic equation, but they are for many reasons preferable. They are described in discrete time units only, because a population is neither a shapeless mass, nor a self-regulatory unit which would immediately react to any increase in its size by reducing its per capita growth. A seasonal environment and the action of each individual to garner as many resources as it requires, if they are available, are much more realistically described by discrete, than by continuous models. In addition, the logistic equation is symmetrical: given that N_t is in both cases equidistant from the carrying capacity K, its rate of growth when $N_t < K$ equals its rate of decline when $N_t > K$, an assumption which can hardly be justified by biological data.

Predictions from the models presented here are intuitively rather obvious. Low stability of uniform forest stands is a well known phenomena. The concepts of scramble and contest competition, as proposed by Nicholson (1954) are very close to the models of equal and unequal resource partitioning, respectively, as presented here. Unfortunately, Nicholson did not define precisely the mechanisms which bring about these two kinds of competition. The problem in the way of partitioning of resources is of importance not only for entire populations but also for every group of individuals which has to survive on limited resources; the obvious example are members of a single brood. If resources are equally divided, then the survival of nestlings in a single brood should be either zero or unity. If, on the other hand, there is extreme inequality in resource intakes, as proposed by the second model presented here, then the number of surviving nestlings should be independent of the brood size. Resources partitioning in single broods fall more or less midway between these two extremes. The concept of group selection is based on the assumption that entire populations are endangered by extinction due to resource depletion, which obviously can be the case if resources are equally partitioned.

If we believe that resource partitioning and individual variation among population members are of crucial importance for population stability, then very little can be learned about ecological processes from theoretical models ignoring individual differences. One should rather expect to learn more about population stability by investigating physiological and behavioural mechanisms which bring about individual variability, as well as ethological mechanisms responsible for its increase and maintenance. If these mechanisms are ignored, ecological theory will appear as if built on shifting sands.

Unequal resource partitioning: its origin and formal description

The existence of individual variation is a phenomenon well known to all field and laboratory ecologists, as well as to botanists and ethologists. The only problem is that, since ecological models largely ignore variation other than that which is related to age, sex, or some hereditary traits, ecological consequences of variation are not taken into account.

The general assumption underlying almost all ecological models is that a population density N_{t+1} is a function of the density N_t of this population at an earlier time. This is obviously the case in an increasing population as shown by equation (1), or in a population with equal or close to equal resource partitioning as shown by equation (2). However, as shown by equation (4) this may not be the case in terrestrial plants where large differences between individuals prevent competition from small seedlings. This is probably the reason why there is so little interest in ecological models among botanists. Individual differences between animals are usually smaller, which can be a reason for large oscillations in population size even in a very stable habitat, as was reported by Nicholson (1957) for blowflies kept in laboratory populations. In animal populations both equal and unequal resource partitioning can be encountered, the latter being due, for example, to a well pronounced dominance hierarchy; the dynamics of such populations would be much like those of plant populations.

When considering hereditary differences among individuals in relation to their survival and reproductive success, the concept of soft selection (Wallace, 1975) must be kept in mind. The fate of an individual is not determined solely by its genotype. The absolute size of the population and its relative frequency will also be important. Genotypes can determine the position of an individual within the population, but as long as these genotypes are not lethal, the ecological conditions determine how many individuals of the highest positions will survive and leave progeny. The same can be said about age, since its effects are also density- and frequency-dependent. At a low density and in the absence of stronger age groups, the weaker one can survive; while at high densities the presence of stronger age groups can result in complete elimination of weak juvenile individuals. Therefore we can learn more about the influence of age structure on population dynamics from a detailed study of a small group of individuals, than from life tables which are highly susceptible to environmental changes.

The existence of individual variation among members of a single brood (e.g. in predatory birds: Lack, 1966) is a well known phenomenon, and it can be of selective advantage for parents if the environment is unpredictable. But even if newborn individuals are identical, random food intakes during early development can bring about large variations in the individual size. If the probability of taking a food item decreases, one can expect, from the properties of the binomial distribution, an increase in variation in cumulative food intake and consequently, in individual size. Since the probability of taking a food item is an increasing function of the size of an individual, at least to a certain point, a skewed log-normal distribution of individual size will result. Both variation and skewness in size have been shown in plants (Harper, 1977), salamander larvae (Wilbur & Collins, 1973), and fish (Rubenstein, 1980). Note that if the probability of taking a food item is an increasing function of the previous food intakes, a stabilization in time of an individual's position within the population is to be expected.

Another important factor that can produce individual variation is related to small-scale variability in timing of seed germination or egg hatching, which at later life stages can bring about disproportionally large differences in individual fitness. The most spectacular data concerning this phenomenon are known for plants (Harper, 1977), but similar phenomena should also occur among animals.

Variation among originally identical individuals can arise during dispersal of young animals away from their parents. As Hamilton & May (1977) showed, dispersing a proportion of one's young can be selectively advantageous for the parent even in a stable and saturated habitat. Individuals that move away from the familiar places where they were born into other crowded sites are in worse positions than those which stay in their places. Although this model assumes that dispersing individuals compete on equal terms with established ones, it allows for mortality during the dispersal phase, which can be considered as similar to obtaining lower status in the population.

Dominance hierarchies, which seem to be much more common among animals than previously supposed and recently have been found even among anthozoan coelenterates (Brace & Pavey, 1978), are probably the final result of the action of all the processes mentioned above. They can result from individual differences in age, hereditary traits, environmental variations in the time of hatching, stochastic growth and dispersal.

This is not to imply that intrapopulation variation is always large enough to assure the population stability. Physiological limits to growth and to the amount of resources an individual can take, resource abundance, and the homogeneity of the resource distribution can promote equality in resource intake. Furthermore, differential mortality which removes the weakest members from a population can mask intrapopulation variation to some extent and make it much less detectable.

For theoretical investigations of population dynamics, the best way to express intrapopulation variation is in terms of the amount of energy or other resources controlled by an individual. Individual resource intake y during a season or throughout the entire life span can be ranked from the highest to the lowest value of y (Fig. 8.2). Ordering all the individual resource intakes y brings about the concept of rank x which is assigned to each individual, but it does not imply the necessity of a well defined linear hierarchy within the population. Such a hierarchy may or may not exist but, for population dynamics, the only important phenomenon is the extent of variation that exists among the way individuals share resources.

An individual resource share y depends not only upon an individual's rank but also upon the amount V of resources available to the entire population and the size N of this population. Given the function $y(x, V, N)$, a general model of population dynamics, with non-overlapping generations in the discrete time can be given by

$$N_{t+1} = \max\left\{0, h\sum_{1}^{L}[y(x, V, N_t) - m]\right\} \qquad (5)$$

where $L = \min(L', N_t)$ and L' is in turn defined by the equation $m = y(L', V, N_t)$. The models presented in section 2 of this chapter are special cases of the model defined by equation (5) for extremely equal and extremely unequal resource partitioning. Note that this model considers three different stages of population growth and regulation: (i) when $y > m$ for each value of y, (ii) when $y > m$ for some values of y, and (iii) when $y < m$ for each value of y. This makes the model discontinuous, but at the same time much more realistic than those based on the logistic equation.

The realism of this model does not imply that any good data are available at present to permit a precise definition of the function $y(x, V, N)$. Nevertheless, it is possible to make inferences about its general properties. By definition, the function $y(x, V, N)$ is (i) a non-increasing function of x, and it follows from other considerations that it is (ii) an increasing function of V, with (iii) an upper limit a of the amount of resources an individual can take, and with (iv) $\sum_{1}^{N} y \leq V$. Since individual variation in resource intake increases with the shortage of resources, $|dy/dx|$ is (v) a decreasing function of V and sometimes also an increasing function of N. For population stability, the most important feature of $y(x, V, N)$ is whether it is (vi) a

Fig. 8.2. Individual resource intakes y as a function of an individual's rank x, for N individuals out of which only L individuals get m or more units of resources. a, upper limit of resources an individual can take per unit of time.

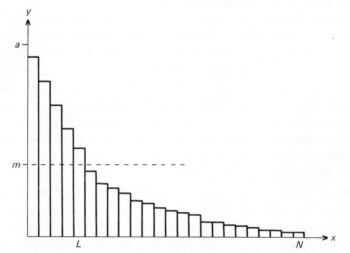

decreasing function of N or independent of N. In a strictly 'free' situation, as defined by Fretwell (1972), with equal or close-to-equal resource partitioning, an increase in the number of low-rank individuals diminishes the resource intake of each population member. This may not be the case in a population with very strong dominance relationships or in a plant population with large variation in individual biomass. In such a despotic situation (Fretwell, 1972), one can expect y to be independent of N, and consequently N_{t+1} to be independent of N_t. This is, for example, the case if y is defined by geometric series, according to the equation

$$y(x, V) = a(1 - a/V)^x. \tag{6}$$

If this is the case, the dynamics of the population are like those described by the equation (4), which are locally and globally stable.

The stabilizing effect that social structure has on population dynamics does not require a group-selectionist explanation. Consider a population with overlapping generations and a strong dominance hierarchy based on age. In dense populations offering very low prospects for successful dispersal, the probability of survival of young individuals is much lower than in the same types of populations without such social structure and where juveniles can compete on equal terms with older individuals. Thus in dense populations, social structuring may result in reduced reproduction in a given season, which is of selective advantage only if the strong dominance hierarchy puts young individuals in inferior positions. Any alteration of the social structure which increases the chances of young individuals in inferior positions relative to the older ones, would result in increased reproduction, followed by population increase. This was experimentally confirmed for laboratory house mouse populations (Petrusewicz, 1957, 1963).

Animal dispersal in relation to unequal resource partitioning

Most animal species live in a heterogeneous environment, with patches of local habitats where their intrinsic rate of natural increase $r > 0$, surrounded by hostile areas where either high mortality occurs or no reproduction is possible and $r < 0$. Some animals leave their local habitats and search for alternatives, while others stay in their places. This is a phenomenon well known to field biologists, although the fate of emigrants and the probability of their survival before reaching another local habitat is rather difficult to determine.

Local habitats are more or less permanent but not eternal: some of them disappear, while others are formed in other parts of the environment. There are also extinctions or partial extinctions of local populations which live in these habitats. One may claim that the probability of a migrant finding a place to live and reproduce can be very low, but higher than zero. There are two kinds of local habitats: those based on renewable resources, which can become extinct due to random events and from which only some population members disperse; others, based on finite amounts of unrenewable resources, which when exhausted can no longer sustain animal populations.

From the standpoint of the population ecology, the questions to be asked about dispersal are: (i) Does dispersal decrease the density of local populations? (ii) Is the survival of migrants lower than that of the non-migrating members of the population? If the answer to either of these questions is no, then dispersal is of little importance for population dynamics and its selective advantage is obvious and does not require any explanation. If dispersal does not bring about a lower population density, the dispersing individuals are those which would die anyway and therefore, dispersal is of no importance for the local population. It only enables colonization of other local habitats. Even though never explicitly stated, this view was and still is widely held in ecology. It implies that a confined laboratory population is a realistic model of natural populations in the field, and that spatial and temporal heterogeneity is of minor importance in regulating populations. If on the other hand one accepts that dispersal can lower the density of a local population but not by increased migrant mortality, then dispersal is a mechanism which would produce an even distribution of animals within the area, the situation described by Fretwell & Lucas (1970) in their model of ideal-free animal distributions.

The problem is whether reductions in the density of local populations and increased mortality of migrants both occur. Even more important is the question how large this density reduction and mortality can be. If population density is decreased by dispersal by an order of magnitude, and migrant mortality is sufficiently high, such that migrants are able to colonize new habitats but are not able to increase the density of local populations reduced by a previous emigration, then emigration can be of crucial importance for population regulation and consequently for many other ecological processes.

The first question to be asked is whether dispersal which brings about reductions in local population densities and migrant survival is theoretically possible. According to Wynne-Edwards (1962), such dispersal can evolve by group selection. Independent investigations of the role of dispersal in regulating populations by Lidicker (1962) and later on, with the application of mathematical models, by Van Valen (1971) and Roff (1975) enumerated a number of theoretical difficulties. Van Valen (1971) did not consider explicitly reductions of population density due to emigration. He only considered emigratory rates from local populations subject to extinction and colonization by migrants. His numerical solutions suggest that emigratory rates will evolve to be roughly equal to the probabilities of extinction of local populations. This provides an explanation for the evolution of dispersal in heterogeneous environments, but not for dispersal which serves as a population-regulatory mechanism.

Roff (1975) took into account not only the evolution of emigratory rates, but also their effects on local population size and survival of neighbouring local populations. The evolution of dispersal combined with reductions in local population sizes and migrant mortality was shown by numerical simulations to be possible, as long as there was temporal and spatial heterogeneity. This heterogeneity was introduced into the model by varying the population's carrying capacity and reproductive rate. The numerical simulations by Roff (1975) show that dispersal will evolve under many different conditions (sets of parameters). But, roughly speaking, the conditions do not allow migrant survival to be lower than 50% and reductions in local population sizes to be larger than 50%. This implies that dispersal can be of considerable importance for population dynamics, but not for population regulation.

The model of ideal-free habitat distribution proposed by Fretwell & Lucas (1970) involving despots has important consequences for the process of population regulation by dispersal. In particular, it provides a mechanism by which low population densities in rich habitats that are hardly colonized by immigrants can be maintained. The mechanism is based on the implication that there are differences among individuals established in the population and those which are newcomers, although these differences are not explicitly presented in the model.

All the theoretical difficulties of accepting emigration as a population-regulatory mechanism disappear if one accounts for individual differences in resource intake within populations. Consider a single local population with unequal resource partitioning, as described earlier and presented in Fig. 8.2, but with an additional assumption that an individual's position at the early stages of its life is strongly correlated with its future position. This implies that the fitness of $(N - L)$ individuals which take less than m units of resources (more precisely, less than $m + 1/h$ units of resources) is equal to zero. If local populations are not eternal but become extinct or reduced in size from time to time, there is always a small chance for a migrant to find a better place in which it can live and reproduce. Therefore given individual variation in fitness, dispersal will be favoured by natural selection. As a consequence, local population size will be reduced and migrant mortality will be high. When the assumption of a strong correlation between the position of young individuals and their future success is relaxed, one can expect the number of emigrants to be smaller than $(N - L)$ individuals: but as long as individual differences in resource intake can be more or less precisely predicted, selection will still favour emigration from crowded populations. It can be concluded that regulation of population density by emigration should not be ignored *a priori* on theoretical grounds. A simple theoretical model of emigration, based on individual variation described by equation (6) demonstrated that emigration reduced local population density and increased food density as well as the reproductive rates of population members (Łomnicki, 1978).

Thus far, the best data concerning population regulation by emigration come from studies on populations of asexual *Hydra* polyps (Łomnicki & Slobodkin, 1966; Ritte, 1969). They confirm that emigration from local laboratory populations can reduce by an order of magnitude the size of these populations. This, in turn, results in more food being left after feeding, and also higher levels of reproduction. In addition, emigrating or floating polyps move to the water surface incurring high mortality levels. Unfortunately this corroboration is inconclusive as it concerns members of a single clone. Therefore, emigration may be a result of kin selection.

As for sexually reproducing animals, large reductions in the density of populations from which animals can emigrate, as compared to confined ones, was found in *Tribolium* (Sokoloff, 1974) and small rodents (Krebs, Keller & Tamarin, 1969). Experiments on emigratory behaviour of the imagines of *Tribolium castaneum* have demonstrated that allowing emigration results in equal numbers of eggs being laid per unit of medium, irrespective of the total amount of medium and the number of beetles placed originally in the vials (Łomnicki & Krawczyk, 1980). This is in contrast to the results of experiments in which emigration was not permitted and in which the number of eggs laid per unit of medium was higher, more variable, and dependent on both the number of original beetles and the amount of medium. An interesting feature of *Tribolium* emigration is that it does not seem to be determined by differences among imagines. Looking for the selective advantage of emigratory behaviour, the following explanation is proposed: the eggs which were laid last and after a critical egg density had been reached had only a small chance of surviving to metamorphosis, since they tended to be cannibalized by previously hatched larvae. Hence, emigration of females when a certain egg density is reached is of selective advantage and it is followed by emigration of males. Emigration is not due to the differences between emigrating individuals but between their progeny. Another feature of local populations of *Tribolium* is that they live on non-renewable resources. In such populations one can expect that the first to emigrate are not the weakest individuals, but the strongest ones, those first to have completed their development. In most *Tribolium* populations this is the case. When the animals are unusually crowded, however, emigration of very small larvae also occurs. The net result of these processes is the regulation of population density in *Tribolium* by emigration. As a consequence, such emigration-regulated populations exhibit lower densities and higher reproductive rates than confined populations.

Survival of migrants away from local habitats can hardly be assessed. The low status of migrants in vertebrate populations is well known (Errington, 1946). Small invertebrates can often be found far away from their natural environment, sometimes in large numbers, with a very low probability of finding an appropriate habitat. This suggests that large reductions in the number of migrants occur in nature. There is a shortage of good quantitative data concerning this phenomenon that is due, in part, to technical difficulties, but also to the present state of ecological theory which does not consider animal dispersion as an important regulatory mechanism.

Concluding remarks

Evolutionary biology matured and developed a solid theoretical base when it confronted ecological questions concerning population self-regulation and group selection. The concepts presented in this chapter which are based on these original questions may appear obvious to ethnologists, but as far as ecological theory is concerned, there is still a strong influence of the holistic approach that tends to ignore important physiological and behavioural properties of individuals.

The models presented here suggest the need for revising simple holistic ecological theories. Higher reproductive rates and their correlates which are presently described in terms derived from the logistic equation, such as r-selected characters (in contrast to K-selected ones), should be explained more explicitly from the properties of individuals in relation to their environment and their physiological limitations. A simple model based on the evolutionarily stable strategy and presented elsewhere (Łomnicki,

1980) shows, independently of the logistic equation, that reproductive rates should be an increasing function of the probability of extinction of local habitats.

If one accepts the mechanism of population regulation by dispersal, there may be far-reaching consequences to ecological theory and its applications in agriculture and forestry. The regulation of population density by dispersal cannot work if the area is homogeneous, i.e. either the entire large area is a single local habitat and consequently dispersal cannot reduce population density, or there are no local habitats for a given species and therefore the species cannot survive. This may be the reason for population outbreaks in homogeneous cultivated fields. It also might explain the apparent correlation between population stability and species diversity, since both the latter characteristics can be brought about by extensive environmental heterogeneity.

Summary

1. The properties of a single species population should be determined by the properties of its members and the habitat in which they live.
2. A simple population model, based on difference equations with survival and reproduction determined by individual differences in resource intake, reveals that variance in the individual resource intake is a necessary condition for population stability.
3. If individual resource intakes are largely independent of the number of individuals of low rank, then local and global population stability, contest competition, and ideal despotic distribution are possible.
4. In patchy environments, differences in the individual resource intake may induce some individuals to leave the population. Under such conditions selection will favour emigration and its regulation of population density, despite high levels of migrant mortality.
5. It is suggested that the variation in the individual resource intake combined with the spatial heterogeneity can be the reason for ecosystem stability.

References

Allee, W.C., Emerson, A.E., Park, O., Park, T. & Schmidt, K.P. (1949). *Principles of Animal Ecology*. Saunders: Philadelphia.
Brace, R.C. & Pavey, J. (1978). Size-dependent dominance hierarchy in the anemone *Actinia equina*. *Nature*, **273**, 752–3.

Errington, P.L. (1946). Predation and vertebrate population. *Quarterly Review of Biology*, **21**, 144–77, 221–45.

Fretwell, S.D. (1972). *Populations in a Seasonal Environment*. Princeton University Press: Princeton.

Fretwell, S.D. & Lucas, H.L. (1970). On territorial behaviour and other factors influencing habitat distribution in birds. I. Theoretical development. *Acta Biotheoretica*, **19**, 16–36.

Hamilton, W.D. (1964). The genetical theory of social behaviour. *Journal of Theoretical Biology*, **7**, 1–52.

Hamilton, W.D. & May, R.M. (1977). Dispersal in stable habitats. *Nature*, **269**, 578–81.

Harper, J.L. (1977). *Population Biology of Plants*. Academic Press: London.

Krebs, C.J., Keller, B.L. & Tamarin, R.H. (1969). *Microtus* population biology: demographic changes in fluctuating populations of *M. ochrogaster* and *M. pennsylvanicus* in Southern Indiana. *Ecology*, **50**, 587–607.

Lack, D. (1966). *Population Studies of Birds*. Clarendon Press: Oxford.

Lidicker, W.Z. (1962). Emigration as a possible mechanism permitting the regulation of population density below carrying capacity. *American Naturalist*, **96**, 29–33.

Łomnicki, A. (1978). Individual differences between animals and natural regulation of their numbers. *Journal of Animal Ecology*, **47**, 461–75.

Łomnicki, A. (1980). Regulation of population density due to individual differences and patchy environment. *Oikos*, **35**, 185–93.

Łomnicki, A. & Krawczyk, J. (1980). Equal egg densities as a result of emigration in *Tribolium castaneum*. *Ecology*, **61**, 432–7.

Łomnicki, A. & Slobodkin, L.B. (1966). Floating in *Hydra littoralis*. *Ecology*, **47**, 881–9.

Matessi, C. & Jayakar, S.D. (1976). Conditions for the evolution of altruism under Darwinian selection. *Theoretical Population Biology*, **9**, 360–87.

Maynard Smith, J. (1964). Group selection and kin selection. *Nature*, **201**, 1145–7.

Maynard Smith, J. & Price, G.R. (1973). The logic of animal conflict. *Nature*, **246**, 15–8.

Nicholson, A.J. (1954). An outline of the dynamics of animal populations. *Australian Journal of Zoology*, **2**, 551–98.

Nicholson, A.J. (1957). The self-adjustment of populations to change. *Cold Spring Harbor Symposia on Quantitative Biology*, **22**, 153–73.

Petrusewicz, K. (1957). Investigations on experimentally induced population growth. *Ekologia Polska seria A*, **5**, 281–309.

Petrusewicz, K. (1963). Population growth induced by disturbance in the ecological structure of the population. *Ekologia Polska seria A*, **11**, 87–125.

Ritte, U. (1969). *Floating an Sexuality in Laboratory Populations of* Hydra littoralis. Ph.D. Thesis, University of Michigan: Ann Arbor.

Roff, D.A. (1975). Population stability and the evolution of dispersal in a heterogeneous environment. *Oecologia*, **19**, 217–37.

Rubenstein, D.I. (1981). Individual variation and competition in the Everglades pygmy sunfish. *Journal of Animal Ecology*, **50**, 337–50.

Sokoloff, A. (1974). *The Biology of Tribolium*, vol. 2. Clarendon Press: Oxford.

Van Valen, L. (1971). Group selection and the evolution of dispersal. *Evolution*, **25**, 591–8.

Wallace, B. (1975). Hard and soft selection revisited. *Evolution*, **29**, 465–73.

Wilbur, H.M. & Collins, J.P. (1973). Ecological aspects of amphibian metamorphosis. *Science*, **182**, 1305–14.

Wynne-Edwards, V.C. (1962). *Animal Dispersion in Relation to Social Behaviour*. Oliver and Boyd: Edinburgh.

III

Evolutionary conflicts of interest

Edited by
R.I.M. DUNBAR

Whenever two individuals interact, a conflict of interest is in principle inevitable at some level since each individual's interests will lie in promoting its own genes and not those of other individuals. This is not, of course, to say that in certain circumstances individuals may not have common interests in some particular respect, nor to say that individuals may not cooperate to further their own long-term interests even if at the expense of some short-term loss. Indeed, the former will often occur in those situations where the successful pursuit of some intermediate goal promotes the evolutionary interests of both parties (as, for example, in the acquisition of more profitable prey through cooperative hunting: see Wrangham, this volume). Rather, as a general principle, we should look to conflicts of interest as the driving force that generates evolutionary change, precisely because the competition so generated will result in individuals pursuing most vigorously those strategies that promote their own genes.

In this section, conflicts of interest of three rather different kinds are examined. These concern (i) conflicts in the conventional sense of direct contests for access to limited resources, (ii) conflicts over the distribution of the costs of reproduction between the members of a reproductive partnership, and (iii) conflicts over the distribution of effort into different reproductive strategies (in this case, the sex ratio of offspring).

In the first paper, Parker examines the effects of phenotypic asymmetries on the evolutionarily stable strategy (ESS) solution to evolutionary conflicts. The ESS approach to evolutionary problems has been thoroughly developed over the past decade. Parker here adds an entirely new dimension to it by considering the effects that phenotypic differences in competitive abilities among individuals will have on the conventional ESS solution to conflicts over access to such evolutionarily desirable resources as mates and territories. Phenotypic differences are those superimposed on the underlying genetic differences by historical accidents that are peculiar to the individual in question. These may be either temporary (e.g. loss of weight due to poor foraging conditions or recent injury) or more permanent (e.g. so called 'transgenerational effects' whereby the mother's inability to provide her offspring with a nutritionally adequate diet results in the latter following a lower life-time growth trajectory than more fortunate competitors). Perhaps the most significant conclusion to emerge from Parker's analyses is that, in scramble competitions, phenotypic differences have proportionately less effect on fitness as group size decreases. Thus, not only are phenotypic effects important in their own right, but other extrinsic factors can influence their severity. This paper heralds a new era of more sophisticated modelling of the evolution of behaviour.

In the second paper, Knowlton considers a more specific conflict of interest: that over how the cost of rearing offspring should be distributed between the parents. The problem of sex role reversal has received surprisingly little attention hitherto. Even though it occurs only rarely in nature, the phenomenon is conspicuous and rather perplexing wherever it does occur, and so far no entirely satisfactory explanation has been given to account for it. Knowlton approaches the problem through simulation, and attempts to determine the conditions required for sex role reversal to become evolutionarily stable. The answer is that the conditions are so extreme that we should expect genuine sex role reversal to occur only rarely. Two key issues emerge from Knowlton's analyses that deserve particular stress, since biologists will be obliged to confront them squarely if any real understanding of the problem is to be achieved. The first is largely a matter of definition: in practice, there is little agreement about what should count as sex role reversal, and hence about which species exhibit it. The second is a matter of fact: even when we can decide whether a particular species shows sex role reversal, we rarely have a sufficient understanding of its biology to hazard more than a passing guess as to why it should have evolved sex role reversal. By crystallising the assumptions underlying existing explanations for the phenomenon, Knowlton has given us a clear indication of what aspects of the biological situation are likely to be important. The next step is up to the field biologists.

The final paper in this section deals with conflicts of interest at a rather deeper level. The conflict here lies less in the kinds of direct competition for resources considered by Parker than in long-term considerations of how to generate more descendants than one's rivals. One important way of doing so is to adjust the sex ratio of offspring in favour of whichever sex will provide the greater benefit. Clutton-Brock & Albon outline the main theories that have been put forward to account for sex ratios, and review at length the mammalian data in an attempt to evaluate the theories produced by Fisher and Trivers & Willard. In the final analysis, the data are equivocal in their support of either theory; indeed, there are instances in which they appear to contradict the predictions of both theories. As Maynard Smith points out in the Introduction to this volume, we face the uninviting prospect of a superfluity of theories, none of which appears to bear any convincing relationship to the facts they purport to explain. This is all the more disturbing since sex ratio is perhaps the one area where we might have expected clear-cut *quantitative* predictions capable of direct empirical verification. In practice, aside from any intrinsic problems in estimating foetal sex ratios, we often lack the background biological information to say anything about how the parents distribute their parental investment; yet convincing explanations for observed departures from predicted sex ratios invariably turn on precisely this point. It is clear that, again, little progress will be made until field biologists are able to provide unequivocal evidence for or against the underlying assumptions of the existing theoretical models. Only then will we know for sure whether the problem lies with bad theory rather than with bad data.

9

Phenotype-limited evolutionarily stable strategies

G.A. PARKER

Introduction

The origin and maintenance of variation between individual organisms has long been an evolutionists' obsession. If all species were ultra-specialists, each would have an almost infinitesimal niche breadth and there would presumably be a near-infinite number. The opposite speculation leads us to imagine an earth populated by a single ultra-generalist, with a protean capacity to assume an almost infinite number of phenotypes, one for each contingency encountered. The observable results of these two extremes might not be altogether dissimilar as judged by the range and types of organism. But whereas the hypothetical ultra-specialist lacks any phenotype plasticity, the ultra-generalist has a genome that encodes for a vast array of strategies and the expression of a particular strategy set is conditional upon environment.

Aside from the fact that our ultra-generalist might need a genome effectively capable of achieving capacities equivalent to the summated genomes of all the ultra-specialists, morphological transformation and plasticity involve energetic costs. A feature of animal behaviour is that a wide range of strategies are possible without the cost of morphological change. Further, certain behaviour strategies are very obviously limited to phenotype – individuals 'play' vastly different strategies conditional upon sex, age, physiological state, etc. If plants appear to overshadow animals in their remarkable phenotypic plasticity of growth form, the balance is more than redressed by animal capacities for (inexpensive) behavioural plasticity. It is tempting to suggest that the reason animals show less morphological plasticity relates directly to this very capacity. But animals do obviously vary in their morphological phenotype; how then should each phenotype behave?

This paper concerns the question of how phenotype will affect competitive strategy. To what extent will an individual's strategy be conditional upon its phenotype, and how will the capacity to adopt phenotype-limited strategies affect the relative fitnesses of individuals? Łomnicki (1978) has investigated effects of competitive differences between individuals in relation to population regulation. I examine phenotype-limited evolutionarily stable strategies (ESS; Maynard Smith & Price, 1973) in three types of competitive interaction that are commonplace in nature. Although the models are phrased specifically in terms of sexual selection, their general solutions should be readily applicable to other forms of intraspecific competition. Firstly, consider the general problem of phenotype limitation of strategy.

Strategies dependent on phenotype

From ESS theory, variation in strategy can come about in two quite separate ways (Parker, 1978; Maynard Smith, 1979; see also the excellent review by Dunbar, 1982).

(i) *Pure ESS, variable conditions.* Here there exists a set of conditions (of phenotype or environment) ordered as A, B, C ... N. The ESS is a pure strategy (e.g. 'when in A play x_A, when in B play x_B, etc.'), so that variation in component strategies comes about by variation in conditions. The fitness payoffs of strategies x_A, x_B etc. will differ. This sort of ESS has been termed 'conditional' by Dawkins (1980).

(ii) *Mixed strategies, fixed conditions.* Sometimes an ESS can be a mixed strategy. That is, when conditions are fixed, individuals show a set of strategies played with specific probabilities. This solution can be summarised as: 'when in A, play x_1 with probability p_1, x_2 with probability p_2,' etc. Variation in strategies arises entirely as a property of the game itself, not through variation in conditions. In this case, the payoffs from x_1, x_2 etc. will be equal. Of course, there is no reason why variation in conditions cannot also occur here; in nature it always will. This acts to increase the variation or to alter the observed frequencies of strategies that will be played overall. But either way, fitness payoffs would differ between, and not within conditions. (A 'condition' can be a particular phenotype that a genome 'finds' itself in, or a particular environmental contingency faced by an individual animal.)

Throughout the paper, we shall be concerned with the problem of strategies that are dependent on condition, i.e. with the problem of linking the correct strategy (pure or mixed) with a particular phenotype or environment. Where strategies are genetic, this depends on the preciseness with which genes can express specific strategies in response to specific cues. To demonstrate the sort of adaptive problem that arises here, imagine the following possibility. An animal has the ability to recognise only cue a, which is present in all conditions A, B, C ... N. It has a single locus L at which a set of alternative alleles are possible, each of which specifies a particular strategy. Ideally, in A, B, ... N the animal would play strategies x_A, x_B ... x_N specified by alleles l_A, l_B, ... l_N. It cannot; assume that selection promotes the fixation of the 'general purpose' allele l_{opt}. Strategy x_{opt} is attained by virtue of its weighted mean effect across conditions A, B ... N. It could be defined as a 'coarse-grained' optimum. There can be no further refinement until the genetic system alters. Note that even this 'imperfect' state demands some complexity; there must be a mechanism for recognising cue α and for playing strategy x_{opt} in association with it.

Advance requires discrimination between A, B, ... N etc., and association of a play of x_A with A, x_B with B, and so on, to produce 'fine-grained' optimisation. There is always a real possibility that perfection cannot occur (at least in the short term) because of limited sensory capacities. However, the much greater problem would seem to be the one of associating cues specific to A, B, etc. with the appropriate play: x_A, x_B etc. When 'conditions' are environmental circumstances, learning provides a ready mechanism. When 'condition' describes a phenotypic state, learning may provide a mechanism, but sometimes less obviously. For genetic determination, one possibility is to have N of the L loci; L_A coding for x_A, L_B for x_B, and so on. Another (and perhaps more likely) possibility is that various modifiers are selected that cause strategy x to range quantitatively in appropriate correlation with some quantitative ranking of the cue for A, B ... N. Although the evolution of strategy refinements seem complex, there is fortunately plenty of evidence from the behaviour of animals in the field to encourage optimism. But equally, some 'imperfection' seems entirely plausible. By reduction, there must always be some subset of conditions (equivalent to α above) within which no strategy refinement can easily occur.

An important aspect of ESS models (particularly those for contests) concerns the degree of 'uncertainty' over conditions. Generally, the occurrence of mixed ESSs relates biologically to this uncertainty. For example, no two contesting individuals can ever have exactly identical amounts to gain from winning, or exactly identical fighting abilities. But there is bound to be a range over which asymmetries cannot be assessed by the combatants. For contests between two individuals, how likely, and how prevalent mixed strategies will be in nature, will depend on how much uncertainty there is. Where individuals 'know' their state accurately, then selection often favours playing a pure strategy dependent on state.

The three examples that follow appear to cover the three main forms of intraspecific competition. In a scramble competition, n competitors compete over a limited resource that is continuously divisible between the competitors. By increasing its competitive expenditure, an individual can increase its share of the resource. In 'alternative strategy' competitions, the fundamental feature is that gains can accrue from two (or more) qualitatively different strategies – interactions between and within strategies may resemble scrambles or contests. Contest competitions classically involve two combatants competing for a non-divisible resource that is exploited by the victor.

For a phenotype-limited strategy to be an ESS, it is assumed that there can be no alternative strategy that can invade *when played by an individual of the same phenotype*. The strategy is therefore derived by a test for stability *within* a particular phenotype (see Bishop, Cannings & Maynard Smith, 1978; Parker & Knowlton, 1980).

Scramble competitions

Consider a scramble in which the amount of resource an individual gains is some increasing function of its expenditure x relative to the strategy played by its competitors. I give a general ESS solution (see also Macnair & Parker, 1979; Parker & Macnair, 1979; Knowlton & Parker, 1979) and then extend it to the case for phenotype-limited ESSs (see also Parker & Knowlton, 1980). To make the arguments more direct, imagine the following sexual advertisement scramble, which is a frequency-dependent version of Andersson's (in press) model. Males attract females by, say, some acoustic or visual signal that makes them noticeable. There is no implication of female choice in the sense that females reject certain males or monitor several males and then move to the one chosen; females are attracted randomly to the advertisement signal. So the louder, say, a male shouts relative to his n competitors, the larger his 'zone of attraction' for females and the greater his relative reproductive success. In a sexual scramble, it seems reasonable to assume that benefits rise linearly with number of matings (though this may be only an approximation due to effects such as sperm depletion). For male i advertising to level x_i, we shall therefore assume that relative number of matings obtained is simply:

$$\left(\frac{x_i}{\bar{x}}\right)^y$$

in which $\bar{x}$ is the mean advertisement level and exponent y simply scales relative benefits (see Fig. 9.1). Where $x_i = \bar{x}$, relative reproductive success is obviously unity, but if a male advertises more than average $(x_i > \bar{x})$ he will obtain a higher than average number of matings, and vice versa.

Assume also that increasing advertisement increases costs; for example by increasing energy expenditure, or (following Darwin, 1871; Fisher, 1930; Endler, 1978, 1980) by increasing predation risk. Let $c(x)$ be the survival probability of a male that advertises to level x; $c(x)$ gives a measure of the costs of advertisement and is expressed as a factor by which gross gains must be multiplied to obtain a value for net gains. We shall assume that c is a monotonic decreasing function of x, declining eventually to zero. Relative reproductive success of a male advertising to level x_i is therefore

$$\left(\frac{x_i}{\bar{x}}\right)^y c(x_i). \tag{1}$$

To establish the ESS level x_*, which is best described as a competitive optimum (see e.g. Oster & Wilson, 1979), we simply assert that no mutant

Fig. 9.1. Gross benefits of an individual: that advertises to level x_m when all others advertise to level $\bar{x}$, in relation to scaling exponent y.

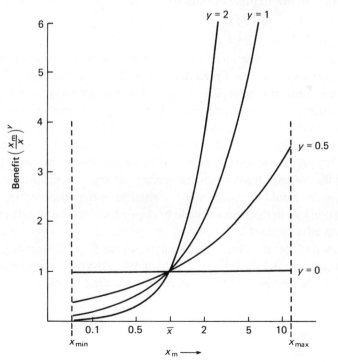

playing $x_m \neq x_*$ can invade in a population fixed to x_*. From (1) we can obtain this ESS by setting

$$\frac{d}{dx_m}\left[\left(\frac{x_m}{x_*}\right)^y c(x_m)\right]\Bigg|_{x_*} = 0, \text{ when } x_m = x_*$$

(for details of this method, see Parker & Macnair, 1979). This gives

$$x_* = \frac{-yc(x_*)}{c'(x_*)}. \tag{2}$$

This gives a positive solution for x_* since the gradient $c'(x)$ is negative. Provided that the costs of shifting from crypsis towards advertisement are not too high (summarised by the gradient $c'(0)$ in the equation), then equation (2) defines the competitive optimum for advertisement that we are seeking.

What if costs accrue through relative (not absolute) expenditure? This might possibly arise if costs are predation risk. Suppose that predators behave like females; i.e. there is a fixed number of them, they specialize entirely on the species we are considering, and they are attracted to attack in proportion to the conspicuousness of a given prey individual relative to others. A suitable cost function for conspicuousness of a given prey individual relative to others would be

$$c(x_m) = 2 - \left(\frac{x_m}{x_*}\right)^z,$$

so that costs are dependent on relative expenditure and at the ESS all individuals sustain equal predation costs. If $y > z$ the ESS will be for maximum advertisement, if $y < z$ it will be for minimum advertisement. Thus an intermediate competitive optimum, x_*, can occur only for scrambles in which expenditure costs have at least some dependence on absolute expenditure. This would always be the case for energetic components of cost; for predation costs there would be an absolute component to costs when the predator feeds on several species – changes in conspicuousness in one species would be independent of changes in the other species, and so predation risk in that species could be dependent on the absolute expenditure on advertisement.

Now consider the effects of phenotype on the ESS. Phenotype could be envisaged to affect the ESS principally in two ways depending on how x is defined. Phenotype could be seen either as scaling benefits, or as scaling costs.

Phenotype scales benefits

If we define strategy x in terms of costs, then it is clear that for the same cost, a strong vigorous individual may advertise to a much higher level than a weaker one. Suppose that individual i invests x_{*i} in advertisement, but receives gains proportional to:

$$\left(\frac{K_i x_{*i}}{K_g x_{*g}}\right)^y$$

in which K is a factor that scales the competitive difference in benefit between phenotypes, and an individual g has a phenotype that, at ESS, will gain an exactly average number of females. Thus if all individuals were to expend equally ($x_a = x_b$, etc.), gains would relate simply to K. Where there is a large population of competing males, the average advertisement level will not be altered significantly if one (mutant) individual deviates from his ESS. When this applies, it is easy to show that the ESS remains as in (2) as $x_{*i} = yc(x_{*i})/c'(x_{*i})$. Since, by definition, all curves $c(x_a)$, $c(x_b)$ etc., are identical, then it follows that all males should proceed to an advertisement level in which each phenotype incurs the same risk or cost, $c(x_*)$.

How is the ESS modified if there is a small number, n, of males in each group of competitors? If we assume for mathematical simplicity that $y = 1$, then from Parker & Knowlton (1980) it follows that the ESS for individual g with an exactly average benefit has

$$x_{*g} = -\frac{(n - 1)c(x_{*g})}{nc'(x_{*g})}$$

and setting $I = nK_g x_{*g} = -\frac{(n - 1)c(x_{*g})K_g}{c'(x_{*g})}$,

the ESS for individual i has

$$x_{*i} = \frac{c(x_{*i})}{[K_i c(x_{*i})/I] - c'(x_{*i})]}. \tag{3}$$

It is obvious from (3) that the ESS for i will converge towards (1) if n is large or if individual i has a phenotype of very low inherent competitive ability with $K_i \ll K_g$; both result in $K_i c(x_{*i}) \ll I$, see Fig. 9.2a. Maximum difference from (1) is obtained by the opposite conditions.

How does the phenotype-limited ESS affect the fitnesses of the phenotypes? Remember that K is defined as the *inherent* difference in competitive ability between phenotypes. At the ESS, is the fitness difference between phenotypes amplified or buffered, relative to the inherent difference? Parker & Knowlton (1980) examined the fitness ratio of the ith phenotype to the gth phenotype (which obtains exactly average benefits; but not necessarily average fitness since this depends on the distribution of K). Using the explicit function $c(x) = \exp(-Cx)$ in which C is a positive constant, the ESS

$$x_{*i} = \frac{K_g(n - 1)}{C[K_i + (n - 1)K_g]}.$$

Fig. 9.2. (a) ESS ratio, x_{*i}/x_{*g}, compared to the phenotypic competitive ratio K_i/K_g. Broken curves for the case where phenotype scales benefits (from Parker & Knowlton, 1980). Solid curves, for case where phenotype scales costs.
(b) Fitness ratio: Fitness of phenotype i/Fitness of phenotype g, compared to K_i/K_g.

In considering the difference between the two sets of curves in (a) it must be remembered that where phenotype scales benefits, the ESS relates only to the cost level. In fact, it is easy to show that the total relative advertisement level is the same for both cases and can be obtained by multiplying the broken curves by K_i/K_g to give the solid curves. Setting $\beta = K_i/K_g$, broken curves $= n/[\beta + (n - 1)]$; solid curves $= \beta n/[\beta + (n - 1)]$.

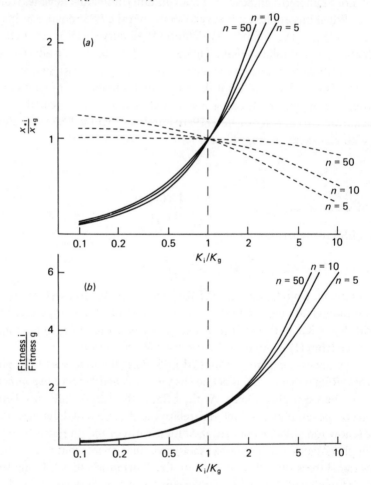

Fig. 9.2 shows how relatives ESSs (x_{*i}/x_{*g}) should vary with relative K (K_i/K_g) in accordance with the rules above. We found that at high n the fitness ratio (i.e. fitness of i/fitness of g) approaches the ratio K_i/K_g. At low n, individuals with low K will gain a fitness ratio marginally greater than K_i/K_g (see Fig. 9.2b). Thus the effect of low n on relative fitnesses in scramble competitions appears to be to buffer the inherent phenotypic difference in competitive ability.

Phenotype scales costs

Suppose we define x in terms of competitive benefits. Thus one unit of extra advertisement will yield markedly different costs to different phenotypes. There is now no single $c(x)$ curve, but $c_a(x)$, $c_b(x)$, etc. We examine this case to establish that the conclusions listed above are robust and not model-specific. In the former model, K was a scale of inherent competitive ability, in the present one it scales inherent survival ability.

For the case where there is a large number of competitors in each group so that a single mutant individual does not affect the mean advertisement level, it is easy to show that the ESS for i will be $x_{*i} = -yc_i(x_*)/c'(x_*)$, following (1). Consider two forms for $c_i(x)$: (1) $= \exp(-x/K_i)$, (2) $= 1 - x/K_i$. K_i is again the factor for inherent scaling due to phenotype; for a tiny unit increases in advertisement, an individual with high inherent survival prospects phenotype (K_i high) sustains less risk ($1/K_i$) than survival prospects (K_i low). Like the former model, we derive the expected conclusion that all phenotypes should stabilise to the same cost level because the cost ESS, $c_i(x_*)$, is constant:

$$c_i(x_*) = \exp\left(-\frac{x_*}{K_i}\right) = \exp(-y), \text{ since } x_* = yK_i$$

and $$c_i(x_*) = 1 - \frac{x_*}{K_i} = 1 - \left(\frac{y}{1+y}\right), \text{ since } x_* = yK_i/(1+y).$$

Now consider the case where there are rather few individuals (n) in each group of competitors, and let us again simplify the maths by assuming that $y = 1$. By applying the technique outlined by Parker & Knowlton (1980), it is easy to show that for the present case where $c_i(x) = \exp(-x/K_i)$,

$$\begin{aligned} x_{*i} &= IK_i/(I + K_i) \\ x_{*g} &= (n - 1)K_g/n \end{aligned} \tag{4}$$

in which phenotype g again obtains an exactly average number of females so that the total advertisement in a group is $I = nx_{*g} = (n - 1)K_g$. Substituting this value for I into (4) gives the result that:

$$x_{*i} = \frac{(n-1)K_g K_i}{K_i + (n-1)K_g}. \tag{5}$$

Defined in this way, it can be seen that if n is high or if $K_i \ll K_g$, an individual should expend on advertisement in direct proportion to its inherent survival ability K_i. When n is low or $K_i \gg K_g$, the advertisement level should be markedly less than the inherent K_i (see Fig. 9.2a). But although this appears to imply a difference from the previous case, the apparent difference in Fig. 9.2a between the two cases stems from the two definitions of x. Any real biological difference will relate to the fitness ratio. It can be calculated that the fitness ratio under both models (phenotype scales benefits *or* costs) is (see Fig. 9.2b):

$$\frac{\text{Fitness of i}}{\text{Fitness of g}} = \frac{K_i n}{[K_i + (n-1)K_g]}$$
$$\cdot \exp\left\{\frac{n-1}{n} - \left[\frac{K_g(n-1)}{K_i + (n-1)K_g}\right]\right\}. \tag{6}$$

Hence the biological conclusions remain identical for both cases; it does not matter whether the inherent phenotypic difference K relates to survivorship or to competitive ability.

Counter selection in sexual advertisement scrambles

If phenotypes 'play' different strategies at an initial ESS, then it seems possible that two further forms of selection may now arise. These concern female choice, and where costs of advertisement are mainly due to predation risk, predator choice.

Female choice. An assumption of the scramble model is that females are attracted *randomly* by advertisement. Remember that intensifying advertisement increases the relative 'domain of attraction' around a given male; a female has highest probability of moving towards the signal she perceives most intensely. Will *active* female choice (in which, say, a female compares the signals of several males and then chooses a particular phenotype) be favoured if there is a correlation between a male's advertisement level and his inherent competitive or survival ability? Active choice (rather than passive attraction to the signal of highest intensity) might involve a number of alternative mechanisms including rejection of all males below a critical threshold (Parker, 1979; Janetos, 1980) and various 'sampling' procedures to take the 'best of n' males encountered (Janetos, 1980). Alexander (1975) has suggested that some male mating swarms and leks may indeed have evolved in response to selective pressures arising from active, female choice; bigger assemblages of males yield better choice prospects to females.

Active female choice has been the subject of considerable controversy since it was first proposed by Darwin (1871). Fisher's (1930) refinements of the theory can (with some licence) be interpreted in the following way. (A rigorous series of genetic models have been developed from Fisher by O'Donald, 1962, 1977, 1980.) A preference gene acting in females for choosing males of higher than average heritable survivorship would spread, because the progeny would inherit the benefit. If females choose males on a relative basis, preferring the maximum measure of some quantitative character, then the character may proceed to an exaggerated level where it actually becomes an impediment to survivorship, and may become sex-limited. This can occur because of a runaway process arising from the competitive benefits to the male, and by virtue of the fact that females with the preference will tend to have sons with the competitive benefit. Zahavi (1975, 1977a) has argued that females will be favoured from the start if they prefer males with exotic characteristics that handicap survival, since this conveys information that the male must in fact be vigorous in order to survive *against* his handicap. This argument has not been widely accepted (Davis & O'Donald, 1976; Maynard Smith, 1976, 1978a).

In the present 'advertisement scramble' models, we assume a slightly different origin from that proposed by Fisher (1930); namely that there is some mechanism by which females recognise males and are attracted to them. From the start, increased expenditure on this male character will have an absolute investment cost in the same sense that any allocation of biological resources can be said to have an absolute fitness cost. The present models can in fact be appropriate for active choice. If females begin to switch from a passive to an active preference, we can represent this by an increase in y in equations (1) and (2), and Fig. 9.1. This will apply if the active choice retains a probabilistic element, i.e. females are more likely to mate with males that they judge to have a relatively high advertisement level (and consequently high competitive ability or survival prospects). But as additive genetic variance in the inherent phenotypic difference (K) diminishes towards zero by selection, then so would benefits via the 'sons effect' to actively choosing females (see Fig. 9.3). (This point has been discussed by various authors since Williams, 1975; see Thornhill, 1980a.) Thus the cost/benefit ratio of the choice (assuming that active choice has costs) will become progressively more unfavourable as heritable variation in K declines. Now, genes for active choice must at some point in evolution crash in favour of passive attraction, since the latter will not incur the costs (time and energy) in discriminating between males, and because the sons of females with passive attraction will experience no disadvantage when there is no genetic component to K. We would therefore expect that the eventual ESS should be the one for which the 'advertisement scramble model' was originally constructed – i.e. females show passive attraction. Parameter y will increase during the phase of selection for active choice, then decline to its original value as active choice crashes. The main effect of the wave of

Fig. 9.3. Changes in distribution of male phenotypes due to active choice. At the start of selection (*a*), the distribution of male phenotypes includes an environmental (unshaded) and a genetic (shaded) component. If benefits to females arise only via the genetic component, and females with the choice have an increasing probability of accepting males with increasing measure of the characteristic, then the benefit/cost ratio will be some function of the frequency of the gene for active choice and the ratio of b/c must become infinitesimal (unless maintained by high mutation pressure) so that the gene for active choice must eventually crash in favour of passive choice.

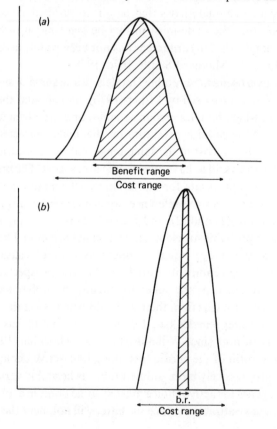

active choice will be to decrease the range of phenotypic variation in *K* by removing the genetic component.

However, there are various circumstances in which a degree of active choice in females might be maintained by selection (see e.g. Maynard Smith, 1978*b*; Thornhill, 1980*b*). The most obvious cases occur when

(i) benefits in choice relate to male genes, but genetic variation in *K* is maintained by recurrent mutation,

and (ii) benefits in choice relate to environmental variation in *K*, e.g. because stronger males can defend bigger territories which allow better feeding prospects for a female and her offspring.

Although female choice based on (ii) could be common, clear examples are rare. However, Thornhill's (1980*a*, *b*, *c*) elegant demonstration of female choice in the mecopteran *Hylobittacus apicalis* probably relate mainly to (ii). Partridge's (1980) experiments on *Drosophila*, however, seem to be a possible candidate for (i).

Where active choice has costs, a possibility here is that selection may produce what is termed a Nash equilibrium (see Maynard Smith, 1978*c*; Oster & Wilson, 1978) in which females exert an ESS arrangement of probabilities for accepting each phenotype. The main effect will again be to scale *y*; at the Nash ESS no mutant male or female will be favoured. This topic would repay further study.

Predator choice. We concluded above that if there is a large group of competing males, all males should show the same risk of predation, independent of phenotype. 'Risk' involves two components; firstly the initial attraction of the predator, and secondly its subsequent success in attack. So one way to interpret the conclusion could be that 'stronger' phenotypes run greater risk of attracting a predator but retain the same total risk by having less risk of subsequent capture. An inverse correlation could therefore exist between advertisement level and attack success. This might have important effects on learning by the predator, which may in turn affect the ESS for advertisement. If a prey item is 'unprofitable' for a predator, it may pay the predator to stop pursuit in favour of withdrawing to find a more 'profitable' item (see Hingston, 1933; Smythe, 1970; Lindroth, 1972; Gibson, 1974; Zahavi, 1977*b*; Baker & Parker, 1979). This effect could theoretically lead to 'active' choice by predators along the lines of discarding high-level advertisers in preference for searching for their more vulnerable competitors. Whether this can happen depends on what numbers and types of other prey item are around at the same time, because it is this that determines whether a given item constitutes an unprofitable prey (see excellent review by Krebs, 1978). Profitability is defined in terms of what a predator should do having perceived a particular prey item.

However, a major problem for active prey choice would concern evolutionary 'cheating'. If a predator can monitor only a prey's advertisement level x and not its inherent value K, then vulnerable individuals that advertise at a high level might, by a form of Batesian mimicry, escape attack from trained predators. Much will depend here on the ratio of naive : non-naive predators, and on the asymmetries between prey in catchability. For example, in our discussion of bird colouration, we (Baker & Parker, 1979) were primarily concerned with sexual dimorphism. In many bird species only the female incubates, and often she must remain cryptic because if a naive predator is attracted, the young will be taken. But if the male advertises conspicuously, even though he might attract naive predators, he has excellent escape prospects. In this situation if a male constitutes an unprofitable prey and the offspring a profitable one, neither females nor offspring can cheat by mimicking the male colouration.

Alternative strategy competitions

In the scramble model there was only one way for a male to obtain a female: by advertising. There is a growing literature on 'alternative mating strategies' in which there may be two or more distinct ways of obtaining matings (see models of Rubenstein, 1981; and the review by Dunbar, 1982). One example, best known to the author, will suffice. Male dungflies may capture females either on the dung surface or in the grass that surrounds the dropping. A male searching in the surrounding grass is most likely to obtain a newly arriving female, but a male searching on the dung surface might (depending on dropping age and competition density) obtain most of his matings by take-overs of females from paired males. On the assumption of no inherent competitive differences between competing males, an ESS distribution can be predicted between the two strategies – grass searching and dung searching. The observed distribution is quite close to this predicted distribution (Parker, 1974a). But large males do better at obtaining take-overs than smaller males (Sigurjónsdóttir & Parker, 1981) and indeed more of them are to be found searching on the dung (Borgia, 1979; Sigurjónsdóttir, 1980). This might therefore distort the ESS distribution for the case where there are no inherent differences in competitive ability between phenotypes.

Once again, I am concerned with the question of phenotype-limited ESSs, and how fitness will vary relative to inherent differences in competitive ability. I first consider a simplistic case where there are just two distinct phenotypes; the conclusions from this model can then be seen to have some generality for the case of a continuous distribution of phenotype.

The discrete-phenotype model. Consider a mating system with the following characteristics:

(a) Alternative mating strategies X and Y are possible, and fitness gains (numbers of matings) per individual in each strategy are inversely proportional to the density of competitors playing that strategy. The system is therefore frequency-dependent in the sense that for a given total number of competitors, the frequency of strategies will set the relative numbers of competitors in X and Y.

(b) Two phenotypes, A and B occur with respective frequencies f and $(1 - f)$. They can arise either through some environmental contingency over which there can be no genetic control (f constant), or else f can be determined genetically (f flexible) and be readily modified by the selective pressures of the mating system. In reality, 'f constant' and 'f flexible' could represent extremes that delimit the ease with which the frequencies of A and B can be altered against some cost constraint. A and B might represent limits within which phenotype limitation can occur, i.e. an animal only 'knows' whether it is 'big' or 'small'. In this case, its concept of its own phenotype will be determined by the threshold explained in the next section; it essentially complies with 'f flexible'.

(c) Phenotypes A and B have different inherent competitive abilities when coexisting in strategy X and/or strategy Y. If f is so flexible that it can be readily modified by selection between 1 and 0, it is obvious that both phenotypes can be maintained only when the competitive interaction reverses between X and Y (e.g. A does better than B in X, but B does better in Y). We will summarise the competitive interactions as follows. Each A gains K times the matings of each B when they occur together in strategy X, and each A gains L times the matings of each B when they coexist in Y. Remember that to maintain both phenotypes in the 'f flexible' case, we need either $K > 1$, $L < 1$; or $K < 1$, $L > 1$. For simplicity, let us assume that $K > L$, i.e. A does best against B in strategy X.

(d) Let the female input into strategy X $= F_X$, and into Y $= F_Y$. Throughout, we call the ratio of females available to the two strategies $= F_X/F_Y = \alpha$.

First consider the ESS where there is no phenotype-limitation, an individual does not 'know' its phenotype. We seek an equilibrium frequency p for playing the X strategy. For p to be an ESS, the overall expectation (per male) from the two strategies must be equal. Allowing that each A phenotype has a competitive 'weighting' of K or L relative to each B phenotype, and that the gains to each male in X or Y are F_X or F_Y multiplied by that male's weighting/total weight of competition, then:

$$\underbrace{\frac{fF_XK + (1-f)F_X}{pfK + p(1-f)}}_{\text{gain per male in X}} = \underbrace{\frac{fF_YL + (1-f)F_Y}{(1-p)(1-f) + (1-p)fL}}_{\text{gain per male in Y}}$$

and if $\alpha = F_X/F_Y$

$$p = \frac{\alpha}{1+\alpha}. \tag{7}$$

In other words, the equilibrium is only dependent on the relative resource availability α, and not on f, the phenotype frequencies. At equilibrium, the fitness ratio of the two phenotypes is as follows:

$$\frac{\text{Fitness of A}}{\text{Fitness of B}} = \frac{\dfrac{pF_XK}{pfK + p(1-f)} + \dfrac{(1-p)F_YL}{(1-p)(1-f) + (1-p)fL}}{\dfrac{pF_X}{pfK + p(1-f)} + \dfrac{(1-p)F_Y}{(1-p)(1-f) + (1-p)fL}}$$

$$= \frac{L(fK + 1 - f) + \alpha K(fL + 1 - f)}{(fK + 1 - f) + \alpha(fL + 1 - f)}. \tag{8}$$

As would be expected, the fitness difference between the phenotypes approaches K when virtually all females are available through strategy X ($F_X \gg F_Y$), and L when conditions are reversed. The ratio is independent of p.

Now consider the evolution of phenotype-limitation. Will a mutant spread that always plays X when it 'estimates' itself to be A. It will spread if its gains in X exceed gains in Y, i.e. if:

$$\frac{F_XK}{p[fK + 1 - f]} > \frac{F_YL}{(1-p)(1-f) + (1-p)fL}$$

i.e. if $p < \dfrac{\alpha K(Lf + 1 - f)}{L(fK + 1 - f) + \alpha K(fL + 1 - f)}$,

and since $p = \alpha/(1 + \alpha)$, this is always true if $K > L$ (A does best against B in X). It follows that the strategy 'play Y when A' spreads but the converse strategy becomes eliminated.

Now consider the phenotype-limited ESSs for the case where the phenotype frequencies cannot readily be altered by selection. There are 3 possible

ESSs if $K \neq L$:

(i) All A individuals play X, B individuals play a mix of X and Y. This will occur when B is so numerous that it pays some of them to 'overflow' into X.

(ii) All B individuals play Y, A plays a mix of X and Y. This is the reverse of (i).

(iii) All A play X, all B play Y.

For ESS (i), let p_B be the mixed ESS for B: 'play X with probability p_B'. Making approximations valid for large numbers of competitors, this requires, for A to stay in X:

$$\frac{F_X K}{fK + p_B(1 - f)} > \frac{F_Y L}{(1 - f)(1 - p_B)} ; p_B < \frac{\alpha K(1 - f) - fKL}{(1 - f)(L + \alpha K)}$$
(9a)

and for p_B to be stable for B:

$$\frac{F_X}{fK + p_B(1 - f)} = \frac{F_Y}{(1 - f)(1 - p_B)} ; \text{i.e. } p_B = \frac{\alpha(1 - f) - fK}{(1 - f)(1 + \alpha)}.$$
(9b)

Equation (9a) is always satisfied if (9b) applies and $K > L$.

For ESS (ii), p_A is the mixed ESS for A: 'play X with probability p_A', and so to keep B in Y:

$$\frac{F_X}{p_A fK} < \frac{F_Y}{(1 - f) + f(1 - p_A)} ; p_A > \frac{\alpha(fL + 1 - f)}{f(\alpha L + K)}$$
(10a)

and for p_A to be stable:

$$\frac{F_X K}{p_A fK} = \frac{F_Y L}{(1 - f) + f(1 - p_A)L} ; p_A = \frac{\alpha(fL + 1 - f)}{fL(1 + \alpha)}.$$
(10b)

Provided $K > L$, there is no contradiction between (10a) and (10b).

It is obvious from conditions 9b and 10b that ESS (iii) must also exist if $K > L$, since for A to begin to play Y needs $f > \alpha/(L + \alpha)$, whereas for B to invade X needs $f < \alpha/(K + \alpha)$. Within this zone of f, both phenotypes play pure strategies.

Fig. 9.4a shows the proportion of the total population that will be found playing X, in relation to f, for the case where $\alpha = 1$, $K = 5$, $L = 1$. This equals $f + (1 - f)p_B$ throughout the range for ESS (i), equals $p_A f$ in ESS (ii), and equals f for ESS (iii). For $K = 5$, $L = 1$, there is the same proportion of X in the ESS (ii) range, but less in the ESS (i) and (iii) range than where there is no limitation.

It is easy to see that the fitness ratio (fitness of A/fitness of B) must be equal to K over the range of f for ESS (i), and that it must be L over the f

range for ESS (ii). In the range for ESS (iii) the fitness ratio is dependent only on α and f (independent of K and L since A and B are not in competition), and is equal to $\alpha(1 - f)/f$ (see Fig. 9.4b). It is interesting that the fitness ratio with perfect limitation sometimes exceeds and sometimes falls below that of the case of no limitation, depending on f. If $K > L$, $L = 1$, greatest fitness differences will be found when B is forced into competition with A in X (f low, α high).

Fig. 9.4. (a) Equilibrium proportion of total population playing strategy X in relation to f, the frequency of phenotype A, for the case where $\alpha = 1$, $K = 5$. Dotted line = no phenotype limitation; solid line = perfect phenotype limitation.
(b) Fitness ratio (Fitness of A/Fitness of B) at the ESS, in relation to f. Otherwise as for (a).

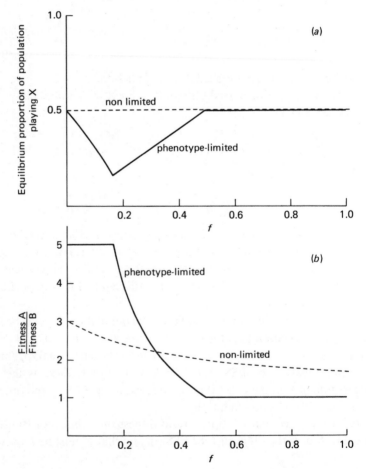

What happens when the proportions of A and B can readily be modified by selection? Coexistence of A and B can exist only when the competitive interaction is reversed in the two strategies. It is clear that selection will then drive f to level $f_* = \alpha/(1 + \alpha)$. Here A plays X, B plays Y, and both have equal fitness. The possibility exists that a difference between A and B may be 'decided' by habits of the mother. For instance, in the bee *Centris pallida*, 'hoverers' wait around shrubs and bushes where virgin females come to feed, whilst larger 'patrollers' search widely and fight over virgin females emerging from burrows (Alcock, 1979). The *C. pallida* system could be 'f flexible' in that the size distribution of males could be modified by changes in the distribution of provisioning habits of mothers. However, for the present model to be applicable, both male phenotypes must be equally expensive to produce. If, say, B costs its mother less than A, it will be 'overproduced' such that, from the point of view of the female parent, the fitness gain due to expenditure over pathway A equals the fitness gain due to expenditure over pathway B. This would result in ESSs of types (i) or (iii), in which the reproductive success of A phenotypes exceeds the reproductive success of B phenotypes.

If one phenotype outcompetes the other in both strategies, then it alone should be produced if f is flexible. Good reasons why this will seldom occur are that 'guarders' will generally be more expensive to produce than 'sneaks' or that they will be produced after growing to a certain critical size, up to which they act as sneaks. This leads to the 'continuous phenotype' model (see below).

The model presented in this section is intended to serve simply to outline the sorts of problem generated by 'alternative strategy' type competitions, in which gains in a given strategy are inversely related to competitor density and there are asymmetries in inherent competitive abilities between phenotypes. For any biological application, the model can be readily modified and complicated. For instance, K and L may be made a function of the total number (rather than frequency) of individuals playing the X strategy. For many systems the number of females available to one strategy may depend on the number of males adopting the alternative strategy (as would be so in dungflies (Parker, 1974a) and toads (Davies & Halliday, 1979). Thus where total females is F_T, we may need, say $F_X = F_T - F_Y(n_Y)$ in which F_Y is a function of the number of competitors adopting Y. These sorts of modification, though essential for applications of the alternative-strategy model, only act to confuse the theoretical issues and have therefore been omitted.

The continuous-phenotype model. A common determinant of phenotype-limited strategy is size, or indirectly age when size relates to age. This and

192   G.A. Parker

most other phenotypic features that may affect inherent competitive abilities will be continuously distributed. Suppose that in strategy X (say guarding), inherent competitive ability increases with size, but that all phenotypes do equally well in Y (sneaking). If there can be perfect phenotype limitation selection will favour a strategy switch at a threshold size T, and the ESS will be to play Y below size T, play X above size T (Fig. 9.5a). Adjustment of T is here equivalent to selective adjustment of f in the last

Fig. 9.5. (a) Frequency distribution $p(s)$ of sizes s in a population of competing males. The size range is $s_{min}-s_{max}$, and below size T, individuals should play strategy Y; above size T, individuals should play X.
(b) Two possible forms of $K(s)$, the 'competitive weighting' of a given phenotype of size s. In (i), a few males have a relatively high inherent advantage (equivalent to low f of the discrete phenotype model); in (ii) a few males have a relatively high disadvantage (equivalent to high f of the discrete phenotype model).

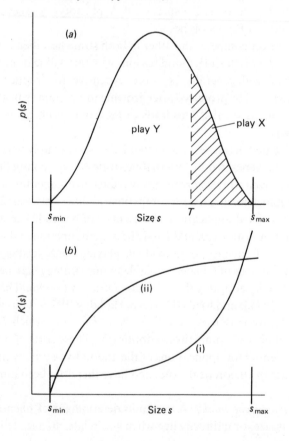

model. From this, calling $p(s)$ the size distribution of the male population and $K(s)$ the inherent competitive ability weighting for a male of size s, it is clear that

$$\frac{F_Y}{\text{total males in Y}} = \frac{F_X(\text{'weight' of smallest male in X})}{\text{total 'weight' of males in X}} \tag{11}$$

$$\therefore \frac{F_Y}{\displaystyle\int_{S_{min}}^{T} p(s)\mathrm{d}s} = \frac{F_X K(T)}{\displaystyle\int_{T}^{S_{max}} p(s)\cdot K(s)\mathrm{d}s}$$

so that T is set by:

$$\alpha = \frac{\displaystyle\int_{T}^{S_{max}} p(s)\cdot K(s)\mathrm{d}s}{K(T)\displaystyle\int_{S_{min}}^{T} p(s)\mathrm{d}s}. \tag{12}$$

From (11) it follows that a strongly increasing $K(s)$ function (very large males do markedly better than smaller ones in X) will push switch point T to a high level, and vice versa. Phenotypic fitness differences will be restricted to individuals playing X, i.e. to the size range T to s_{max}. Relative fitnesses will equal $K(s)$ over this range, and $K(T)$ for all Y strategists. If α is relatively large, fitness differences will be wide, as in the previous model. If the system proceeds from no phenotype-limitation to the perfect state with switch point T, then whether the range of fitnesses will increase or decrease will depend on the rules we deduced in the previous model. Translating, if $K(s)$ increases sharply towards s_{max} (curve (i), Fig. 9.5b; equivalent to low f), then the effect of phenotype limitation is likely to be to increase the range of fitnesses; if $K(s)$ is initially steep, then flattens (curve (ii), Fig. 9.5b; equivalent to high f) it will decrease fitness differences. Similarly if for a given $K(s)$, α is high, phenotype limitation will tend to *increase* fitness differences, and vice versa.

Thus we can formulate the general conclusion that for alternative strategy competitions obeying the sorts of rules outlined in this section, that the effect of phenotype limitation will be: to *increase* fitness differences when the ratio α ($=$ females available to the strategy in which a high competitive interaction exists/females available to alternative strategy where phenotypes do equally well) is high and where a few males have a marked advantage over the rest; and to *reduce* fitness differences when α is low and when a few males have a marked competitive disadvantage relative to the others.

For species in which reproductive adults can grow continuously, the switch point T may be determined by a particular age (equivalent to a threshold size). For instance, red deer (Clutton-Brock, Albon, Gibson & Guiness, 1979), elephant seal (LeBoeuf, 1974), impala (Jarman, 1973) and bluegill sunfish (Gross & Charnov, in press) would fit this pattern. Here it may be necessary to include survival probability as a cost in pursuing a particular strategy. Rather surprisingly, if we call $p(s)$ the probability of surviving to age s, and allow again that $K(s)$ is the competitive weighting factor for an individual age s, then the switch age T is given by equation (12) exactly as before (see Fig. 9.6a). This can be again deduced by substituting appropriately into (11).

Suppose that the inherent competitive differences in strategy X are very small. Then $K(s) \simeq 1$. Let the probability of being alive at age s when playing Y be $p_Y(s) = \exp(-C_Y s)$; and let $p_X(s) = \exp(-C_Y T) \cdot \exp(-C_X s)$, since there will be a proportion $\exp(-C_Y T)$ of individuals that survive to make the switch. Then, assuming there is no maximum age limit,

$$\frac{F_Y}{\int_0^T \exp(-C_Y s)\mathrm{d}s} \simeq \frac{F_X}{\exp(-C_Y T) \int_T^\infty \exp(-C_X s)\mathrm{d}s}$$

which eventually gives:

$$\alpha \cdot \frac{C_X}{C_Y} \simeq \frac{\exp(-C_X T)}{[\exp(C_Y T) - 1]}. \tag{13}$$

From (13) it is easy to iterate switch age T. Some results are shown in Fig. 9.6b. T will be highest when α is low and C_X/C_Y is high; in biological terms this means that the switch to the 'guarder' strategy will be delayed most when relatively few females are available to guarders, and where the costs of the guarding strategy are high relative to those of the sneak strategy (see also Rubenstein, 1980).

Rather similar techniques to those used in this section have been used by Hamilton (1979) and Gross & Charnov (in press).

Contest competitions

I include this sort of competition mainly for completeness and to give a brief review of current theory as it relates to phenotypic differences.

A contest consists of a battle between, say, two males over a female. The important distinction from the two previous competitions is the characteristic that the 'winner takes all'. Thus one individual emerges as victor and mates with the female, and the other retreats. ESSs for contests can be markedly influenced by phenotype. Maynard Smith (1974) showed that in a symmetric (i.e. no differences between contestants) 'war of attrition' in which the winner is he who is prepared to persist longer, the result is a mixed ESS where the 'bids' (choices of persistence times, and hence of maximum costs an opponent is prepared to pay out to win) follow a negative exponential distribution. An arbitrary asymmetry between contestants, uncorrelated to payoff, can make a vast difference to this ESS. Two pure ESSs were thought to be possible when individuals have perfect

Fig. 9.6. (*a*) Probability $p(s)$ of surviving to age s (and hence of attaining size s). With continuous breeding and random, overlapping generations, this should also be the distribution of size in the competing population of males. At age $s = T$, individuals should switch from Y to X.
(*b*) Switch point T for various values of α plotted against C_X/C_Y. It is assumed that inherent competitive weightings $K(s)$ exert minor effects. $C_Y = 1$ throughout.

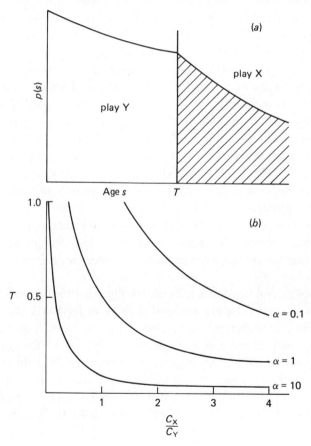

information about the asymmetry (Maynard Smith, 1974; Maynard Smith & Parker, 1976): 'when in role A, be prepared to escalate to cost $-M > V$; when in B, retreat', and vice versa. Roles A and B are specified by the asymmetry between contestants.

Of special importance are 'payoff relevant' asymmetries such as differences in inherent fighting ability or resource holding power (RHP), and differences in the resource value V to the two contestants (Parker, 1974b). The alternative ESSs relating to payoff relevant asymmetries were termed 'commonsense' solutions (smaller individual, or individual with least to gain retreats) and 'paradoxical' solutions (large individual or individual with most to gain retreats). In general, paradoxical solutions appeared possible but less likely to evolve (Maynard Smith & Parker, 1976), a conclusion that has been reinforced recently by Hammerstein (1981) for 'hawk/dove' games ('hawks fight at an escalated level and retreat only if injured, 'doves' retreat if they meet 'hawk', or settle arbitrarily with minimal cost in contests between themselves). For 'war of attrition' games, Parker & Rubenstein (1981) and Hammerstein & Parker (in press) showed that a paradoxical solution cannot persist in the presence of rare mistakes about role or rare recurrent mutation for convention breaking. The ESS approximates to the commonsense one in which individuals retreat in role B specified by $V_A/K_A > V_B/K_B$, where V_A and V_B are the resource values for A and B, and K_A and K_B are the rates at which costs would be expended if the opponents were to fight (i.e. K relates to the difference in fighting ability). This corresponds to the 'optimal assessor' rule (Parker, 1974b) that the individual should retreat who would first begin to experience a negative payoff, were the contest to continue indefinitely. In summary, where strategies cannot be regulated continuously (e.g. hawks/doves game) paradoxical solutions are theoretically possible; where strategies can be regulated continuously (e.g. war of attrition), only commonsense solutions can be ESSs (Hammerstein & Parker, in preparation).

One problem still outstanding concerns the relationship between an individual's resource value and his fighting ability or RHP. V is strictly the fitness benefit due to winning, not including contest costs. A case can be made that V may increase as RHP decreases (Parker, 1974b; Parker & Rubenstein, 1981). Thus it becomes rather difficult to establish the range of fitness differences in a population with continuous variation in RHP. However, assume for simplicity that V is symmetric ($V_A = V_B$ for all contests), and call the distribution of RHP (? equivalent to the distribution of size, Fig. 9.6a) $p(s)$. It is then obvious, if the 'optimal assessor' rule holds, that the distribution $F(s)$ of fitness in relation to RHP must be

$$F(s) = \int_{s_{min}}^{s_{max}} p(s)ds;$$

since individual i of RHP s_i will win all contests with smaller individuals and lose those with larger individuals, so that he wins a proportion $\int_{s_{min}}^{s_i} p(s)ds$ of all contests. Biggest fitness differences will exist when the range of RHP is greatest, and $F(s)$ depends entirely on $p(s)$.

A major complication occurs if information concerning payoff-relevant asymmetries in contests is not perfect or almost so, as we assumed above. If individuals make mistakes concerning their payoff-relevant role, increasing amounts of escalation will occur (Hammerstein & Parker in press). This will greatly complicate any calculation of fitness differences because the probability of making a mistake will increase as the RHP disparity between opponents decreases. For contests in which an individual can 'know' perfectly only his own resource value V, but not at all that of his opponent, there will always be some escalation. Bishop *et al.* (1978) have shown for the war of attrition that if V is continuously distributed the ESS is to select a pure strategy bid m_i that increases with V_i, so that the opponent with the higher V will always win, but at a cost dependent on the V of his opponent.

Summary
1. In competitive games, ESSs will generally be phenotype-limited. This is to say that where phenotypes differ in their inherent competitive abilities, individuals will play strategies that are conditional upon their phenotype. *Inherent competitive abilities* are best defined in terms of the benefits (or costs) that would accrue competitively if individuals were all to play an identical strategy. A 'coarse-grained' optimum is defined as an optimum that is averaged over a set of conditions of environment or phenotype, as distinct from 'fine-grained' optima to each condition. Phenotype limitation represents a trend towards fine-grained optimization.
2. It is of interest to establish the fitness differences that will exist between phenotypes at the ESS for a particular game, and to compare this with the inherent difference in competitive ability. It is also instructive to compare fitness differences that would exist in a hypothetical ancestral population in which strategies are not phenotype-limited with a similar one in which they are. To this

end, I discuss three general forms of competitive game: (i) 'scramble' competitions in which there are *n* competitors and benefits accrue in proportion to an individual's *relative* investment in a particular strategy; (ii) 'alternative strategy' competitions in which there are again *n* competitors; benefits are inversely proportional to competitor density and can accrue by playing either of two (or more) quite separate alternative strategies; and (iii) 'contest' competitions in which two individuals compete over an unsharable resource that will be exploited by the winner of the contest. The formal models presented are framed in terms of intrasexual competitions between males for access to females.

3. In 'sexual advertisement scrambles' to attract females, the amount of advertisement may become phenotype-limited (see also Andersson, 1981). For scrambles that involve large aggregations of males, all phenotypes should generally proceed to the same level of costs, and fitness ratios will be close to the inherent competitive (or survival) difference between phenotypes. But when the competitive group is small, 'strong' individuals will experience a relative fitness that is markedly less than their relative competitive ability (judged against an arbitrary 'standard' phenotype). In contrast, 'weak' individuals experience a marginally higher relative fitness than their relative competitive ability. The evolutionary effects of active female choice are complex, but may be significant ultimately only if advantages in the choice to the female accrue through environmentally-determined components of a male's phenotype.

4. In models of 'alternative mating strategy' competitions, I assumed that mating opportunities per male in each of two strategies decline with competitor density. In many cases (e.g. 'sneaks' and 'guarders'), inherent competitive differences between phenotypes will exert a major effect only within one strategy. Depending on conditions, fitness differences between phenotypes will either be equal to or less than the inherent competitive difference. The effects of phenotype limitation (compared to the case of no limitation) will be to *increase* fitness differences when the ratio α (= females available to the strategy in which the competitive interaction is marked/females available to the alternative strategy) is high and where a few males have a relatively marked competitive advantage, but to *reduce* fitness differences when α is low and where a few males have a relatively marked competitive disadvantage.

5. In contests where two males fight for the right to mate with a female, and both contestants have near-perfect information about each other's fighting abilities, the distribution of phenotype fitnesses will equal the integral of the distribution of fighting abilities, provided that the value of victory is equal for the two opponents.

The year I spent in the Research Centre, King's College, was extremely stimulating and rewarding. It is a pleasure to thank those who made it possible and who made the experience so pleasant. I am indebted to Anthony Arak, Robin Dunbar and Dan Rubenstein for discussions, and to Anita Callaghan for typing.

References

Alcock, J. (1979). The evolution of intraspecific diversity in male reproductive strategies in some bees and wasps. In *Sexual Selection and Reproductive Competition in Insects*, ed. M.S. Blum & N.A. Blum, pp. 381–402. Academic Press: New York.

Alexander, R.D. (1975). Natural selection and specialised chorusing behaviour in acoustical insects. In *Insects, Science and Society*, ed. D. Pimentel, pp. 35–77. Academic Press: New York.

Andersson, M. (1981). Sexual selection, natural selection and quality advertisement. (In press.)

Baker, R.R. & Parker, G.A. (1979). The evolution of bird colouration. *Philosophical Transactions of the Royal Society*, B, **287**, 63–130.

Bishop, D.T., Cannings, C. & Maynard Smith, J. (1978). The war of attrition with random rewards. *Journal of Theoretical Biology*, **74**, 377–88.

Borgia, G. (1979). Sexual selection and the evolution of mating systems. In *Reproductive Competition and Sexual Selection in Insects*, ed. M.S. Blum & N.A. Blum, pp. 19–80. Academic Press: New York.

Clutton-Brock, T., Albon, S.D., Gibson, R.M. & Guinness, F.E. (1979). The logical stag: adaptive aspects of fighting in red deer (*Cervus elephas* L.). *Animal Behaviour*, **27**, 211–25.

Darwin, C. (1871). *The Descent of Man and Selection in Relation to Sex*. John Murray: London.

Davies, N.B. & Halliday, T.R. (1979). Competitive mate searching in common toads, *Bufo bufo*. *Animal Behaviour*, **27**, 1253–67.

Davis, J.W.F. & O'Donald, P. (1976). Sexual selection for a handicap: a critical analysis of Zahavi's model. *Journal of Theoretical Biology*, **57**, 345–54.

Dawkins, R. (1980). Good strategy or evolutionarily stable strategy? In *Sociobiology: Beyond Nature/Nurture?* ed. G.W. Barlow & S. Silverberg, pp. 331–67. Westview Press: Boulder, Colorado.

Dunbar, R.I.M. (1982). Intra-specific variations in mating strategy. In *Perspectives in Ethology*, vol, **5**, ed. P.P.G. Bateson & P. Klopfer, (in press). Plenum Press: New York.

Endler, J. (1978). A predator's view of animal color patterns. *Evolutionary Biology*, **11**, 319–64.

Endler, J. (1980). Natural selection on color patterns in *Poecilia reticulata*. *Evolution*, **34**, 76–91.

Fisher, R.A. (1930). *The Genetical Theory of Natural Selection*. Clarendon Press: Oxford.

Gibson, D.O. (1974). Batesian mimicry without distastefulness? *Nature, London*, **250**, 77–9.

200   G.A. Parker

Gross, M.R. & Charnov, E.L. (1981). Alternative male life histories in bluegill sunfish. (In press.)

Hammerstein, P. (1981). The role of asymmetries in animal contests. *Animal Behaviour*, **29**, 193–205.

Hammerstein, P. & Parker, G.A. (1982). The asymmetric war of attrition. *Journal of Theoretical Biology* (in press).

Hamilton, W.D. (1979). Wingless and fighting males in fig wasps and other insects. In *Sexual Selection and Reproductive Competition in Insects*, ed. M.S. Blum & N.A. Blum, pp. 167–220. Academic Press: New York.

Hingston, R.W.G. (1933). *The Meaning of Animal Colouration and Adornment*. Edward Arnold: London.

Janetos, A.C. (1980). Strategies of female mate choice: a theoretical analysis. *Behavioural Ecology and Sociobiology*, **7**, 107–12.

Jarman, M. (1975). The quintessential antelope: a study of the behaviour of the impala. *African Wildlife Leadership Federation News*, **8**, 2–7.

Knowlton, N. & Parker, G.A. (1979). An evolutionarily stable strategy approach to indiscriminate spite. *Nature*, **279**, 419–21.

Krebs, J.R. (1978). Optimal foraging: decision rules for predators. In *Behavioural Ecology: an Evolutionary Approach*, ed. J.R. Krebs, & N.B. Davies, pp. 23–63. Blackwells: Oxford.

LeBoeuf, B.J. (1974). Male–male competition and reproductive success in elephant seals. *American Zoologist*, **14**, 163–77.

Lindroth, C.H. (1972). Disappearance as a protective factor. A supposed case of Batesian mimicry among beetles (Coleoptera: Carabidae and Chrysomelidae). *Entomologica Scandinavica*, **2**, 41–8.

Łomnicki, A. (1978). Individual differences between animals and natural regulation of their number. *Journal of Animal Ecology*, **47**, 461–75.

Macnair, M.R. & Parker, G.A. (1979). Models of parent–offspring conflict. III. Intrabrood conflict. *Animal Behaviour*, **27**, 1202–9.

Maynard Smith, J. (1974). The theory of games and the evolution of animal conflicts. *Journal of Theoretical Biology*, **47**, 209–21.

Maynard Smith, J. (1976). Sexual selection and the handicap principle. *Journal of Theoretical Biology*, **57**, 239–42.

Maynard Smith, J. (1978a).The handicap principle – a comment. *Journal of Theoretical Biology*, **70**, 251–2.

Maynard Smith, J. (1978b). *The Evolution of Sex*. Cambridge University Press: Cambridge.

Maynard Smith, J. (1978c). Optimization theory in evolution. *Annual Review of Ecology and Systematics*, **9**, 51–6.

Maynard Smith, J. (1979). Game theory and the evolution of behaviour. *Proceedings of the Royal Society of London*, B, **205**, 475–88.

Maynard Smith, J. & Parker, G.A. (1976). The logic of asymmetric contests. *Animal Behaviour*, **24**, 159–75.

Maynard Smith, J. & Price, G.R. (1973). The logic of animal conflict. *Nature, London*, **246**, 15–18.

O'Donald, P. (1962). The theory of sexual selection. *Heredity*, **17**, 541–52.

O'Donald, P. (1977). Theoretical aspects of sexual selection. *Theoretical Population Biology*, **12**, 298–334.

O'Donald, P. (1980). *Genetic Models of Sexual Selection*. Cambridge University Press: Cambridge.

Oster, G. & Wilson, E.O. (1978). *Caste and Ecology in the Social Insects*. Princeton University Press: Princeton.

Parker, G.A. (1974*a*). The reproductive behaviour and the nature of sexual selection in *Scatophaga stercoraria* L. (Diptera: Scatophagidae). IX. Spatial distribution of fertilization rates and evolution of male search strategy within the reproductive area. *Evolution*, **28**, 93–108.

Parker, G.A. (1974*b*). Assessment strategy and the evolution of animal conflicts. *Journal of Theoretical Biology*, **47**, 223–43.

Parker, G.A. (1978). Evolution of competitive mate searching. *Annual Review of Entomology*, **23**, 173–96.

Parker, G.A. (1979). Sexual selection and sexual conflict. In *Sexual Selection and Reproductive Competition in Insects*, ed. M.S. Blum & N.A. Blum, pp. 123–66. Academic Press: New York.

Parker, G.A. & Knowlton, N. (1980). The evolution of territory size: some ESS models. *Journal of Theoretical Biology*, **84**, 445–76.

Parker, G.A. & Macnair, M.R. (1979). Models of parent–offspring conflict, IV. Suppression: evolutionary retaliation by the parent. *Animal Behaviour*, **27**, 1210–35.

Parker, G.A. & Rubenstein, D.I. (1981). Role assessment, reserve strategy, and the acquisition of information in asymmetric animal conflicts. *Animal Behaviour*, **29**, 221–40.

Partridge, L. (1980). Mate choice increases a component of offspring fitness. *Nature*, **283**, 290–1.

Rubenstein, D.I. (1980). On the evolution of alternative mating strategies. In *Limits to Action: the Allocation of Individual Behavior*, ed. J.R. Staddon. Academic Press: New York.

Sigurjónsdóttir, H. (1980). *Evolutionary Aspects of Sexual Dimorphism in Size; Studies on Dungflies and Three Groups of Birds*. Ph.D thesis, University of Liverpool.

Sigurjónsdóttir, H. & Parker, G.A. (1981). Dung fly struggles: evidence for assessment strategy. *Behavioral Ecology and Sociobiology*, **8**, 219–30.

Smythe, N. (1970). On the existence of "pursuit invitation" signals in mammals. *American Naturalist*, **104**, 491–4.

Thornhill, R. (1980*a*). Mate choice in *Hylobittacus apicalis* (Insecta: Mecoptera) and its relation to some models of female choice. *Evolution*, **34**, 519–38.

Thornhill, R. (1980*b*). Competitive, charming males and choosy females: was Darwin correct? *Florida Entomologist*, **63**, 5–30.

Thornhill, R. (1980*c*). Sexual selection in the Black-tipped Hangingfly. *Scientific American*, **242**, 162–72.

Williams, G.C. (1975). *Sex and Evolution*. Princeton University Press: Princeton.

Zahavi, A. (1975). Mate selection – a selection for a handicap. *Journal of Theoretical Biology*, **53**, 205–14.

Zahavi, A. (1977*a*). The cost of honesty. (Further remarks on the handicap principle). *Journal of Theoretical Biology*, **67**, 603–5.

Zahavi, A. (1977*b*). Reliability in communication systems and the evolution of altruism. In *Evolutionary Ecology*, ed. B. Stonehouse & C.M. Perrins, pp. 253–9. MacMillan: London.

10

Parental care and sex role reversal

N. KNOWLTON

Parents do not send their descendants into the world as naked DNA. The unfertilized egg is rich in nutrients, and the zygote and developing offspring may be cared for in a number of ways. This care represents a commitment of time, energy, and risk.

It is generally the female who provides most or all of the nourishment which goes into the egg. This initial discrepancy between the sexes in parental commitment is often maintained or exaggerated by subsequent parental care by the female. As a result, the availability of females is generally rate limiting for reproduction within a population. This situation leads, through the process of sexual selection, to the well-known differences between the sexes in sex roles – namely, that males are typically more conspicuous and aggressive in courtship interactions than females (Darwin, 1871; Fisher, 1930; Bateman, 1948; O'Donald, 1962, 1973; Williams, 1966; Trivers, 1972; Dawkins & Carlisle, 1976; Emlen & Oring, 1977; Parker, 1974, 1979).

In some species, however, paternal care is substantial and maternal care slight or nonexistent (see review by Ridley, 1978). In a few of these there appears to be genuine sex role reversal, i.e. females show the typically male characteristics associated with competition for mates. This role reversal stems from a reversal from female to male in the sex which limits the population's reproductive rate (Williams, 1966; Trivers, 1972; Emlen & Oring, 1977).

Examples of such high levels of paternal commitment are extremely rare among animals. The purposes of this paper are to review the natural history patterns of extensive male parental care and the theory which attempts to explain them, and to present results of a computer simulation designed to explore conditions which favour increased paternal commitment. The results suggest that high levels of male parental care evolve most readily when (1) a mutation in females gives males the option of providing care, (2) failure by males to provide care results in lower offspring survivorship, and (3) the frequency of males potentially willing to provide care is already high.

Natural history patterns

Sex role reversal is best documented in several species of birds, and jacanas represent the extreme case (Jenni, 1974). In *Jacana spinosa* (Jenni & Collier, 1972) the female defends a large territory which contains the smaller territories of her harem of males. The males build the nests, incubate the eggs and raise the young. Although the plumages of males and females are similar, the females are on average over one and a half times heavier than males. In other sex role-reversed birds such as the phalaropes, males provide most or all of the parental care, but polyandry is less well developed; females typically have a more conspicuous breeding plumage than males but differ less from them in size. In the majority of bird species, in contrast, parental care is provided jointly by males and females (Lack, 1968).

In mammals the presence of mammary glands restricts early feeding of the young to females. In only a few species do males provide large amounts of care (Kleiman, 1977), and there are no known examples of sex role reversal.

In both fishes and anuran amphibians, care by the male alone is more common than exclusively female or joint care, although most often neither sex cares for the young (Ridley, 1978). Among the fishes only the pipefish and seahorses (Syngnathidae) show clear evidence for sex role reversal. In all members of this family the males brood the eggs under the abdomen, sometimes in a brood pouch. In several species the females are bigger, more brightly coloured, and more aggressive in courtship (Fiedler, 1954; T. Lim, personal communication). Possible herpetological examples of sex role reversal (some of the dendrobatid frogs in which the male carries the young on his back) have not been rigorously confirmed (Ridley, 1978; Wells, 1981).

Among the invertebrates, species with parental care, particularly male care, are relatively rare (Ridley, 1978; Smith, 1980b). The best studied and most striking examples of paternal care are some of the giant water bugs (Belostomatidae) (Smith, 1976, 1979, 1980a). In the Belostomatidae, females lay the fertilized eggs on the backs of males, who brood them. Even here, however, there is no unambiguous evidence for sex role reversal, although Smith (1980*a*) believes that the backs of males may limit the reproductive rate of populations he has studied during certain seasons. In a number of insects, males may contribute substantially to the energetic costs of egg production through courtship feeding (Thornhill, 1976), but in none of these do the sexes appear to be role reversed.

Sex role reversal is so rare that it is difficult to correlate it with ecological, behavioural or reproductive features. Looking more broadly at species with exclusively male parental care, there is a general tendency for such species to be externally fertilizing (Dawkins & Carlisle, 1976; Ridley, 1978). One may contrast, for example, fish and anuran amphibians with birds, mammals and insects, or note that the only salamanders with paternal care are found in the few families with external fertilization (Ridley, 1978). There is also a loose correlation between paternal care and male territoriality (Ridley, 1978).

Previous theoretical contributions

As Trivers (1972), Dawkins (1976) and Parker (1979) have argued, the members of a mating pair are often in conflict over how much each should invest in the offspring. Once fertilization has occurred, each would usually enjoy a higher reproductive success if the other would care for the offspring until further care would be ineffective. Thus one theoretical approach is to specify the conditions which permit or encourage sex role reversal as the evolutionary resolution of this conflict.

Females generally lack the ability to force males by physical means to care for the offspring. As the limiting sex, females can, however, use 'strategies' of timing (e.g. synchrony) to prevent male desertion when males would otherwise find it advantageous to desert. But the potential for the trait of reproductive synchrony to spread through the females of a population decreases as the male to female potential reproductive rate ratio approaches unity (Knowlton, 1979). Thus sex role reversal cannot be achieved through such a mechanism. There are probably similar constraints which limit the precopulatory demands (e.g. courtship feeding) which females can make.

Several verbal models have been suggested for the evolution of sex role reversal, particularly as associated with polyandry in birds (see Emlen & Oring, 1977). Jenni (1974) proposed an evolutionary sequence running from (1) monogamy with care of the offspring by both parents through (2) 'double clutching', in which the male cares for the first clutch his mate lays and the female cares for the second, to (3) systems in which females lay clutches for a number of males, never attending any of the offspring in the most extreme case. Jenni hypothesized that males as well as females might benefit from female emancipation from care if it allowed females to lay additional clutches for their mates, or replacement clutches (should the original clutch fail).

Smith (1980b) suggested that paternal care in the giant water bugs might have evolved because females laying eggs on the backs of males avoided competition for oviposition sites and perhaps egg cannibalism. He noted that males were likely to be available and receptive because of their tendency to guard females to prevent sperm competition.

Ridley (1978) has reviewed a number of features which have been proposed to facilitate the evolution of paternal care: the potential for increasing female fecundity (described above), male territoriality, external fertilization, and female preference for caring males. He also suggested that the condition of 'isoinvestment' might be more susceptible to destabilizing evolutionary forces than conditions where the sexes differed greatly in parental investment (and thus potential reproductive rate). If the direction of destabilization were random, then sex role reversal would be the outcome in some cases. This idea, based on Parker, Baker & Smith's (1972) analysis of the evolution of anisogamy, has merit. The Fisher effect (Fisher, 1930), for example, is a kind of positive feedback loop which results in increasingly intense selection on one sex for characteristics which indicate ability to attract mates, potentially at the expense of ability to care for offspring.

Several analytic models for the evolution of paternal care have also been put forward. All of these have been based on the concept of the evolutionarily stable strategy (or ESS; Maynard Smith & Price, 1973) – a strategy which once established is stable against invasion by all other mutant strategies. Also assumed is that the ESS for each sex will be that which maximizes the number of surviving offspring produced per unit time given the ESS characteristic of the opposite sex.

Dawkins (1976) presented a simple analysis for the case when males can either desert or be faithful and females can either be coy or indiscriminate in their mating preferences. Drawing on this, Maynard Smith (1977) analysed the case when both males and females have the options of guarding or deserting, and offspring survival is a function of the number of parents guarding. The model assumes that if females do not care for the young then they are potentially able to lay more eggs, while if males desert they have a constant probability of obtaining a second mate. Male care and female desertion were found to be favoured when (1) the probability of the male's finding a second mate is low, (2) female fecundity increases with desertion, and (3) care by one parent greatly increases offspring survival but the addition of a second parent has a much smaller positive effect. For some parameter values, both male care/female desertion and female care/male desertion are ESSs.

Although supportive of Jenni's (1974) verbal model, the analysis has several limitations. The probability of offspring survival with single parent care is not dependent on which sex provides the care (although this feature could be easily added to the model). More seriously, males have a constant probability of obtaining a second mate. This probability should be a function of the proportion of males which desert their mates (as in Rubenstein's (1980) model for the evolution of territoriality as a reproductive strategy). Females are also not given the option of mating again (an option which they clearly have in polyandrous species), so that males always directly benefit through the increased fecundity of their mates.

Later in the same paper, Maynard Smith escaped the latter two problems in a model for a continuously breeding population. The analysis specifies the ESS for the amount of time each sex should spend with the offspring (i.e. both males and females have an infinite number of potential strategies). He again reached the conclusion that there may sometimes be two ESSs for single parent care, even when one alternative would result in a higher average reproductive rate for the population than the other. He stressed that starting conditions would be expected to influence critically the outcome whenever two ESSs are theoretically possible.

The continuous strategy set model of Grafen & Sibly (1978) provides the most precise predictions for the evolution of parental care. They explored in detail the consequences of the following special assumption: 'The rate of increase of expected benefit from a brood at any one time depends only on the expected benefit from the brood at that time (in other words, the current state of development of the brood) and on whether the male, or the female, or neither has already been deserted'. With this assumption they were able to conclude that

$$\text{for } t_1 < t_2 \quad h(g)/h_2(g) = (1/r) + 1$$
$$\text{and} \quad \text{for } t_2 < t_1 \quad h(g)/h_1(g) = r + 1$$

where t_1 and t_2 are the times when males and females desert the young, respectively; $h(g)$, $h_1(g)$ and $h_2(g)$ are the rates at which benefit from the brood increases with time spent caring, for joint care, male care, and female care, respectively; and r is the number of breeding males per breeding female.

These are powerful predictions. For a 1 : 1 sex ratio, for example, they imply that desertion will first occur when for one member of the pair, the rate of benefit increase from joint parental care falls below twice that which would result from care by the mate alone. This suggests that the evolution of parental care is very conservative. Once one sex becomes parental, it is likely to be more efficient in providing care than the other sex and thus be the one to be deserted, since the less efficient sex is the one which will desert first unless the breeding sex ratio is strongly skewed towards an excess of the less-efficient sex. This would tend to make the evolution of sex role reversal extremely difficult, a finding not inconsistent with the rarity of the phenomenon.

It is important to examine the biological implications of their special assumption, however. Fig. 10.1 illustrates the relationship between benefit from the brood and time spent caring when benefit is a function of the number of eggs laid times the probability of the egg producing a surviving offspring, and when the probability of survival is directly related to the time for which they are cared. The differences in clutch size between the two cases presented are assumed to result from differences in the amount of care initially provided by the male. This example violates the special assumption of Grafen & Sibly (1978) because the rate of increase of benefit at any one time depends not only on the benefit achieved and who will provide the care, but also on the past history of caring for the brood through its effect

Fig. 10.1. The expected number of surviving offspring from a clutch as a function of the number of eggs laid times the probability (P) of each egg producing a surviving offspring. This number is assumed to be a function of the time (T) for which the eggs are cared. For $T \leq 10$, $P = T/10$; for $T > 10$, $P = 1$. The curves represent the hypothetical case of clutch size being doubled if males help in the caring during the early stages of clutch deposition.

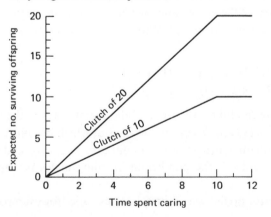

on brood size. When an expected benefit of ten offspring has been achieved, for example, the first female may still expect a positive rate of benefit increase, while the second female can expect no further benefit. Thus their special assumption appears to exclude from consideration that feature which many believe to be the most potent force favouring the evolution of high levels of male parental care.

In summary, the available analytic ESS models for the evolution of parental care are of only partial value in understanding sex role reversal. In addition to their individual weaknesses, they also fail by definition to examine whether strategies, which though stable when established, can spread when rare.

A computer simulation

These limitations inspired the writing of a computer program capable of simulating changes in the frequencies of parental strategies. As in the first of the Maynard Smith (1977) models, each sex has only two behavioural options. Both sexes have the potential for multiple matings, however, and the simulation is also capable of examining the influence of starting conditions on the final outcome.

The original design was influenced by Smith's (1980*a*) scenario for the evolution of male parental care in the giant water bugs: a population consisting of normal females, who lay their eggs on vegetation; mutant females, who attempt to lay their eggs on the backs of males; tolerant males, who allow mutant females to lay eggs on their backs; and intolerant males, who refuse to accept the eggs of mutant females. Thus there are four types of matings, but only three different sets of consequences: normal female/tolerant or intolerant male (in either case the eggs receive the same treatment), mutant female/intolerant male, and mutant female/tolerant male. In more general terms, this model describes the fate of mutations which cause females to provide males with the opportunity to care for the offspring, and mutations in males which govern their response to this opportunity.

Each of the three mating types has associated with it three parameters: (1) the cost to the female (in terms of the percentage of her reproductive effort which the mating represents), (2) the cost to the male, and (3) the proportion of the offspring produced which survive. The simulations fell into two broad classes as a function of whether or not mutant females had lower reproductive costs than normal females. Other parameters were varied to determine the effects of (1) increasing the cost to tolerant males who mate with mutant females, (2) increasing the probability of survival of eggs from tolerant male/mutant female matings, (3) decreasing the probability of survival of eggs from intolerant male/mutant female matings, and (4) changing the discrepancy between males and normal females in reproductive costs. For all simulations the starting frequency of mutant females was set at 2%. Two starting frequencies for tolerant males, 2 and 98%, were tried for all combinations of parameter values.

The bulk of the program consists of two nested, iterative loops. Each passage through the outer loop generates the numbers of the four adult types for the next generation from their relative proportions in the previous generation. This is done by standardizing these proportions against a population consisting of 100 females and 100 males.

The inner loop simulates mating and production of offspring within each generation. The loop repeats until the reproductive potential of the males or the females is exhausted. At each iteration, the number of matings between males and females of each type is equal to the proportion of females available of that type times the proportion of males available of that type times the number of available males or females, whichever is smaller. Thus there is no potential for random mating effects, and the population simulated is effectively infinite. The number of available individuals of each type for the next iteration is reduced by substracting the cost of each mating in which individuals of that type participated. The number of matings of each type is stored cumulatively.

After mating is completed, the total number of matings of each type is multiplied by the probability for that mating type of offspring survival. Half of this number are designated females of the mother's type and half males of the father's type. These numbers are then summed for each of the four types of individuals, and the sums standardized for the next generation as described above. The Appendix outlines the statements of the program.

Results

The results of the simulations are presented in a series of seven figures. In each, the left-hand (L) pair of graphs shows the outcome when tolerant males started out at 98%, and the right-hand (R) pair when they started out at 2%. In each graph, the effects of increasing costs for tolerant males mating with mutant females (from 0.1 to 0.5 and 0.9, except in Fig. 10.7) are represented as families of curves. The two sets of simulations (Figs. 10.2–10.5, Figs. 10.6–10.8) distinguish between situations when mutant females save nothing directly by leaving their eggs with males (as would be the case, perhaps, if they simply shifted their oviposition sites), and situations when mutant females decrease their costs (by, for example, caring less for the offspring).

Mutant and normal female costs equal

If the offspring from matings between mutant females and tolerant males did not have a higher survivorship than offspring produced by normal females, then mutant females never increased in frequency. This was expected. Mutant and normal females had identical costs in these simulations, and thus mutant females could only do better than normal females if survivorship from some of their matings were higher.

Increasing tolerant male costs always lowered the rate of increase or increased the rate of decrease in the frequency of tolerant males and generally mutant females. Some of these rate alterations were very slight, however. The final equilibrium frequencies of tolerant males were also lowered in some simulations (especially Figs. 10.2, 10.3L, 10.4). Again, this

Fig. 10.2. Simulations when mutant female costs = 0.5, and the probability of their offspring surviving = 1.0 for matings with tolerant males and 0.5 for matings with intolerant males. Normal females have a reproductive cost of 0.5 and a probability of offspring survival of 0.5. Curves represent outcomes, from lowest to highest, when costs to tolerant males from matings with mutant females are 0.9, 0.5, and 0.1; the two upper curves or all three curves are sometimes indistinguishable. Costs to intolerant males and tolerant males mating with normal females = 0.1.

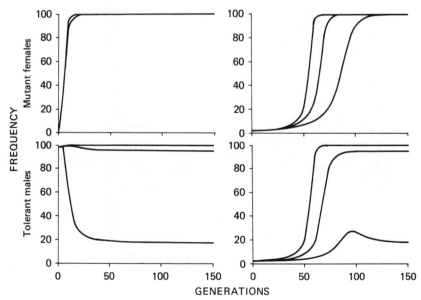

Fig. 10.3. Simulations as in Fig. 10.2, except that the probability of offspring surviving for mutant female/intolerant male matings was lowered to 0.25.

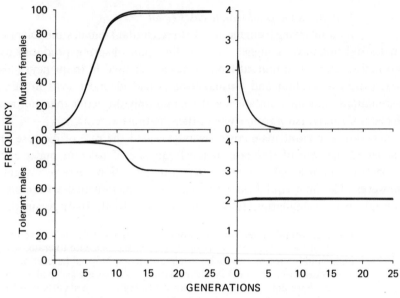

Fig. 10.4. Simulations as in Fig. 10.2, except that mutant and normal female costs were raised to 0.75.

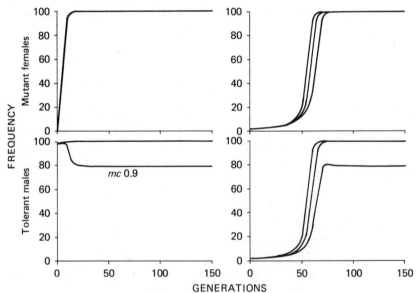

was not unexpected. It should be noted that there appeared to be no evidence for boundary conditions surrounding the point where tolerant male costs equalled female costs. For example, in the simulations illustrated by Fig. 10.2, the point where tolerant males did not increase to fixation occurred when their costs, when mated with mutant females, were approximately 0.48.

Increasing the baseline level of female costs (from 0.5 to 0.75) increased the equilibrium frequency of tolerant males when the equilibrium frequency was originally less than 100% (compare Figs. 10.2 and 10.4, and Figs. 10.3L and 10.5L). Thus the greater the cost discrepancy between intolerant males and females, the more likely was the establishment of higher levels of paternal care.

The starting frequency of tolerant males sometimes, but not always, had an effect on the final outcome. This frequency dependence was established by lowering the probability of survival of the offspring produced from mutant female/intolerant male matings (from 0.5 to 0.25). For example, Figs. 10.2L and 10.2R show the same equilibrium results while those of Figs. 10.3L and 10.3R differ dramatically. A similar comparison can be made between Figs. 10.4 and 10.5. A low probability of survival of offspring from mutant female/intolerant male matings made a high starting frequency of tolerant males necessary for tolerant males to increase in frequency. Given a high starting frequency, however, the final equilibrium frequency of tolerant males was higher when survivorship of mutant female/intolerant male offspring was lower (compare Figs. 10.2L and 10.3L, Figs. 10.4L and 10.5L).

Mutant female costs lowered

In some respects this set of simulations resembled those described above. Increasing tolerant male costs, for example, lowered their final equilibrium frequency for at least some cost levels in all simulations. In one case mutant female equilibrium frequency was also lowered (Fig. 10.8L). Decreasing the probability of survival of offspring from mutant female/intolerant male matings again created an initial frequency dependence effect and raised the final equilibrium frequency of tolerant males when their starting frequency was high (compare Figs. 10.7 and 10.8).

There were important differences, however. First, it was no longer necessary for the probability of survival of mutant female/tolerant male offspring to exceed that of offspring produced by normal females. This was not surprising, for mutant females had lower reproductive costs than normal females in all cases. Second, raising the baseline cost level of normal

Fig. 10.5. Simulations as in Fig. 10.3, except that mutant and normal female costs were raised to 0.75.

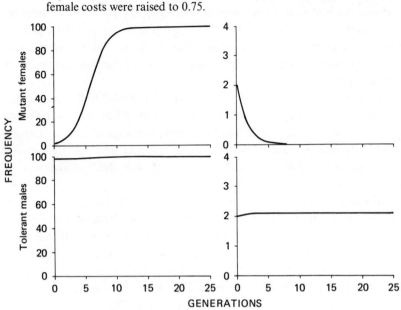

Fig. 10.6. Simulations as in Fig. 10.3, except that mutant female costs were lowered to 0.2.

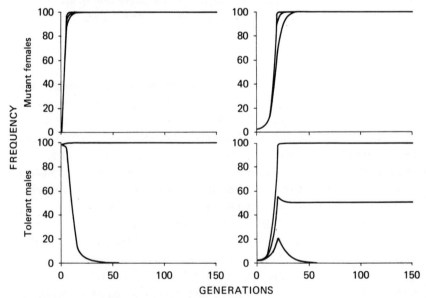

females from 0.5 to 0.75 had little effect; when simulations were run with parameter values otherwise equal to those run for Fig. 10.7, results were very similar with identical equilibrium values. Finally, the equilibrium levels of tolerant males were changed in several ways. Fig. 10.6 can be compared to Fig. 10.3, where starting conditions were identical except for the mutant female costs. When starting frequencies of tolerant males were high, then costly forms of male care were less likely to evolve than they were when mutant female costs remained unchanged. When starting frequencies were low, mutant females increased instead of rapidly disappearing, and tolerant males as a consequence became established at levels determined by the cost of male care.

A more biologically realistic picture of the effects of a cost decrease for mutant females is presented in Figs. 10.7 and 10.8, however. In these simulations, there was no difference in offspring survivorship between matings involving normal females and those involving mutant females and tolerant males (i.e. tolerant males merely compensated for the effort not expended by mutant females). A comparison of Figs. 10.3 and 10.7 illustrates the difficulty in establishing male parental care under these con-

Fig. 10.7. Simulations as in Fig. 10.6, except that the probability of offspring surviving for mutant female/tolerant male matings was lowered to 0.5. The results when costs to tolerant males mating with mutant females = 0.25 are also shown (curve with second highest values).

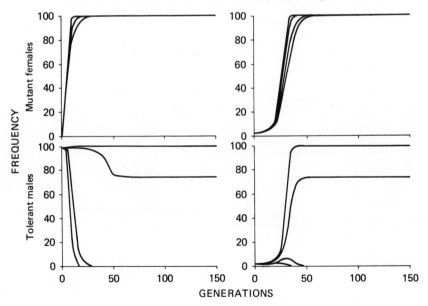

ditions. Even moderate levels of paternal care seemed unlikely to evolve unless the probability of survival of offspring from mutant female/intolerant male matings was quite low and the starting frequency of tolerant males high (Fig. 10.8L).

Discussion

The simulations presented here are limited in scope; a variety of assumptions (more complex modes of inheritance, variations in clutch size and sex ratio, etc.) and intermediate parameter values have yet to be tried. Within the context of these limitations, however, several results which were not derived from earlier models deserve mention.

First, a large initial discrepancy between the sexes in reproductive costs favours increases in male parental care if female care is not at the same time reduced. In essence, this feature tends to stabilize, or decrease up to a point, differences between the sexes in potential reproductive rate and hence the intensity of sexual selection. This tendency opposes the Fisher effect, which acts as a positive feedback loop in the sexual selection process.

The simulations in which females save nothing also show that mutations in females which give males the option of providing additional care can

Fig. 10.8. Simulations as in Fig. 10.6, except that the probabilities of offspring surviving for mutant females were lowered to 0.5 for matings with tolerant males and 0.125 for matings with intolerant males.

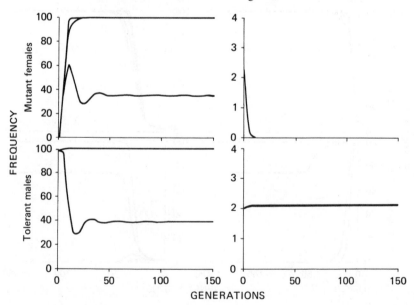

result in higher levels of paternal care than mutations in males alone. This is seen in the effect of lowering offspring survivorship from mutant female/intolerant male matings. When there is no lowering of survival, the situation is logically equivalent to one in which males simply vary in the amount of care they provide. (Logical equivalence was verified by a modified simulation.) Decreasing the survivorship of offspring from mutant female/intolerant male matings allowed higher levels of male care to evolve, provided the starting frequency of tolerant males was high.

Interestingly, Smith's (1980*b*) assessment of the conditions which led to the evolution of male care in giant water bugs parallels these simulation results. He stressed two features: (1) females changing their oviposition site from emergent vegetation to the backs of males (which would certainly involve the potential for poor survivorship if males discarded or otherwise mistreated the eggs), and (2) a high probability of male acceptance of these eggs because of their tendency to guard females in an effort to avoid sperm competition. His discussion also points up the need for simulations in which females test male willingness to care by a preliminary investment in a small number of eggs. This might reduce the starting frequency of tolerant males needed for the evolution of paternal care.

A parallel effect is seen in the simulations in which mutant females do save in reproductive costs (i.e. mutations in both sexes are by definition involved). If offspring survivorship is lowered, as is likely, when females provide less care and males provide no additional care, then the highest levels of male care occur when survivorship is considerably impaired and males willing to provide extra care occur at high frequency. This accords very well with Jenni's (1974) linking of double clutching and sex role reversal in birds. In all birds, offspring survivorship is very low if neither sex cares, but in species with a history of double clutching there is likely to be the necessary high starting frequency of males willing to care for the young without female help.

The relationship between territoriality and male parental care (Ridley, 1978) makes sense in light of these simulation results. As Ridley argued, the extra costs to males for guarding eggs on their territories might be low (provided defence against egg predators was not particularly costly). In addition, territoriality could be viewed as a preadaptation which results in a high starting frequency of tolerant males.

Interpreting the general relationship between external fertilization and care by the male alone is more complex. This complexity stems partly from the fact that costs to males vary widely within this category of parental care. In addition, internal fertilization can act in two ways with respect to the parameters of these simulations. First, it would increase the baseline discrepancy between the sexes in reproductive costs if internal fertilization represented a more substantial commitment for females than external fertilization. Second, it might increase the potential for loss in offspring survivorship in matings between mutant females and intolerant males. This would be very likely if mutant females retained the fertilized eggs for a shorter time. The consequences of this might help to explain the apparent rarity of transitions from internal to external fertilization (in sessile invertebrates, Ghiselin, 1974, p. 120; in fishes, J. Gittelman, personal communication).

Even if mutant females simply changed their oviposition sites (i.e. no direct savings), the change might be more likely to affect adversely offspring survivorship in mutant female/intolerant male matings when fertilization is internal. Externally fertilizing females would be expected to leave their eggs in the vicinity of males in any case, because the male must fertilize them. Internally fertilizing females are not normally under this constraint, and thus a mutation for leaving eggs with males might involve a more radical change in oviposition site. For the parameter values tried, decreases in offspring survivorship necessitated high starting frequencies of tolerant males, even when the initial discrepancy between the sexes in reproductive cost was increased. This suggests that moderate increases in male parental care would be expected to evolve more readily in species with external fertilization, because there would be a less-stringent prerequisite for a high starting frequency of tolerant males.

Finally, it should be noted that the conditions which make the regular evolution of some male parental care probable (no decrease in female costs, or other features likely to require a high starting frequency of tolerant males) do not facilitate the evolution of the highest levels of paternal care. This may explain why a number of the extreme cases which approach or achieve sex role reversal (e.g. jacanas, giant water bugs) are found in groups where exclusively male paternal care is atypical.

While the details of these simulations may later be shown to be limited by their assumptions, the sensitivity of the outcome to the initial frequencies of the strategies is likely to be a general phenomenon in the evolution of parental care. Analyses based only on the concept of the ESS cannot examine this problem because they consider only the stability of strategies once they are established.

The theory for the evolution of mating and parental care strategies has many potential directions for growth. Analytic methods should be directed at the situations examined here. More unusual forms of sex role reversal also need to be explored. Hatziolos (1979), for example, has demonstrated that in a species of mantis shrimp in which only the female cares for the eggs, males are coy and females actively court them. She suggested that matings are relatively risky for males (mantis shrimp are extremely aggressive and effective predators and females are generally larger than males), and thus that males should only mate with females of the highest quality (large females produce much larger clutches). It would be interesting to model the evolution of complex systems of this type.

All of the theoretical approaches outlined and used here share a common microevolutionary bias, based essentially on the principles (though not the elegant mathematics) of population genetics. The substantial developments in macroevolutionary theory (Gould, 1977; Stanley, 1979) have had almost no influence on sociobiological issues (the evolution of sex being a notable exception (Stanley, 1975)). The relationship between parental care strategies and speciation and extinction rates, for example, and the influence such a relationship might have on the patterns we observe (e.g. the rarity of male parental care) remain to be explored.

Ultimately, however, our theories are only as good as the assumptions on which we base them, and these assumptions are largely drawn from our knowledge of natural history. The diversity of male parental care types in tropical frogs, cichlids, and wading birds invites further careful study. Equally fascinating on a more fine-grained level, is the variation among pipefish in the degree to which females compete for males as mates (T. Lim, personal communication). Although the ancestral conditions for the situations studied will often have been obscured by subsequent evolutionary events, partial knowledge is clearly preferable to none.

Summary
1. The natural history of and earlier models for the evolution of paternal care and sex role reversal are reviewed.
2. The fate of mutations in females which give males the opportunity to care for the offspring (mutant *vs.* normal), and mutations in males which govern their response to that opportunity (tolerant *vs.* intolerant) are examined with computer simulations.
3. The evolution of modest amounts of male care can be expected to occur regularly when there is no loss in offspring survivorship for matings between mutant females and intolerant males.
4. The evolution of costly forms of male care typically requires the

more stringent conditions of a loss in offspring survivorship for mutant female/intolerant male matings, coupled with a high starting frequency of tolerant males.

5. These results are used to interpret previously documented natural-history patterns, including the associations between paternal care and territoriality, external fertilization, and double clutching.

The King's College Research Centre and the Sub-Department of Animal Behaviour at Madingley, Cambridge University, generously accepted me as a visitor while I was on a NATO Postdoctoral Fellowship working with G.A. Parker. Members of the King's College Research Centre Sociobiology Group L. Buss, J. Gittleman, J.B.C. Jackson, B. Keller, T. Lim, J. Maynard Smith, G.C. Williams, J. Wulff, and many others helped in the development of this paper. I was supported by grant BNS-7904747 from the National Science Foundation.

Appendix
Outline of computer program

I. Read in values for (1) numbers of mutant females, normal females, tolerant males, intolerant males; (2) the reproductive costs and probabilities of offspring survival for the mutant female/tolerant male, mutant female/intolerant male, and normal female matings; (3) the number of generations to be simulated. The total number of males and the total number of females always equalled 100.

II. Outer loop

    II 1. For each of the four mating types, set the total number achieved to zero.

    II 2. Set numbers of available mutant females, normal females, tolerant males, and intolerant males to their initial values.

III. Inner loop

    III 1. Calculate the total number of available females and the total number of available males.

    III 2. If the number of available individuals of either sex is less than one, exit from inner loop and go to II3.

    III 3. Calculate the proportion each type represents of its sex (e.g. number of available normal females/total number of available females).

    III 4. Set the number of members of the limiting sex to the number of available males or the number of available females, whichever is smaller.

    III 5. Calculate for this passage through the loop the number of matings of the four types. Do this by multiplying the proportion of males of a given type by the proportion of females of a given type by the number of members of the limiting sex.

III 6. Recalculate the numbers of the two types of available females and the two types of available males. Do this by subtracting from the current value for each, the product of the number of matings and their cost for each of the two relevant mating types.

III 7. Recalculate the total number of matings of each type achieved by adding to the current number the number achieved in this passage through the loop.

III 8. Return to III 1.

II 3. Calculate for each of the four mating types the number of offspring produced. Do this by multiplying the number achieved by the probability of survival.

II 4. Calculate the total number of offspring produced.

II 5. Recalculate the initial values for the number of mutant females, normal females, tolerant males and intolerant males. For each, (1) add the number of offspring produced from the two types of matings, (2) multiply this sum by 100, (3) divide this product by the total number of offspring produced.

II 6. If the desired number of generations has been reached, stop simulation.

References

Bateman, A.J. (1948). Intra-sexual selection in *Drosophila. Heredity*, **2**, 349–68.

Darwin, C. (1871). *The Descent of Man and Selection in Relation to Sex*. John Murray: London.

Dawkins, R. (1976). *The Selfish Gene*. Oxford University Press: Oxford.

Dawkins, R. & Carlisle, T.R. (1976). Parental investment, mate desertion and a fallacy. *Nature*, **262**, 131–3.

Emlen, S.T. & Oring, L.W. (1977). Ecology, sexual selection, and the evolution of mating systems. *Science*, **197**, 215–23.

Fiedler, K. (1954). Vergleichende Verhaltensstudien an Seenedeln, Schlangennalden und Seepferdchen (Syngnathidae). *Zeitschrift für Tierpsychologie*, **11**, 358–416.

Fisher, R.A. (1930). *The Genetical Theory of Natural Selection*. Clarendon Press: Oxford.

Ghiselin, M.T. (1974). *The Economy of Nature and the Evolution of Sex*. University of California Press: Berkeley.

Gould, S.J. (1977). *Ontogeny and Phylogeny*. Belknap Press: Cambridge.

Grafen, A. & Sibly, R. (1978). A model of mate desertion. *Animal Behaviour*, **26**, 645–52.

Hatziolos, M.E. (1979). *Ecological Correlates of Aggression and Courtship in the Stomatopod* Pseudosquilla ciliata. Ph.D. dissertation, University of California, Berkeley.

Jenni, D.A. (1974). Evolution of polyandry in birds. *American Zoologist*, **14**, 129–44.

Jenni, D.A. & Collier, G. (1972). Polyandry in the American Jacana (*Jacana spinosa*). *Auk*, **89**, 743–65.

Kleiman, D. (1977). Monogamy in mammals. *Quarterly Review of Biology*, **52**, 39–69.

Knowlton, N. (1979). Reproductive synchrony, parental investment, and the evolutionary dynamics of sexual selection. *Animal Behaviour*, **27**, 1022–33.

Lack, D. (1968). *Ecological Adaptations for Breeding in Birds*. Oxford University Press: Oxford.

Maynard Smith, J. (1977). Parental investment: a prospective analysis. *Animal Behaviour*, **25**, 1–9.

Maynard Smith, J. & Price, G.R. (1973). The logic of animal conflict. *Nature*, **246**, 15–18.

O'Donald, P. (1962). The theory of sexual selection. *Heredity*, **17**, 541–52.

O'Donald, P. (1973). Models of sexual and natural selection in polygamous species. *Heredity*, **31**, 145–56.

Parker, G.A. (1974). The reproductive behaviour and the nature of sexual selection in *Scatophaga stercoraria* L. (Diptera: Scatophagidae). IX. Spatial distribution of fertilization rates and evolution of male search strategy within the reproductive area. *Evolution*, **28**, 93–108.

Parker, G.A. (1979). Sexual selection and sexual conflict. In *Sexual Selection and Reproductive Competition in Insects*, ed. M.S. & N.A. Blum, pp. 123–66. Academic Press: New York.

Parker, G.A., Baker, R.R. & Smith, V.G.F. (1972). The origin and evolution of gamete dimorphism and the male-female phenomenon. *Journal of Theoretical Biology*, **36**, 529–53.

Ridley, M. (1978). Paternal care. *Animal Behaviour*, **26**, 904–32.

Rubenstein, D.I. (1980). On the evolution of alternative mating strategies. In *Limits to Action: The Allocation of Individual Behavior*, ed. J.E.R. Staddon, pp. 65–99. Academic Press: New York.

Smith, R.L. (1976). Male brooding behavior of the water bug *Abedus herberti* (Hemiptera: Belostomatidae). *Annals of the Entomological Society of America*, **69**, 740–7.

Smith, R.L. (1979). Paternity assurance and altered roles in the mating behaviour of a giant water bug, *Abedus herberti* (Heteroptera: Belostomatidae). *Animal Behaviour*, **27**, 716–25.

Smith, R.L. (1980a). Daddy water bugs. *Natural History*, **89**(2), 56–63.

Smith, R.L. (1980b). Evolution of exclusive postcopulatory paternal care in the insects. *Florida Entomologist*, **63**, 65–78.

Stanley, S.M. (1975). Clades versus clones in evolution: why we have sex. *Science*, **190**, 382–3.

Stanley, S. (1979). *Macroevolution: Pattern and Process*. W.H. Freeman & Co: San Franciso.

Thornhill, R. (1976). Sexual selection and paternal investment in insects. *American Naturalist*, **110**, 153–63.

Trivers, R.L. (1972). Parental investment and sexual selection. In *Sexual Selection and the Descent of Man: 1871–1971*, ed. B. Campbell, pp. 136–79. Aldine Publishing Co: Chicago.

Wells, K.D. (1981). Parental behaviour of male and female frogs. In *Natural Selection and Social Behavior: Recent Research and New Theory*, ed. R.D. Alexander & D.W. Tinkle, pp. 184–97. Chiron Press: New York.

Williams, G.C. (1966). *Adaptation and Natural Selection: A Critique of Some Current Evolutionary Thought*. Princeton University Press: Princeton.

11

Parental investment in male and female offspring in mammals

T.H. CLUTTON-BROCK AND S.D. ALBON

'Among innumerable Footsteps of Divine Providence to be found in the Works of Nature, there is a very remarkable one to be observed in the exact Ballance that is maintained, between the Numbers of Men and Women; for by this means it is provided, that the Species may never fail, nor perish, since every Male may have its Female, and of a proportionable Age. This Equality of Males and Females is not the Effect of Chance but Divine Providence, working for a good End....

From hence it follows, that Polygamy is contrary to the Law of Nature and Justice, and to the Propagation of Human Race; for where Males and Females are in equal number, if one Man takes Twenty Wives, Nineteen Men must live in Celibacy, which is repugnant to the Design of Nature; nor is it probable that Twenty Women will be so well impregnated by one Man as by Twenty.'

Arbuthnott (1710)

Introduction

Few sociobiologists today would be quite so sure as John Arbuthnott that mammalian sex ratios were distributed so as to provide for the greatest satisfaction of the greatest number. However, it is not uncommonly argued that mammals allocate their investment to their male and female progeny in a way that is consistent with current evolutionary theory (Trivers & Willard, 1973; Maynard Smith, 1978). In this paper, we examine the extent to which two principal theories – the first concerning the allocation of parental resources to individual sons and daughters, the second the numbers of each sex that parents should produce – predict the distribution of parental investment in mammals.

The central theories

The first theory, which was originally formulated by Trivers & Willard (1973) and subsequently developed by other authors (Reiter, Stinson & Le Boeuf, 1978; Dittus, 1979; Maynard Smith, 1980) predicts that where reproductive success varies more widely among offspring of one sex and is influenced by parental investment (Trivers, 1972), parents should invest more heavily in individuals of that sex. This could be accomplished either by allocating a higher proportion of available resources to individual sons than to daughters (Reiter *et al.*, 1978) or, as Trivers & Willard originally suggested, by adaptive modification of the sex ratio leading to an increase in the proportion of sons produced by mothers who could afford to invest heavily.

The basis for this argument is obvious. Suppose that variance in lifetime reproductive success is greater among males than females and that an individual's breeding success as an adult increases with the amount of investment it received during the first months of its life. Under such circumstances, parents that invested more heavily before weaning in individual sons than individual daughters would be survived by a greater number of grandchildren than those that invested equally in offspring of each sex (Trivers & Willard, 1973).

This situation is probably not uncommon in mammals. Since the majority of mammalian species are polygynous, it is likely that variance in reproductive success is usually greater among males than females (Trivers, 1972; Clutton-Brock, Harvey & Rudder, 1977) and long-term studies of reproductive success in wild populations have so far confirmed this suggestion (Le Boeuf, 1974; Clutton-Brock, Albon, Gibson & Guinness, 1979). In several species where contests involve grappling, pushing or charging, there is evidence that reproductive success among males is related to body size (Geist, 1971; Le Boeuf, 1972, 1974; Clutton-Brock *et al.*, 1979), which is usually well correlated with early growth rates, maternal milk yields and maternal body condition (Gunn, 1964a, b, 1965, 1967; Fraser & Morley-Jones, 1975; Schinkel & Short, 1961; Russell, 1976; Sadleir, 1969; Gosling & Petrie, 1981; Clutton-Brock, Guinness & Albon, 1982). In such cases, it seems likely that a male's reproductive success is strongly influenced by maternal investment before weaning and parents should invest more heavily in their sons than their daughters during this stage.

However, two additional complications need to be considered. Which sex the parents should invest more heavily in will depend on the *effects* of parental investment on the reproductive success of male and female offspring rather than on variance in reproductive success per se. For example, in situations where parental investment has a greater effect on the eventual reproductive success of daughters than sons, selection may prefer mothers who invest more heavily in individual daughters, even if reproductive success varies more widely among their sons. In practice, parental investment may usually have a greater effect on the reproductive success of the sex that shows the greater variance in reproductive success, but this may not always be the case. Secondly, although Trivers & Willard's argument (1973) is principally concerned with investment prior to weaning, post-weaning investment must also be taken into account. As we argue below, it seems likely that selection may sometimes favour increased investment in sons prior to weaning and increased investment in daughters afterwards, making it difficult to compare the costs of producing sons versus daughters.

The second theory, which was originally outlined by Darwin (1871) and first stated formally by Fisher (1930), predicts that the average parents should divide their total investment equally between their male and female progeny. Fisher's theory is based on the fact that the mean reproductive success of members of each sex is inversely related to their frequency in the population. It can be understood intuitively, though it is usually expressed in mathematical terms (e.g. MacArthur, 1965; Eshel, 1975; Charnov, 1975, 1979; Charlesworth, 1977). Suppose that a gene which caused its carriers to produce an excess of females had spread through a population as a result of some chance event. Because the population would include a high proportion of females, the mean reproductive success of individual males would exceed that of females. Consequently, selection would favour genes (or individuals) that produced a higher proportion of male offspring. As male-producing genes spread, their advantage would decline and, when the population contained a preponderance of males, there would again be selection for genes producing female-biased sex ratios. Fisher concluded that, where the costs of producing sons and daughters were the same, the average parent should produce equal numbers of each sex. However, as he pointed out, where offspring of one sex cost more to produce, the benefits in producing that sex have to be modified by the extra costs, and the sex ratio of progeny should be biased against the more expensive sex by the end of the period of investment. It is important to notice that this does not mean that sex ratios should necessarily be biased in the same direction from birth if differences in mortality are involved – for example, if the costs of rearing sons and daughters are the same but sons are more likely to die before the end of investment, the average cost to the parents per son *conceived* will be less than per daughter (because investment in sons is more frequently terminated before completion) but the cost per son *reared* will be greater (on account of the 'wasted' investment in sons that died). In such circumstances, parents should produce more males at birth, but the sex ratio should be female biased by the end of the investment period. Fisher supported this suggestion by pointing out that the sex ratio in human progeny showed precisely this pattern.

Three points concerning Fisher's theory should be noticed. Firstly, although sex differences in mortality that occur during the process of investment will affect the optimal sex ratio of progeny, differences expressed after the end of investment will not do so – since any tendency for members of one sex to show higher mortality will be counterbalanced by increased reproductive success among the survivors (see Leigh, 1970; Maynard Smith, 1978). However, there is one important exception to this argument. If mortality after the end of parental care is higher in one sex than the other and *survival* is influenced by parental investment, selection will favour mothers that invest more heavily in the sex that shows higher mortality, these offspring will cost more to rear and fewer of them should be produced. For example, if offspring of one sex disperse at the end of parental care, mortality is high during the dispersal phase and is related to early parental investment, mothers should invest more in individuals of the dispersing sex but should produce fewer of them.

Second, it is important to notice that Fisher's theory applies to the average parent: equal investment in male and female offspring would be achieved if fifty percent of parents invested only in males and fifty per cent invested only in females as well as by a situation in which each parent allocated half its investment to sons and half to daughters (Crow & Kimura, 1970; Williams, 1979) though selection may tend to favour the latter situation, especially in small populations (Verner, 1965; Taylor & Sauer, 1980).

Third, Fisher's theory depends on several assumptions which will not necessarily hold in all species. In particular, it assumes that competition between relatives is no more common than between individuals selected at random from the population. If relatives of one sex commonly compete with each other for food or breeding access, the optimal strategy will be for parents to invest less in the sex where competition between relatives is more intense (Hamilton, 1967; Clark, 1978; Dittus, 1979).

In the following sections, we examine three questions: (1) Do mammalian mothers allocate a greater proportion of their resources to offspring of one sex? (2) Does the sex ratio of progeny vary with the parent's ability to invest? And (3) Do parents divide their total investment equally between their male and female progeny?

Do mammalian mothers invest more heavily in offspring of one sex?

Evidence for increased investment in sons before weaning

In strongly polygynous mammals where a male's competitive success depends on contests in which physical strength is important, we might expect mothers to invest more heavily in their sons than their daughters before weaning (see above). Recent work on two polygynous species, the northern elephant seal and the red deer, is consistent with this prediction.

Among elephant seals, male pups are born heavier and grow faster and larger than females. Males are also weaned later and tend to be more persistent in their attempts to steal milk from females other than their mothers after weaning (Reiter *et al.*, 1978). However, though this study strongly suggests that females invest more in their sons, evidence that rearing sons affects the mother's subsequent reproductive performance more than rearing daughters is missing.

This objection is covered in studies of parental investment in red deer (Clutton-Brock, Albon & Guinness, 1981). In this species, the gestation length and birth weight of male calves are significantly greater than those of females, males grow faster and suckle significantly more frequently. These differences apparently affect the mother's future reproductive potential: mothers that rear male calves successfully in one year are significantly less likely to calve again the following year compared to mothers that rear females (Guinness, Albon & Clutton-Brock, 1978; Clutton-Brock *et al.*, 1981). Moreover, hinds calve (on average) 11 days later than in seasons following years when they have reared a female calf. Since late birth dates are associated with low calf survival (Guinness, Clutton-Brock & Albon, 1978), the cost of rearing males is presumably higher than the difference in fecundity would suggest.

Examination of the literature suggests that increased investment in male offspring may occur in a variety of other dimorphic ungulates. Male offspring commonly have longer gestation lengths, heavier birth weights and faster growth rates (Defries, Touchberry & Hays, 1959; Short, 1970; Glucksman, 1974; Nordan, Cowan & Wood, 1970; Krebs & Cowan, 1962; Robbins & Moen, 1975; McEwan & Whitehead, 1972; Benedict, 1938), and their food intake is greater both in absolute terms (McEwan, 1968; McEwan & Whitehead, 1971, 1972) and per unit body weight (Morrison, 1948). In addition, some evidence supports the suggestion that males cost more to rear: two studies of Indian cattle have shown a (non-significant) tendency for mothers that produce male calves to show a longer interval between parturition and conception than those that produce females (Dhillon, Acharya, Tiwana & Aggarwal, 1970; Singh, Singh & Srivastava, 1965); and , in sheep, lambs born co-twin with females have higher birth weights, grow faster and are more likely to survive than those born co-twin with males (Burfening, 1972).

Post-weaning investment

The evidence we have described above only concerns investment prior to weaning. Is it safe to assume that this will reflect total investment? The answer is often no, for in many terrestrial mammals, daughters adopt home ranges overlapping those of their mothers or join the same social group, while sons disperse (Lockie, 1966; Geist, 1971; Loudon, 1979; Clark, 1978; Bertram, 1975; Dittus, 1979; Kurland, 1977; Greenwood, 1980). It is conceivable that the presence of mature daughters and their dependants may reduce the abundance of resources available to the mother and her future offspring (Clark, 1978; Dittus, 1979). In this case, by permitting daughters to share their home range, mothers are continuing to invest in them after weaning and the total costs of producing daughters may equal or even exceed those of producing sons.

Moreover, there are theoretical reasons why selection might be expected to favour increased early investment in sons and increased later investment in daughters. Where the reproductive success of sons is affected by their body size, strong selection pressures will favour early investment in males (see above), while the potential for post-weaning investment in sons is often limited by the fact that they disperse from their mother's home range as well as by sex differences in food requirements (e.g. Watson & Staines, 1978; Staines & Crisp, 1978; Clutton-Brock *et al.*, 1981). In contrast, the advantages of heavy early investment in daughters are probably reduced in many species because increased adult body size is unlikely to improve a female's reproductive success to the same extent as that of a son: for example, in red deer, the skeletal size of hinds is not significantly related to their fecundity, or to the body condition or skeletal size of their calves (Mitchell & Lincoln, 1973; Mitchell & Brown, 1974; Mitchell, McCowan & Nicholson, 1976; Clutton-Brock *et al.*, 1981). Providing mature daughters with access to assured food supplies may have a major influence on their ability to undergo the strains of lactation (see Pond, 1977) and may increase their reproductive success to a greater extent than would similar assistance to mature sons.

The argument that the presence of mature daughters within a mother's home range constitutes an extension of parental investment depends on two assumptions: (1) that if daughters were ejected, the resources saved would be available to the mother and would not be eaten by unrelated animals, and (2) that the costs of the daughters' continued presence to the mother's future breeding potential is not outweighed by any benefits (for example in terms of reduced liability to predation). Both assumptions are more likely to apply in species where individuals or groups occupy discrete territories (see Clark, 1978) than to animals which range widely and do not defend feeding territories.

In red deer, recent evidence shows that the reproductive success of hinds declines with the size of their matrilineal group and the extent to which their home-ranges are used by relatives: compared to members of small matrilineal groups, members of large ones start breeding later, their fecundity tends to be lower and their calves have an increased chance of dying in their first year of life (Clutton-Brock *et al.*, 1982). Consequently, it is possible that the increased costs of pre-weaning investment in sons are balanced or even exceeded by the heavier costs of post-weaning investment in daughters. However, in elephant seals, pups are abandoned on the breeding beaches by their mothers and there is no evidence of any continuing social relationship between mothers and their offspring after pups are weaned (Le Boeuf & Briggs, 1977; Reiter *et al.*, 1978).

Evidence for increased pre-wearing investment in daughters
In apparent contrast to the studies described above, recent research on captive groups of macaques indicates that the costs of rearing female infants may exceed those of rearing males (Simpson, Simpson, Hooley & Zunz, 1981). Though males are typically slightly heavier than females at birth and are more active thereafter, rhesus macaque mothers that produce and rear sons are significantly more likely to conceive another infant in the following year than those that rear daughters. Similar results have been found in the free-ranging macaque population of Cayo Santiago (Colvin, quoted in M.J.A. Simpson *et al.*, in preparation) and in captive groups of stumptail macaques whose infants were removed at birth (Chamove, quoted in M.J.A. Simpson *et al.*, in preparation) but not in two other free-ranging rhesus populations or in baboons (Altmann, 1980).

Simpson and his colleagues suggest two causal explanations. Mothers may monitor the development rates of their offspring and terminate investment in males earlier in response to their higher activity levels and faster development. Alternatively (or additionally), the responses of other group members may be involved: in the rhesus group studied by Simpson, mothers pregnant with female foetuses were more frequently threatened, chased or attacked than mothers pregnant with male foetuses while, in a captive colony of pigtail macaques, the former were more frequently wounded than the latter (Sackett, Holm, Davis & Fahrenbuch, 1975). In support of this rather surprising result, adult group members of toque macaques are known to be less tolerant of female than male infants, possibly because the former represent future competitors for their own offspring (Dittus, 1977, 1979).

Neither of these theories accounts for the difference between the macaque studies and those of other mammals. There are at least two possible explanations. All populations which show delayed reproduction after a female has been produced are provisioned and their nutritional plane is probably superior to that of wild populations. Under these circumstances, it is conceivable that any increase in the energetic costs of rearing males may affect the mother's food intake rather than her body condition and reproductive performance. This may allow the effects of differences in development between male and female infants to be revealed: for example more frequent or protracted periods spent on their mother's nipples by female infants might lead to a longer period of post-partum amenorrhea after daughters are born. Moreover, it is possible that these effects might be exaggerated by confined conditions or high population density.

Alternatively, the difference between macaques and other mammals may have adaptive origins. In all the species of macaques studied so far, daughters typically remain in their natal troop throughout their lives, inheriting their mother's social rank and assisting her in competitive encounters between matrilineal groups within the troop (e.g. Kurland, 1977). Sons disperse to other troops and their breeding success may be less closely related to body size than in deer and seals since supportive coalitions between males are often important. Consequently it is conceivable that the benefits of extra investment to daughters may exceed those of extra investment to sons, even if variance in reproductive success is greater among the latter. An adaptive interpretation is supported by comparisons between dominant and subordinate macaque mothers: dominants, whose daughters are likely to inherit high ranks and will be able to assist them effectively in competition between kin groups, show substantially longer interbirth intervals after they have produced daughters versus sons while subordinates do not (M.J.A. Simpson *et al.*, unpublished data). However, the fact that male infants tend to be heavier than females at birth (M.J.A. Simpson, unpublished) is difficult to resolve with this explanation. Further detailed studies of natural populations are required and the energetic costs of rearing females need to be examined.

Does the sex ratio of progeny vary with the parent's ability to invest?

Adaptive modification of progeny sex ratios is widespread among invertebrates (Hamilton, 1967; Trivers & Hare, 1976; Charnov, Hartogh,

Jones & van den Assem, 1981) and would, on theoretical grounds, be expected among mammals (Trivers & Willard, 1973; Williams, 1979). However, recent studies have raised the possibility that it may be prevented by physiological constraints imposed by the process of sex determination (Beatty, 1970; Williams, 1979; Maynard Smith, 1980). This section considers three related questions: Is adaptive, modification of progeny sex ratios possible in mammals? Do birth sex ratios vary with environmental conditions? And is this variation likely to be adaptive?

Is adaptive modification of progeny sex ratios possible in mammals?

The sex ratio of progeny at birth might be modified adaptively either by distortion of the sex ratio at conception or through differential mortality during the period of parental investment. In the first case, the question at issue is whether modification is possible – for if so, there is no reason why selection should not exploit this potential. In the second, it is whether modification is likely to be favoured by selection, for differential mortality both before and after birth is known to occur widely in mammals.

Evidence concerning variation in primary sex ratios is equivocal. There is no known mechanism by which conception sex ratios can be manipulated and detailed studies have shown that they are close to unity in some mammals, including the laboratory mouse (Vickers, 1967, 1969; Kaufman, 1973) and the rabbit (Fechheimer & Beatty, 1974). In addition, there is relatively little evidence for intraspecific genetic effects on progeny sex ratios despite the persistent efforts of animal breeders (Maynard Smith, 1978; Williams, 1979).

However, these arguments do not exclude the possibility of variation in conception sex ratios. X- and Y-bearing spermatozoa may differ in motility and this could lead to consistent variation in conception ratios (Roberts, 1972, 1978). Moreover, high rates of sperm loss are known to occur immediately prior to fertilization (Cohen, 1975; Cohen & McNaughton, 1974) and it is possible that differential loss of X- and Y-bearing sperm could occur (Guerrero, 1975). The fact that sex ratios at conception are close to unity in the mouse and the rabbit cannot be taken to indicate that species with contrasting breeding systems will necessarily show the same pattern.

Several lines of evidence are difficult to reconcile with the suggestion that the primary sex ratio is immutably fixed at unity. Both foetal and birth sex ratios commonly show some degree of male bias – among large samples, statistically significant biases are not uncommon (see Table 11.1) – and foetal mortality is also typically higher among males (man: McMillen, 1979; fur seals: U.S. Department for Game & Fisheries; rats: Weisner & Sheard, 1935; whales: R.L. Trivers, R. Seger & H. Hare, unpublished data; mule deer: Robinette, Baer, Pillmore & Knittle, 1957; cows: Chapman, Cassida & Cote, 1938). As Craft (1938) has argued, it is difficult to reconcile both trends with an equal conception ratio unless there is a higher incidence of mortality among female zygotes shortly after conception. Although it is possible that errors in sexing or the allocation of a greater proportion of females to 'unsexed' categories may contribute to male-biased foetal ratios (Keller, 1969), detailed consideration of the data indicates that it is most unlikely that such errors explain all observed cases and birth sex ratios

Table 11.1. *Mammal species in which progeny sex ratios differ significantly from unity in any recorded sample excluding known cases of meiotic drive*

FOETAL SEX RATIOS
  Male-biased
    Rattus exulans 133.0 (424)** Harrison, 1955
    Suncus murinus 193.9 (194)** Harrison, 1955
    Physter catodon 128.3 (1118)*** Ohsumi, 1965
    Balaenoptera physalus 108.3 (13054)*** Mackintosh, 1942
    Megaptera novaengliae 134.6 (1717)*** Mackintosh, 1942
    Sibbalolus musculus 111.5 (10195)*** Mackintosh, 1942
    Sus scrofa 131.3 (583)** Henning, 1939
    Cervus elaphus 148.6 (271)** Miller, 1932
    Odocoileus hemionus 111.0 (2299)* Robinette *et al.*, 1955; Taber, 1953
    Bos domesticus 123.2 (1000)** Chapman *et al.*, 1938
    Raphicerus campestris 191.4 (102)** Wilson & Kerr, 1969
  Female-biased
    None located

BIRTH SEX RATIOS
  Male-biased
    Galago crassicaudatus 131 (122)* Clark, 1978
    Canis lupus 111.4 (1368)* Mech, 1975
    Halichoerus grypus 107.5 (2959)* Coulson & Hickling 1961, 1964
    Odocoileus hemionus 121 (808)** Robinette *et al.*, 1955, 1957
    Rangifer tarandus 108.7 (3459)* Nowosad, 1975: Taber, 1953
    Giraffa camelopardalis 160 (117)* Asdell, 1964
    Bos domesticus 110 (157, 255)*** Bar-Anan & Robertson, 1975

  Female-biased
    Dicotyles tajacu 67.0 (147)* Sowls, 1974

Figures shown are the numbers of males per 100 females with sample size in parentheses. *$P < 0.05$; **$P < 0.01$; ***$P < 0.001$.

should be relatively free from this problem. In addition, there is some evidence that genetic factors can influence sex ratios within species (see Weir, 1962; Bar-Anan & Robertson, 1975; Hasler & Banks, 1975; Fredga, Gropp, Winking & Frank, 1977; Myers & Krebs, 1971; Gini, 1951) and sex ratios within litters are sometimes more even than would be expected by chance (James, 1975). Finally, both foetal and birth sex ratios apparently differ between species and within species (see below).

Nor do theoretical considerations rule out the possibility that parents manipulate sex ratios after conception by selective abortion or resorption of one sex. If foetuses (or neonates) can be rejected while the parent's investment is still low, or if the zygotes' chances of successfully reproducing are close to zero (as may often be the case), adaptive manipulation of sex ratios by parents would be expected. Evidence of adaptive manipulation is available from recent studies of coypu (*Myocastor coypu*) and woodrats (*Neotama floridana*). In coypu, females with larger than average fat reserves show a statistically significant tendency to abort small, female-biased litters between the fourteenth and nineteenth week of gestation (Gosling & Petrie, 1981; L.M. Gosling, unpublished data) and there appears to be little alternative to the explanation offered by Gosling – that females whose potential for investment is high during the breeding season are likely to increment their reproductive success by abandoning small, female-biased litters and producing a larger litter, later in the season, because the benefits of heavy investment in individual females are low. As Gosling points out, sample sizes were unusually large in his study and it is possible that similar effects may have been overlooked in other species. In woodrats, experimental restriction of food availability leads to an increase in the frequency with which mothers ignore male offspring, to a decline in the weight of sons compared to daughters and to increased mortality among males (McClure, 1981).

Thus while, as Maynard Smith (1980) suggests, there are grounds for thinking that adaptive variation of sex ratios in mammals may be unlikely to occur, there are also reasons for believing that sex ratios can vary adaptively in some cases. In these circumstances, it would be premature to exclude the possibility that sex ratios can vary adaptively.

Do birth sex ratios vary with environmental conditions?

If adaptive modification of progeny sex ratios in mammals cannot be precluded, what grounds are there for thinking that it exists? Although Trivers & Willard (1973) originally claimed that mammalian mothers in good body condition tended to produce relatively more sons than those in poor condition, several of their examples were unconvincing and their empirical conclusions have been disputed (Myers, 1978; Williams, 1979).

Examination of the published literature shows that most of the suggested correlations between environmental factors and birth sex ratios do not reach statistical significance. Moreover, since evidence that sex ratios vary is more likely to be published than evidence that they do not, a considerable proportion of significant results are probably fortuitous. Nevertheless, both experimental results and the recurrence of similar relationships between birth sex ratios and environmental factors in different species suggest that sex ratios can be influenced by external circumstances – though there is no consistent tendency for circumstances likely to increase the mother's potential for investment to be associated with either male- or female-biased sex ratios at birth.

The following sections review the relevant data on relationships between progeny sex ratios and different factors that might affect the parent's potential for investment, including maternal nutrition, environment, previous reproductive status, age, dominance and sex of previous offspring. To standardize figures, all measures have been converted into the number of males per 100 females. Cases where males outnumber females are referred to as high sex ratios and those where females outnumber males as low sex ratios.

Maternal nutrition. Experiments with laboratory mice have shown that the imposition of low fat diets reduces the number of males born and causes a decline in the birth sex ratio (Rivers & Crawford, 1974). The decline in this case was striking (from 101.5 : 100 in the control group to 32.2 : 100 in those maintained on a low fat diet) and highly significant. However a similar experiment with white-tailed deer (Verme, 1969) produced significant results in the opposite direction: in this case, prime-aged females maintained on a low plane of nutrition showed a birth sex ratio of 230 : 100 whereas animals maintained on a high plane of nutrition showed a ratio of 87.5 : 100 and tendencies for birth sex ratios to be inversely related to maternal nutrition have been found in other cervid populations (Verme, 1965; Robinette *et al.* 1973; McCullough, 1979) as well as in some other mammals (Mech, 1975; Sachdeva, Sengar, Singh & Lindahl, 1973).

*Weather.*After harsh winters, mule deer have been reported to produce fewer males than after mild ones (Robinette, Gashwiler, Jones & Crane, 1957) though differences were not significant. In contrast, studies of roe deer show an increase in sex ratios after hard winters (Borg, 1971) while, in red deer, no effects of weather on birth sex ratio are evident (Clutton-Brock *et al.*, 1981).

Maternal environment. Most attempts to compare foetal or birth sex ratios between populations of mammals living in different environments have been based on data sets too small either to show statistically significant differences or to provide a reliable indication that no difference was present. Both tendencies for populations showing high reproductive performance to show higher than average sex ratios and tendencies for them to show lower than average sex ratios have been recorded (Jones, Robinette & Julander, 1956; Robinette *et al.*, 1957; Brohn & Robb, 1955; Mech, 1975; Flook, 1970; Kittams, 1953). Among humans, statistically significant differences exist both between societies (Parkes, 1926) and between socio-economic classes (Teitelbaum, 1970, 1972; Rostron & James, 1977) but may be caused by variation in sexual behaviour (James, 1971).

Mother's age. In most natural mammalian populations, the body condition of females declines with increasing age (Sadleir, 1969; Clutton-Brock *et al.*, 1981). In several mammals the sex ratio of a female's progeny also tends to decline as she ages (dogs: Ludwig & Bost, 1951; roe deer: Borg, 1971; white tailed deer: Mangold, 1958; Verme, 1969: Dapson, Ramsey, Smith & Urbston, 1979; mule deer: Robinette *et al.*, 1957; wapiti: Flook, 1970; red deer: Lowe, 1969; Clutton-Brock *et al.*, 1981; cattle, pigs and horses: Kamaljan, 1962; humans: Teitelbaum, 1972; James, 1975; Rostron & James, 1977), though the majority of these results are not statistically significant (see Caughley, 1971). Some studies have also shown a tendency for sex ratios to increase towards the end of the mother's lifespan (mule deer: Robinette *et al.*, 1957; cattle, pigs and horses: Kamaljan, 1962; red deer: Lowe, 1969; humans: Hylton & Leitch, 1964; Teitelbaum, Mantel & Stark, 1971).

Maternal dominance. In wild populations of yellow baboons (Altmann, 1980) and captive groups of rhesus and bonnet macaques (M.J.A. Simpson & A.E. Simpson, unpublished data; Silk, Samuels & Rodman, 1980) dominant females produce significantly more daughters than subordinates. This difference has been interpreted as adaptive (Altmann, 1980): since mothers and daughters assist each other in competitive encounters and daughters (but not sons) inherit their mother's rank, it may be advantageous for dominant mothers to produce more daughters than subordinates – though, under these conditions, subordinate females might be expected to produce no daughters at all. An alternative explanation is that subordinate mothers carrying female foetuses are particularly likely to lose their infants as a consequence of harassment by other group members (see p. 230).

Mother's previous reproductive status. In mammals where all females do not breed every year, body condition at the time of conception is usually poorer among mothers that bred successfully in the previous season compared with those that did not. Several studies have compared foetal sex ratios between these two categories: in a sample of two-year-old mule deer, first breeders showed significantly higher sex ratios (194 : 100, $n = 50$) than females that had bred previously (78 : 100, $n = 132$; Robinette *et al.*, 1957). In contrast, in larger samples of wapiti and red deer, differences tended in the opposite direction (wapiti: 112.5 : 100 in lactating females versus 107 : 100 in non-lactating females, $n = 238, 199$ (Flook, 1970); red deer: 182 : 100 in lactating females versus 137 : 100 in non-lactating females, $n = 79, 192$ (Miller, 1932)).

Sex of previous offspring. On the grounds that a mother's potential for investment is likely to be similar from one conception to another, Williams (1979) predicts that the sex ratio of successive births should be positively correlated. However, where the costs of rearing one sex exceed those of rearing the other, a negative correlation between the sex ratio of successive offspring might be expected. There are few samples of data for which the sexes of consecutive offspring are known. Results for humans are conflicting (see Edwards, 1966; Greenberg & White, 1967) and may be affected by cultural differences. In wild red deer there is no evidence of any association between the sex of consecutive progeny (Clutton-Brock *et al.*, in 1981) but in one population of chimpanzees a significant tendency for consecutive offspring to alternate in sex has been found (C. Tutin, unpublished data).

Date of birth. In at least three species of seals (grey seals, Weddell seals and Australian fur seals) there is a strongly significant tendency for males to be born (and, presumably, conceived) earlier than females, with the effect that birth sex ratio declines during the course of the breeding season (Coulson & Hickling, 1961; Boyd & Campbell, 1971; Stirling, 1971*a*, *b*). Similar, though less pronounced, trends have been found in red deer (Clutton-Brock *et al.*, 1981), whales (R.L. Trivers, R. Seger & H. Hare, unpublished) and bats (Fisler, 1971).

Litter size. Mothers that produce large litters can presumably afford to invest less heavily in each offspring. In dogs (Ludwig & Bost, 1951), mink

(Apelgren, 1941; Enders, 1952), mule deer (Robinette *et al.*, 1957), white-tailed deer (Mangold, 1958; Verme, 1969), horses (Platt, 1978), common marmosets (Herschkowitz, 1977) and humans (Scheinfeld, 1943) the highest sex ratios are found in the smallest litters, though most samples do not show statistically significant differences. No obvious trend is apparent among roe deer (Borg, 1971) or cotton-top tamarins (Herschkowitz, 1977).

Timing of fertilisation. Studies of humans suggest that sex ratios may be influenced by the timing of fertilisation relative to ovulation. The sex ratio is higher when natural insemination occurs three or more days before ovulation compared to when it occurs at or after ovulation (Guerrero, 1974, 1975). In contrast, experiments with white-tailed deer suggest that inseminations substantially before ovulation tend to produce low sex ratios: animals mated late in their oestrous period produced more males than those mated early (Verme & Ozoga, 1981). The mechanism underlying these results is not known, though it could involve differential motility of X- and Y-bearing sperm (Roberts, 1972, 1978).

Is such variation adaptive?

With the data currently available, it is impossible to determine whether or not particular examples of sex ratio variation in mammals are adaptive. It is conceivable that most intraspecific differences in birth sex ratios are caused by physiological mechanisms which are either resistant to evolutionary change or are maintained by selection for some other attribute, and which affect the sex ratio at conception or influence survival during gestation. For example, male foetuses and neonates may be less likely to survive very stressful environments – both on account of the effects of their unguarded X chromosome (see Haldane, 1922; Craft, 1938; Myers, 1978) and because sexual selection favours faster growth rates and higher metabolic rates in males than females (see Latham, 1947; Lack, 1954; Ralls, Brownell & Ballou, 1980; Clutton-Brock *et al.*, 1982) – and this could explain why birth sex ratios in harsh environments are sometimes female-biased. Alternatively, such mechanisms may, themselves, be consequences of selection favouring the ability of parents to manipulate the sex ratio of their offspring and the majority of observed trends may be adaptive.

Since virtually all individual examples of sex ratio variation in mammals can be explained either under an adaptive hypothesis or under a non-adaptive one, firm evidence of adaptation must rely on the confirmation of quantitative predications concerning the distribution of biased sex ratios (see, for example, Trivers & Hare, 1976). Such predictions will need to be based on accurate knowledge of the factors affecting the parent's ability to invest and of the consequences of investment for their offspring. At present, this information is scarce and definite predictions can seldom be made. For example, the common suggestion that mothers should produce relatively more sons in their prime years would be reversed either if old mothers proved to invest more heavily than prime ones because their reproductive value was low (see Clutton-Brock *et al.*, 1981) or if investment influenced the survival or reproductive success of daughters more than of sons (see p. 230). In these circumstances, little reliance can be placed on post-hoc explanations of particular examples of biased sex ratios.

Is total investment divided equally between male and female progeny?

In that the numbers of sons and daughters produced by most mammals are approximately equal, the available evidence conforms to Fisher's prediction that parents should divide their investment equally between their male and female progeny. However, his hypothesis has two more specific predictions: (1) that where mortality rates are particularly high in one sex during the period of parental investment, the sex ratio at the start of investment should be biased towards that sex; (2) that where offspring of one sex cost more to produce (either because they are more likely to die during the period of investment or because parents invest more heavily in them) sex ratios at the end of the period of investment should be biased against the more expensive sex.

Comparisons of data from different mammalian species provide some support for the first prediction. Across three species of whales (humpback, blue and fin), analysis of large data sets shows that the degree of male bias in foetal ratios is related to the degree of differential male mortality (R.L. Trivers, J. Seger and H. Hare, unpublished). In addition, the highest foetal ratios tend to be found in mammal species showing the biggest difference in sex ratios between foetal and birth samples (Clutton-Brock & Albon, in preparation). However, both results should be regarded with some scepticism because of the possibility that systematic sexing errors can lead to inflated foetal ratios and, in the second case, the danger that variation in the age at which foetal ratios were collected could have contributed to the correlation.

Data to provide a conclusive test of the second prediction are currently unavailable. In neither of the two species where increased investment in individual sons is implicated does the weaning sex ratio show any evidence of being female-biased (see Table 11.2). In red deer, as we have already argued, this may be because the total costs of producing females equal or exceed those of producing males as a result of post-weaning investment in daughters. In elephant seals, this seems unlikely and some constraint on adaptation may be involved. As Maynard Smith (1980) has shown, if conception sex ratios were immutably fixed at unity, subsequent alteration through differential mortality was selected against, and increased investment in individuals of one sex was favoured, heavier total investment in the same sex would be expected. But, as we have argued above, there are no conclusive grounds for believing that conception ratios are immutably fixed, while some evidence suggests that adaptive modification of sex ratios can occur after conception. Further studies are clearly necessary.

Conclusions

The most obvious conclusion to be drawn from this survey of parental investment in mammals is that the problems are more complex than is generally realized and relevant data are sparse. No conclusive answers can yet be given to any of the three questions we have examined. As would be predicted, mothers invest more in sons prior to weaning in some polygynous species but this trend may be reversed in others and the situation is complicated by the possibility of increased post-weaning investment in daughters. Within species, birth sex ratios appear to vary in relation to environmental factors – but effects apparently differ between species and cannot easily be accommodated with a single adaptive explanation. Finally, in neither of the two cases where males apparently cost more to rear is the weaning sex ratio female-biased, though, in one of these, investment in daughters but not in sons may continue after weaning.

Table 11.2. *Sex ratios at birth and weaning in two polygynous mammals (males per 100 females)*

	Birth	12 months (approx. 6 months post weaning)
Red deer (from Clutton-Brock *et al.*, 1981)	132 *n* = 423	115 296
	Birth	1 month (shortly after weaning)
Northern elephant seal (Le Boeuf & Briggs, 1977)	107 *n* = 2396	105 2052

Nevertheless, enticing glimpses of potentially adaptive effects suggest that further research may well be rewarding. In particular, it would be valuable to examine the costs of producing males in species, like elephant seals, where post-weaning investment can be firmly excluded. Further attempts are also needed to measure the costs to mothers of post-weaning investment in daughters in species which form matrilineal social groups – while investment in male and female offspring by fathers has yet to be examined.

To determine whether or not patterns of sex-ratio variation are adaptive, future studies will need to test specific hypotheses, use larger samples and validate the accuracy of their sexing techniques. In particular, it would be valuable to determine whether or not sex ratios early in gestation differ from unity in species which typically show imbalanced birth sex ratios.

Finally, underlying many of the problems we have discussed, is our current ignorance of the effects of parental investment on the reproductive success of male and female offspring. It is only through an understanding of these relationships – and of the extent to which they differ between species – that it will be possible to generate firm predictions concerning the allocation of parental investment to sons and daughters.

Summary

1. Current evolutionary theories predict that parents should invest more heavily in individual sons than daughters (either by allocating a greater proportion of their resources to individual sons or by producing relatively more male offspring at times when their own investment potential is high) but that they should adjust the sex ratio of their progeny so as to divide their total investment equally between their male and female progeny. This paper compares these predictions with the available evidence from studies of mammals.

2. In at least two polygynous mammals, mothers appear to invest more heavily in individual sons prior to weaning. However, in other species, pre-weaning investment may favour daughters – possibly because parental investment can have a stronger effect on the reproductive success of daughters than of sons where daughters inherit their mothers' rank.

3. Evidence that the sex ratio of progeny varies with the parents' ability to invest is inconclusive, though there are no conclusive reasons for believing that it cannot occur.

4. As evolutionary theory would predict, most parents produce ap-

proximately similar numbers of sons and daughters and there is some evidence that in species where sons are especially likely to die before the end of investment, birth sex ratios show a particularly strong male bias.

We should like to thank Dr Robin Dunbar, Dr Paul Harvey, Dr Richard Wrangham, Dr Dafila Scott, Professor R.V. Short, F.R.S., Professor John Maynard Smith, F.R.S., Dr C.R. Packer, Mr M. Reiss and Dr A. Carothers for advice, comments and criticism; Dr M. Gosling, Drs A. and M.J. Simpson for permission to quote unpublished results.

References

Altmann, J. (1980). *Baboon Mothers and Infants*. Harvard University Press: Cambridge, Massachusetts.

Apelgren, R. (1941). Kullstorleken och dräktighetstidens längd hos misk. *Vara Pälsdynr*, **12**, 349.

Arbuthnott, J. (1710). An argument for Divine Providence, taken from the Constant Regularity observed in the Births of both sexes. Quoted in *Philosophical Transactions of the Royal Society*, **27**, 186–90.

Asdell, S.A. (1964). *Patterns of Mammalian Reproduction*. 2nd edn. Cornell University Press.

Bar-Anan, R. & Robertson, A. (1975). Variation in sex ratio between progeny groups in dairy cattle. *Theoretical and Applied Genetics*, **46**, 63–5.

Beatty, R.A. (1970). Genetic basis for the determination of sex. *Philosophical Transactions of the Royal Society London*, B **259**, 3–13.

Benedict, F.G. (1938). *Vital Energetics: a Study in Comparative Basal Metabolism*. Carnegie Institute: Washington.

Bertram, B.C.R. (1975). Social factors influencing reproduction in wild lions. *Journal of Zoology, London*, **177**, 463–82.

Borg, K. (1971). *On Mortality and Reproduction of Roe Deer in Sweden during the Period 1948–1969*. Viltrevy: Stockholm.

Boyd, J.M. & Campbell, R.N. (1971). The grey seal (*Halichoerus grypus*) at North Rona 1959–68. *Journal of Zoology, London*, **164**, 469–512.

Brohn, A. & Robb, D. (1955). *Age Composition Weights, and Physical Characteristics of Missouri's deer, 1944–1951*. Missouri Conservation Commission, P-R Series No. 13, 28 pp.

Burfening, P.J. (1972). Parental and postnatal competition among twin lambs. *Animal Production*, **15**, 61–6.

Caughley, G. (1971). Offspring sex ratio and age of parents. *Journal of Reproduction and Fertility*, **25**, 145–7.

Chapman, A.B., Casida, L.E. & Cote, A. (1938). Sex ratios of fetal calves. *Proceedings of the American Society of Animal Production, 1938*, 303–4.

Charlesworth, B. (1977). Population genetics, demography and the sex ratio. In *Measuring Selection in Natural Populations*, ed. F.B. Christiansen & T.M. Fenchel, pp. 345–63. Springer-Verlag: Berlin.

Charnov, E.L. (1975). Sex ratio selection in an age-structured population. *Evolution*, **29**, 366–8.

Charnov, E.L. (1979). The genetical evolution of patterns of sexuality: Darwinian fitness. *American Naturalist*, **113**, 465–80.

Charnov, E.L., Hartogh, R.L.L., Jones, W.T. & van den Assem, J. (1981). Sex ratio evolution in a variable environment. *Nature*, **289**, 27–33.

Clark, A.B. (1978). Sex ratio and local resource competition in a prosimian primate. *Science*, **201**, 163–5.

Clutton-Brock, T.H. & Albon, S.D. (in preparation). Do mammalian sex ratios vary adaptively?

Clutton-Brock, T.H., Albon, S.D., Gibson, R.M. & Guinness, F.E. (1979). The logical stag: adaptive aspects of fighting in red deer (*Cervus elaphus* L.). *Animal Behaviour*, **27**, 211–25.

Clutton-Brock, T.H., Albon, S.D. & Guinness, F.E. (1981). Parental investment in male and female offspring in a polygynous mammal. *Nature*, (in press).

Clutton-Brock, T.H., Guinness, F.E. & Albon, S.D. (1982). *Red deer: the Behavior and Ecology of Two Sexes*. University of Chicago Press: Chicago.

Clutton-Brock, T.H., Harvey, P.H. & Rudder, B. (1977). Sexual dimorphism, socionomic sex ratio and body weight in primates. *Nature*, **269**, 797–9.

Cohen, J. (1975). Gamete redundancy – wastage or selection? In *Gamete Competition in Plants and Animals*, ed. D.L. Mulcahy, pp. 99–112. North-Holland Publishing: Amsterdam.

Cohen, J. & McNaughton, D.C. (1974). Spermatozoa: the probable selection of a small population by the genetical tract of the female rabit. *Journal of Reproduction and Fertility*, **39**, 297–310.

Coulson, J.C. & Hickling, G. (1961). Variation in the secondary sex-ratio of the grey seal *Halichoerus grypus* during the breeding season. *Nature*, **190**, 281.

Coulson, J.C. & Hickling, G. (1964). The breeding biology of the grey seal *Halichoerus grypus* on the Farne Islands, Northumberland. *Journal of Animal Ecology*, **33**, 485–512.

Craft, W.A. (1938). The sex ratio in mules and other hybrid mammals. *Quarterly Review of Biology*, **13**, 19–40.

Crow, J. & Kimura, M. (1970). *An Introduction to Population Genetics Theory*. Harper & Row: New York.

Dapson, R.W., Ramsey, P.R., Smith, M.H. & Urbston, D.F. (1979). Demographic differences in contiguous populations of white-tailed deer. *Journal of Wildlife Management*, **43**, 889–98.

Darwin, C. (1871). *The Descent of Man and Selection in Relation to Sex*, 1888 edn. John Murray: London.

Defries, J.C., Touchberry, R.W. & Hays, R.L. (1959). Heritability of the length of the gestation period in dairy cattle. *Journal of Dairy Science*, **42**, 598–606.

Dhillon, J.S., Acharya, R.M., Tiwana, M.S. & Aggarwal, S.C. (1970). Factors affecting the interval between calving and conception in Hariana cattle. *Animal Production*, **12**, 81–7.

Dittus, W.P.J. (1977). The social regulation of population density and age-sex distribution in the Toque monkey. *Behaviour*, **63**, 281–322.

Dittus, W.P.J. (1979). The revolution of behaviour, regulating density and age-specific sex ratios in a primate population. *Behaviour*, **69**, 265–301.

Edwards, A.W.F. (1966). Sex ratio data analysed independently of family limitation. *Annals of Human Genetics, London*, **29**, 337–47.

Enders, R.J. (1952). Reproduction in the mink *Mustella vison*. *Proceedings of the American Philosophical Society*, **96**, 691–755.

Eshel, I. (1975). Selection on sex ratio and the evolution of sex-determination. *Heredity*, **34**, 351–61.

Fechheimer, N.S. & Beatty, R.A. (1974). Chromosome abnormalities and sex ratio in rabbit blastocysts. *Journal of Reproduction and Fertility*, **37**, 331–41.

Fisher, R.A. (1930). *The Genetical Theory of Natural Selection*. Oxford University Press: Oxford.

Fisler, G.F. (1971). Age structure and sex ratio in populations of *Reithrodontomys*. *Journal of Mammalogy*, **52**, 653–62.

Flook, D.R. (1970). A study of sex differential in the survival of Wapiti. *Canadian Wildlife Service Reports*, Series No. 11.

Fraser, D. & Morley-Jones, R. (1975). The 'teat order' of suckling pigs. I. Relation to birth weight and subsequent growth. *Journal of Agricultural Science, Cambridge*, **84**, 387–91.

Fredga, K., Gropp, A., Winking, H. & Frank, F. (1977). A hypothesis explaining the exceptional sex ratio in the wood lemming (*Myopus schistocolar*). *Hereditas*, **85**, 101–4.

Geist, V. (1971). *Mountain Sheep: A Study in Behaviour and Evolution*. University of Chicago Press: Chicago.

Gibson, R.M. & Guinness, F.E. (1980). Differential reproductive success in red deer stags. *Journal of Animal Ecology*, **49**, 199–208.

Gini, C. (1951). Combinations and sequences of sexes in human families and mammalian litters. *Acta Genetica et Statistica Medica*, **2**, 220–44.

Glucksman, A. (1974). Sexual dimorphism in mammals. *Biological Reviews*, **49**, 423–75.

Gosling, L.M. & Petrie, M. (1981). The economics of social organisation. In *Physiological Ecology: an Evolutionary Approach*, ed. P. Calow & C.R. Townsend. Blackwells: Oxford. (In press.)

Greenberg, R.A. & White, C. (1967). The sexes of consecutive sibs in human sibships. *Human Biology*, **39**, 374–404.

Greenwood, P.J. (1980). Mating systems, philopatry and dispersal in birds and mammals. *Animal Behaviour*, **28**, 1140–62.

Guerrero, R. (1974). Association of the type and time of insemination within the menstrual cycle with the human sex ratio at birth. *New England Journal of Medicine*, **29**, 10–56.

Guerrero, R. (1975). Type and time of insemination within the menstrual cycle and the human sex ratio at birth. *Studies in Family Planning*, **6**, 367–71.

Guinness, F.E., Albon, S.D. & Clutton-Brock, T.H. (1978). Factors affecting reproduction in red deer (*Cervus elaphus*) hinds on Rhum. *Journal of Reproduction and Fertility*, **54**, 325–34.

Guinness, F.E., Clutton-Brock, T.H. & Albon, S.D. (1978). Factors affecting calf mortality in red deer. *Journal of Animal Ecology*, **47**, 817–32.

Gunn, R.G. (1964a). Levels of first winter feeding in relation to performance in Cheviot Hill ewes. I. Body growth and development during treatment period. *Journal of Agricultural Science, Cambridge*, **62**, 99–122.

Gunn, R.G. (1964b). Levels of first winter feeding in relation to performance of Cheviot Hill ewes. II. Body growth and development during the summer after treatment. *Journal of Agricultural Science, Cambridge*, **62**, 123–49.

Gunn, R.G. (1965). Levels of first winter feeding in relation to performance of Cheviot Hill ewes. III. Tissue and joint development to 12–18 months of age. *Journal of Agricultural Science, Cambridge*, **64**, 311–21.

Gunn, R.G. (1967). Levels of first winter feeding in relation to performance in Cheviot Hill ewes. IV. Body growth and development from 18 months to maturity. *Journal of Agricultural Science, Cambridge*, **69**, 341–4.

Haldane, J.B.S. (1922). Sex ratio and unisexual sterility in hybrid animals. *Journal of Genetics*, **12**, 101–9.

Hamilton, W.D. (1967). Extraordinary sex ratios. *Science*, **156**, 477–88.

Hamilton, W.D. (1971). Geometry of the selfish herd. *Journal of Theoretical Biology*, **31**, 295–311.

Harlap, S. (1979). Gender of infants conceived on different days of the menstrual cycle. *New England Journal of Medicine*, **300**, 1445–8.

Harrison, J.L. (1955). Data on the reproduction of some Malayan mammals. *Proceedings of the Zoological Society, London*, **125**(2), 445–60.

Hasler, J.F. & Banks, E.M. (1975). Reproductive performance and growth in captive collared lemmings (*Dicrostonyx groenlandicus*). *Canadian Journal of Zoology*, **53**,

777–87.

Henning, W.L. (1939). Prenatal and postnatal sex ratios in sheep. *Journal of Agricultural Research*, **58**, 560–80.

Herschkowitz, P. (1977). *Living New World Monkeys 1*. University of Chicago Press: Chicago.

Hylton, F.E. & Leitch, R.I. (1964). *The Physiology of Human Pregnancy*. Blackwells: Oxford.

James, W.H. (1971). Cycle day of insemination, coital rate and sex ratio. *Lancet*, (1), 112.

James, W.H. (1975). The distributions of the combinations of the sexes in mammalian litters. *Genetical Research*, **26**, 45–53.

Jones, D.A., Robinette, W.L. & Julander, O. (1956). Influence of summer range conditions on mule deer reproduction in Utah. Paper presented at *3rd Annual Conference of Western Association*, 8 pp. State Game & Fisheries Commissioners: Vancouver.

Kamaljan, V.S. (1962). The effect of parental age on the sex ratio of offspring. *Zhurnal Obshcheĭ Biologii*, **23**, 455.

Kaufman, M.H. (1973). Analysis of the first cleavage division to determine the sex ratio and incidence of chromosome anomalies at conception in the mouse. *Journal of Reproduction and Fertility*, **35**, 67–72.

Keller, C.A. (1969). *Embryonal Sex Ratios of Animals and Man*. Ph.D. thesis, University of California, Berkeley.

Kittams, W.H. (1953). Reproduction of Yellowstone elk. *Journal of Wildlife Management*, **17**, 177–83.

Krebs, C.J. & Cowan, I.McT. (1962). Growth studies of reindeer fawns. *Canadian Journal of Zoology*, **40**, 863–9.

Kurland, J.A. (1977). Kin selection in the Japanese monkey. *Contributions to Primatology*, **12**, 1–145.

Lack, D. (1954). *The Natural Regulation of Animal Numbers*. Oxford University Press: Oxford.

Latham, R.M. (1947). Differential ability of male and female game birds to withstand starvation and climatic extremes. *Journal of Wildlife Management*, **11**, 139–49.

Le Boeuf, B.J. (1972). Sexual behaviour in the northern elephant seal, *Mirounga angustirostris*. *Behaviour*, **41**, 1–26.

Le Boeuf, B.J. (1974). Male–male competition and reproductive success in elephant seals. *American Zoologist*, **14**, 163–76.

Le Boeuf, J.L. & Briggs, K.T. (1977). The cost of living in a seal harem. *Mammalia*, **41**, 169–95.

Leigh, E.G. (1970). Sex ratio and differential mortality between the sexes. *American Naturalist*, **104**, 205–10.

Lockie, J.D. (1966). Territory and small carnivores. *Symposium of the Zoological Society, London*, **18**, 143–65.

Loudon, A.S.I. (1979). *Social Behaviour and Habitat in Roe Deer (Capreolus capreolus)*. Unpublished Ph.D. thesis, University of Edinburgh.

Lowe, V.P.W. (1969). Population dynamics of the red deer (*Cervus elaphus* L.) on Rhum. *Journal of Animal Ecology*, **38**, 425–57.

Ludwig, W. & Bost, C. (1951). Über Bezietngen zwischen Elternalten, Wurfegrösse und Geschlechsverhättnis bei Hunden. *Zeitschrift für Induktive Abstammungs- und Vererbungslehre*, **83**, 383.

MacArthur, R.H. (1965). Ecological consequences of natural selection. In *Theoretical and Mathematical Biology*, ed. T. Waterman & H. Morowitz, pp. 388–97. Blaisdell: New York.

Mackintosh, N.A. (1942). The southern stocks of whalebone whales. *Discovery Reports*, **22**, 197–300.

Mangold, R.E. (1958). A report on the age and sex of deer killed in the Harbowton area. *New Jersey Outdoors*, **9**, 2–11.

Maynard Smith, J. (1978). *The Evolution of Sex*. Cambridge University Press: Cambridge.

Maynard Smith, J. (1980). A new theory of sexual investment. *Behavioural Ecology and Sociobiology*, **7**, 247–51.

McClure, P.A. (1981). Sex-biased litter reduction in food-restricted woodrats (*Neotama floridana*). *Science* (in press).

McCullough, D.R. (1979). *The George Reserve Deer Herd: Population Ecology of a K-selected species*. University of Michigan Press: Ann Arbor.

McEwan, E.H. (1968). Growth and development of barren ground caribou. II. Postnatal growth rates. *Canadian Journal of Zoology*, **46**, 1023–9.

McEwen, E.H. & Whitehead, P.E. (1971). Measurement of the milk intake of reindeer and caribou calves using tritiated water. *Canadian Journal of Zoology*, **49**, 443–7.

McEwen, E.H. & Whitehead, P.E. (1972). Reproduction in female reindeer and caribou. *Canadian Journal of Zoology*, **50**, 43–6.

McMillen, M.M. (1979). Differential mortality by sex in fetal and neonatal deaths. *Science*, **204**, 89–91.

Mech, L.D. (1975). Disproportionate sex ratios of wolf pups. *Journal of Wildlife Management*, **39**, 737–40.

Miller, W.C. (1932). A preliminary note upon the sex ratio of Scottish red deer. *Proceedings of the Royal Physiological Society, Edinburgh*, **22**, 99–101.

Mitchell, B. & Brown, D. (1974). The effects of age and body size on fertility in female red deer (*Cervus elaphus* L.). *Proceedings of the International Congress of Game Biology*, **11**, 89–98.

Mitchell, B. & Lincoln, G.A. (1973). Conception dates in relation to age and condition in two populations of red deer in Scotland. *Journal of Zoology, London*, **171**, 141–52.

Mitchell, B., McCowan, D. & Nicholson, I.A. (1976). Annual cycles of body weight and condition in Scottish red deer. *Journal of Zoology, London*, **180**, 107–27.

Morrison, F.B. (1948). *Feeds and Feeding*. 21st edn. Morrison Publishing: Ithaca, New York. 1207 pp.

Myers, J.H. (1978). Sex-ratio adjustment under food stress: maximisation of quality or numbers of offspring. *American Naturalist*, **112**, 381–8.

Myers, J.H. & Krebs, C.J. (1971). Sex ratios in open and enclosed vole populations: demographic implications. *American Naturalist*, **105**, 325–44.

Nordan, H.C., Cowan, I.McT. & Wood, A.J. (1970). The feed intake and heat production of the young black-tailed deer (*Odocoileus hemionus columbianus*). *Canadian Journal of Zoology*, **48**, 275–82.

Nowosad, R.F. (1975). Reindeer survival in the Mackenzie delta herd, birth to 4 months. *Proceedings of the 1st International Reindeer/Caribou Symposium, Biological Papers, University of Alaska*. Special Report No. 1, 199–208.

Ohsumi, S. (1965). Reproduction of the sperm whale in the N.W. Pacific. *Scientific Reports of the Whaling Research Institute, Tokyo*, **17**, 1–35.

Parkes, A.S. (1926). The mammalian sex-ratio. *Biological Reviews*, **2**, 1–51.

Platt, H. (1978). *A Survey of Perinatal Mortality and Disorders in the Thoroughbred*. Publication of the Animal Health Trust.

Pond, C.M. (1977). The significance of lactation in the evolution of mammals. *Evolution*, **31**, 177–99.

Ralls, K., Brownell, R.C. & Ballon, J. (1980). Differential mortality by sex and age in mammals with specific reference to sperm whales. *Reports of the International Whaling Commission*, **2**, 233–43.

Reiter, J., Stinson, N.L. & Le Boeuf, B.J. (1978). Northern elephant seal development: the transition from weaning to nutritional development. *Behavioural Ecology and Socio-*

biology, **3**, 337–67.

Rivers, J.P.W. & Crawford, M.A. (1974). Maternal nutrition and the sex ratio at birth. *Nature*, **252**, 297–8.

Robbins, C.T. & Moen, A.N.M. (1975). Milk consumption and weight gain of white-tailed deer. *Journal of Wildlife Management*, **39**, 355–60.

Roberts, A.M. (1972). Gravitational separation of x and y spermatozoa. *Nature*, **238**, 223–5.

Roberts, A.M. (1978). The origins of fluctuations in the human secondary sex ratio. *Journal of Biosocial Science*, **10**, 169–82.

Robinette, W.L., Baer, C.H., Pillmore, R.E. & Knittle, C.E. (1973). Effects of nutritional change on captive mule deer. *Journal of Wildlife Management*, **37**, 312–26.

Robinette, W.L., Gashwiler, J.S., Jones, D.A. & Crane, H.S. (1955). Fertility of mule deer in Utah. *Journal of Wildlife Management*, **19**, 115–36.

Robinette, W.L., Gashwiler, J.S., Low, J.B. & Jones, D.A. (1957). Differential mortality by sex and age among mule deer. *Journal of Wildlife Management* **21**, 1–16.

Rostron, J. & James, W.H. (1977). Maternal age, parity, social class and sex ratio. *Annals of Human Genetics, London*, **41**, 205–17.

Russell, W.S. (1976). The effects of twin birth on the growth of cattle. *Animal Production*, **22**, 167–73.

Sachdeva, K.K., Sengar, O.P.S., Singh, N. & Lindahl, I.L. (1973). Studies on goats: 1: Effect of plane of nutrition on the reproductive performance of does. *Journal of Agricultural Science, Cambridge*, **80**, 375–9.

Sackett, G.P., Holm, R.A., Davis, A.E. & Farenbuch, C.E. (1975). Prematurity and low birth weight in pigtail macaques: incidence, prediction, and effects on infant development. In *Symposium of the 5th Congress of International Primate Society*, ed. S. Kondo, M. Kawai, E. Ehara & S. Kawamura, pp. 189–205. Japan Science Press: Tokyo.

Sadleir, R.M.F.S. (1969). *The Ecology of Reproduction in Wild and Domestic Mammals*. Methuen: London.

Scheinfeld, A. (1943). Factors influencing the sex ratio. *Human Fertility*, **8**, 33–42.

Schinkel, P.G. & Short, B.F. (1961). The influence of nutritional level during pre-natal and early post-natal life on adult fleece and body characteristics. *Australia Journal of Agricultural Research*, **12**, 176–202.

Short, C. (1970). Morphological development and ageing of mules and white-tailed deer fetuses. *Journal of Wildlife Management*, **34**, 383–8.

Silk, J.B., Samuels, A. & Rodman, P.S. (1980). Rank, reproductive success, and skewed sex ratio in *Macaca radiata*. *American Journal of Physical Anthropology*, **52**, 279.

Simpson, M.J.A., Simpson, A.E., Hooley, J. & Zunz, M. (1981). Infant related influences on inter-birth intervals in rhesus monkeys. *Nature* (in press).

Singh, O.N., Singh, R.N. & Srivastava, R.R.P. (1965). Study in post-partum interval to first service in Tharparkar cattle. *Indian Journal of Veterinary Science*, **35**, 245–8. I.U.C.N.: Morges, Switzerland.

Sowls, L.K. (1974). Social behaviour of the collared peccary *Dicotyles tajacu*. In *The Behaviour of Ungulates and its Relation to Management*, ed. V. Geist & F. Walther, pp. 144–65.

Staines, B.W. & Crisp, J.M. (1978). Observations on food quality in Scottish red deer (*Cervus elaphus*) as determined by chemical analysis of the rumen contents. *Journal of Zoology, London*, **185**, 253–9.

Stirling, I. (1971*a*). Studies on the behaviour of the South Australian fur seal, *Arctocephalus forsteri* II. Adult females and pups. *Australian Journal of Zoology*, **19**, 267–73.

Stirling, I. (1971*b*). Variation in sex ratio of newborn Weddell seals during the pupping season. *Journal of Mammalogy*, **52**, 842–4.

Taber, R.D. (1953). The secondary sex ratio in *Odocoileus*. *Journal of Wildlife Management*, **17**, 95–7.

Taylor, P.D. & Sauer, A. (1980). The selective advantage of sex ratio homeostasis. *American Naturalist*, **116**, 305–10.

Teitelbaum, M.S. (1970). Factors affecting the sex ratio in large populations. *Journal of Biosocial Science, Supplement*, **2**, 61–71.

Teitelbaum, M.S. (1972). Factors associated with the sex ratio in human populations. In *The Structure of Human Populations*, ed. G.A. Harrison & A.J. Boyce, pp. 90–109. Clarendon Press: Oxford.

Teitelbaum, M.S., Mantel, N. & Stark, C. (1971). Limited dependence of the human sex ratio on birth order and parental ages. *American Journal of Human Genetics*, **23**, 271–80.

Trivers, R.L. (1972). Parental investment and sexual selection. In *Sexual Selection and the Descent of Man*, ed. B. Campbell, pp. 136–79. Aldine: Chicago.

Trivers, R.L. & Hare, H. (1976). Haplodiploidy and the evolution of the social insects. *Science*, **191**, 249–63.

Trivers, R.L. & Willard, D.E. (1973). Natural selection of parental ability to vary the sex ratio. *Science*, **179**, 90–2.

Verme, L.J. (1965). Reproduction studies on penned white-tailed deer. *Journal of Wildlife Management*, **29**, 74–9.

Verme, L.J. (1969). Reproductive patterns of white-tailed deer related to nutritional plane. *Journal of Wildlife Management*, **33**, 881–7.

Verme, L.J. & Ozoga, J.J. (1981). Influence of temporal relationships during oestrus on deer sex ratio. *Journal of Wildlife Management* (in press).

Verner, J. (1965). Selection for sex ratio. *American Naturalist*, **99**, 419–21.

Vickers, A.D. (1967). A direct measurement of the sex-ratio in mouse blastocysts. *Journal of Reproduction and Fertility*, **13**, 375–6.

Vickers, A.D. (1969). Delayed fertilization and the prenatal sex-ratio of the mouse. *Journal of Reproduction and Fertility*, **13**, 375–6.

Vickers, A.D. (1969). Delayed fertilization and the prenatal sex-ratio of the mouse. *Journal of Reproduction and Fertility*, **20**, 63–8.

Watson, A. & Staines, B.W. (1978). Differences in the quality of wintering areas used by male and female red deer (*Cervus elaphus*) in Aberdeenshire. *Journal of Zoology, London*, **286**, 544–50.

Weir, J.A. (1962). Hereditary and environmental influences on the sex ratio of PHH and PHL mice. *Genetics*, **47**, 881–97.

Weisner, B.P. & Sheard, N.M. (1935). The duration of life in an albino rat population. *Proceedings of the Royal Society, Edinburgh*, **55**, 1–22.

Williams, G.C. (1979). The question of adaptive sex ratio in outcrossed vertebrates. *Proceedings of the Royal Society, London*, B **205**, 567–80.

Wilson, V.J. & Kerr, M.A. (1969). Brief notes on reproduction in steenbok *Raphicerus campestris*, Thunberg. *Arnoldia*, **5**(23), 1–5.

Wrangham, W.R. (1980). An ecological model of female-bonded primate groups. *Behaviour*, **75**, 262–99.

IV

Sociality

Edited by
BRIAN C.R. BERTRAM

The three chapters in this section all deal with relationships within societies, between individuals who provide assistance for one another. The emphasis is on societies which are long-lived and in which individuals have opportunities to interact repeatedly. In these circumstances an extra level of complexity is introduced, which becomes the more apparent as we progress through the chapters and roughly up the phylogenetic tree.

The concept of altruism crops up repeatedly here, as it does widely elsewhere in this book and in sociobiology in general. Bertram's chapter reveals a wide and apparently accidental divergence in the ways in which altruism has been defined, and proposes and attempts to justify a much more explicit definition. He considers that this clarification of the definition is required before it is practicable to understand the evolutionary maintenance of altruistic behaviour in particular circumstances. Maynard Smith in chapter 2 (this volume) emphasised kin selection and explored models of its role in the evolution of altruism. Bertram emphasises the combined action of different selection pressures in favouring altruistic behaviour in the examples he quotes.

Some altruistic acts may have negligible cost, and some are quickly repaid by a reciprocally altruistic act. Both could almost be considered to be mutualistic rather than altruistic. In chapter 13, Wrangham explores the topic of mutualism which in close-knit communities of animals interacting frequently with one another is likely to be of great importance. A mutualistic relationship may include a whole string of exchanges of altruistic acts, or in other cases it may consist of relatively short-term cooperative interactions. In either case both participants in the mutualistic relationship benefit. Their gain may or may not be at the expense of other members of the species. Wrangham suggests that the distribution of resources, whether food or mates, should determine whether or not the mutualism reduces the fitness of these conspecifics and hence should determine whether the species lives in groups of related individuals. On the whole it appears to.

The intertwining of altruism and mutualism becomes more complex as societies become more complex, and their interaction itself adds yet further layers of complexity. This interaction is well shown in Chagnon's chapter which is based on the study of a human culture, that of the Yanomamö Indians. Chagnon shows that kinship is of tremendous importance and interest in this society, particularly because of its influence on the number of allies an individual can muster. Human beings are clearly able to comprehend a great deal of kinship information and to make use of it in interactions with other humans, even manipulating it in certain circumstances to the advantage of themselves or their relatives. As human beings, we are uniquely well equipped to measure the advantages and costs of our actions. As sociobiologists we can see that altruism, mutualism and kin selection have all been involved together in the evolution of human societies. And we can see too that we are a far cry from the level of the genes and alleles discussed in the early chapters of this book.

12

Problems with altruism

BRIAN C.R. BERTRAM

Introduction

A lioness lies on her side and allows her companions' cubs as well as her own to suckle from her. A wild dog regurgitates food for another hungrier individual. A chaffinch seeing a hawk emits an alarm call which warns other chaffinches of danger. A worker honeybee stings an animal threatening its hive and dies as a result. In each case, the lioness, the wild dog, the chaffinch or the bee loses rather than benefits from its action while other individuals do benefit. Such actions come within the general category of altruistic behaviour.

In a human context, altruism means 'doing something for someone else' (Ruse, 1979) or 'unselfish regard for others' (Davies & Krebs, 1978). Dictionary definitions are similar but longer; for example the Oxford English Dictionary defines altruism as 'regard for others, as a principle of action; opposed to egoism or selfishness'. Chambers' English Dictionary defines it as 'the principle of living and acting for the interest of others'.

Animals in some circumstances help others, and rightly or wrongly in the past 15 years the term 'altruism' has become used to cover such behaviour. The term is now so widely applied that it is too late, even if it were considered desirable, to substitute a different word. Nonetheless, it is important to bear in mind that the phenomenon under consideration in this chapter is altruism *in its biological sense*, not in a moral or ethical sense nor as relevant to human beings.

Altruism in biology is of interest particularly because its evolution is not easy to explain. We understand the way in which natural selection has generally favoured the evolution of traits which cause the actor to leave more offspring but it is less clear how natural selection could favour traits which apparently are likely to cause him or her to leave fewer offspring.

Two main possible mechanisms have been proposed, which I will loosely label 'kin effects' and 'delayed benefits' and will discuss below.

The aim of this chapter is to clarify the general subject of altruism in biology, its definition, its causation, its effects, and associated problems which cannot be satisfactorily resolved.

Definition of altruism

Some of the problems in considering altruism have arisen because of surprisingly different definitions and therefore understandings of the term. In what follows I aim to draw attention to the current diversity of opinion as to what the term 'altruism' means and is taken to include, rather than to criticise these definitions. However, as a vehicle for doing this, I propose, and I justify below, the following definition:

'*Altruism in biology is defined as behaviour which is likely to increase the reproductive output of another member of the same species who is not a descendant of the actor, and which at least in the short term is likely also to reduce the number of the actor's own descendants.*'

The features of this definition, and some of the problems associated with this and other definitions of altruism, are the following:

Altruism in relation to human altruism

In general it is probably desirable for the concept of altruism in biology to be similar to that used for human beings. It is inevitable, and indeed it has already happened (e.g. Trivers, 1971; Wilson, 1978), that the principles postulated to be involved in the evolution of altruism in animals will be applied to humans. Unless there are good reasons to the contrary, the closer the definitions the better, since one would hope that less confusion should then arise.

Not benefiting other species

The recipient benefiting from the altruism must be a member of the same species as the altruist.

I do not want to say that a cow is indulging in altruism towards mosquitoes if it walks unnecessarily, expending energy but also leaving extra footprints in which more mosquitoes can breed. I do not want to say that a reed warbler (*Acrocephalus scirpaceus*) foster parent is behaving altruistically when it feeds a nest-parasitic cuckoo (*Cuculus canorus*). The fairly arbitrary reasons for my reluctance are threefold. First, the restriction is necessary to prevent the whole concept of altruism from becoming meaninglessly large: we would have to say that almost all animals were behaving altruistically to innumerable others almost all the time – witness the cow and the mosquitoes it helps. Second, the genes of members of two different species are not usually in reproductive competition with one another in nearly as direct a way as are those of members of a single species. And third, the concept of altruism as applied to human beings does not generally include being kind to animals – St. Francis of Assisi is rarely quoted as being a supreme altruist.

Interactions between species are of course of considerable interest, and the evolution of the cuckoo–foster parent relationship, for example, is certainly worthy of study (Lack, 1968). Nonetheless, to widen the concept of altruism to include such relationships is scarcely useful. Trivers (1971) gave as an example of altruism the restraint shown by the grouper (*Epinephelus striatus*) towards the wrasses (*Labroides dimidiatus*) which cleaned it and which it could have eaten; such an instance would not come within the definition of altruism used in this chapter. The definitions used by Wilson (1971, 1975), Alexander (1977), West Eberhard (1975), Lin & Michener (1972), and Emlen (1978) do not specifically exclude nor include the possibility of altruism towards other species. Ridley & Dawkins (1980) specifically include it.

Not benefiting offspring

Parental care is not included within the definition of altruism, or again the concept becomes so wide as to be almost useless.

In general it is easy to see how parental care has evolved, since the genes which contribute towards successful rearing of offspring are obviously likely to be passed on to those offspring. I accept that the behaviour involved when a wild dog (*Lycaon pictus*) regurgitates food is the same whether the recipient is her own offspring or another's; nonetheless, the evolution of caring for animals other than own offspring involves an extra complexity as will be discussed. I have excluded 'descendants' rather than excluding 'offspring' because the evolution of grandparental care is a straightforward (if rare) extension of parental care.

Even if parental care were not specifically excluded from the definition of altruism, in many cases it would not fall within it anyway. For an animal of a species which regularly produces only one litter of young in its lifetime, the parental care bestowed on those offspring would not reduce the number of that animal's future offspring or the total number of its descendants; thus there would be no 'cost' of the parental care, which would consequently not be considered to be an example of altruism. By contrast, an animal of a species which produced many successive litters might, by bestowing excessive parental care on the first, reduce the number or success of its future litters; it would thus be in a position to incur a cost, and therefore be eligible to be considered as at least partly altruistic. But an extra and unnecessary complication is introduced if the behaviour of parental care is, in some cases only, partly, but only partly, altruistic. The anomaly is best removed by excluding all parental care from being treated as altruism. This also corresponds with the general understanding of the meaning of altruism as applied to human behaviour – the self-sacrificing mother is labelled as maternal, not as altruistic.

Wilson's (1971) definition of altruism (p. 321) apparently includes parental care: 'Altruism is self-destructive behaviour performed for the benefit of others', where the self-destructive behaviour can range in intensity all the way from total bodily sacrifice to a slight diminishment of reproductive powers. It is commonplace in the responses of parents towards their young'. Trivers' (1971) definition specifically excludes all close relatives (including offspring) as recipients: 'Altruistic behaviour can be defined as behaviour that benefits another organism, not closely related, while being apparently detrimental to the organism performing the behaviour, benefit and detriment being defined in terms of contribution to inclusive fitness'. The definitions of Wilson (1975) and of Emlen (1978) are not explicit on this point but probably could include parental behaviour in some cases. I accept that 'parental care is only a special case of caring for close relatives' (Dawkins, 1979), yet it is a special case.

Other relatives may benefit

The recipient of the altruistic act may be a close relative other than a descendant. One mechanism by which altruism benefiting close relatives can evolve has been elaborated by Hamilton (1963, 1964) and others (Maynard Smith, 1964; Dawkins, 1976). It is the process often known as kin selection which is discussed further below. Other mechanisms may also be important too.

I include as altruistic the caring for close relatives, but not the caring for own offspring. Otherwise, because some relatives are closer than others, we would have to draw a completely arbitrary line somewhere, on no logical basis in principle and usually with no way in practice of determining on which side of this arbitrary relatedness figure a recipient of altruism lay. The offspring/not-offspring division is completely clear in principle and usually in practice. The relative/non-relative boundary line cannot be defined clearly in the same way.

Only Trivers' (1971) definition of altruism (in 'Not benefiting offspring' above) excludes close relatives, but does not try to specify how close. The other definitions of altruism already referred to would include the caring for relatives who are not descendants. So does the customary use of the term as applied to human altruism.

Not an explanation

The definition of altruism should be distinct from the explanation of how it may have evolved. This is particularly the case when, as discussed below, there are a number of different possible mechanisms involved. To incorporate an explanation of the phenomenon into the definition of it is to risk circularity and to invite further problems of definition later when our explanation turns out to be inadequate.

The definition by Alexander (1977, p. 294) incorporates an explanation – 'Altruism ... may be described as phenotypically (or self) sacrificing but genotypically selfish' – which we may not want to accept in all cases. Similarly, Lin & Michener (1972, p. 133) define altruism as 'activity that promotes the perpetration of an individual's genes ... not directly ... but via another individual'. Suppose however that we find instances of apparently altruistic activity which do *not* promote the perpetration of an individual's genes. We would not want to have to say that they were not examples of altruism after all merely because our explanation of them was faulty.

Time scale and net cost

The donor of an altruistic act may benefit in the long term from his altruism – such cases are considered below. It may be only in the short term that there is an apparent drop in his probable reproductive output (as in the case of reciprocal altruism – Trivers, 1971), or it may be in the long term as well (as in some cases of altruism towards his kin). Thus in some cases there is a net cost to the donor in terms of his own fitness while in other cases there is not. The definition of altruism by Wilson (1975, p. 117) – 'When a person (or animal) increases the fitness of another at the expense of his own fitness, he can be said to have performed an act of altruism' – does not make clear whether the reduction in the altruist's fitness is a net reduction or any reduction. The same point applies to Emlen's (1978) definition (see below).

Currency of cost and benefit

The cost and benefit to the altruist and to the recipient respectively are measured in terms of the probable reproductive output of those individuals, not in terms of their inclusive fitness. The definition by Emlen (1978, p. 245) 'Altruism is here defined as any behaviour performed by an individual that benefits a recipient while incurring a cost to the donor' implies but does not specify that cost and benefit are to be measured in terms of reproductive output or fitness. Trivers' (1971) definition of altruism (in 'Not benefiting offspring' above) measures cost and benefit in terms of inclusive fitness, whereas Wilson's (1975) definition (see above) uses individual fitness.

Motive

The definition of altruism makes no reference to the motive of the altruist. To do so would raise considerable problems concerning the altruistic organism's mental capacity to experience such intentions; it would also make it impossible to recognize an altruistic act, for we cannot even question animals about their motives. None of the definitions of altruism in biology refers to the altruistic animal's motives, and it is in this way that they differ most importantly from the concept of altruism in human behaviour.

The definition I have given at the start of this section is more explicit than previous definitions in what it includes or excludes; therefore inevitably it is more cumbersome. It is basically in general agreement with previous definitions, but is contrary to certain aspects of some of them. This is a reflection of previous contradictions between definitions which passed either unnoticed or at least unremarked upon at the time of their formulation. Such large disparities have a number of unfortunate results. They cause great waste of time, they cause considerable mistrust of sociobiological concepts, and they make more difficult the more interesting task of trying to understand at an evolutionary level the existence of altruistic behaviour in animals.

Explanations of the evolutionary existence of altruism

There are four main ways of explaining how altruism (as defined above) in animals continues 'despite natural selection', i.e. despite the fact that by definition it apparently reduces the reproductive output of the altruist. Briefly these are the following. First, that because of the effects of the altruism on close relatives, the inclusive fitness of the altruist is increased. Second, that the reduction of the probable reproductive output of the altruist is only temporary and that he benefits at a later date. Third, that altruism is imposed on the altruist by the group in which he lives. And fourth, that some altruistic behaviour may be nonadaptive. I shall deal with each of these categories of explanation in turn, and will then consider some examples.

Effects on close relatives

Hamilton (1964) first demonstrated that altruistic behaviour among close relatives can be selected for by natural selection because the gene or genes responsible for the altruistic behaviour are likely to be present not only in the altruist's offspring but also in his close relatives. Altruistic genes will obviously be selected if the altruism they produce results in there being more of them in subsequent generations, regardless of whether they are in the bodies of the offspring of the altruist or in the bodies of the offspring of his relatives. They are less likely to be in the body of a relative the less closely related he or she is; therefore more extra distant relatives need to be produced to compensate for each of his own offspring which the altruist has foregone. The algebra of cost and benefit is simple (Hamilton, 1964; Wilson, 1975; Davies & Krebs, 1978). Altruistic genes will spread if $K > 1/r$, where K is the ratio of the recipient's benefit to the altruist's cost, and where r is the coefficient of relatedness between the altruist and the recipient; cost and benefit are measured in terms of individual fitness.

Changes in the frequency of a gene in the population due to the effects of that gene on the reproductive output of relatives (other than descendants) of the bearer of the gene are attributed to 'kin selection' (Maynard Smith, 1964). I do not wish to use the term except to connote that part of natural selection which operates by means of effects on relatives other than descendants.

Merely to demonstrate that in a particular context the altruist and the recipient are generally close relatives does not adequately explain the evolution of altruism in that context, for two main reasons. The first is that the way in which 'favours' (whether food, care, or protection) are distributed among descendants and other kin is extremely complicated, as discussed later. The second reason is that there may be other benefits to the altruist in these circumstances; such benefits will be discussed next.

Delayed benefit

There is a wide variety of ways in which an altruist may reap a reproductive benefit from, but long after, his altruistic act. The range of such delayed benefits have been examined particularly in the case of bird species in which nest helpers occur (Emlen, 1978); the altruism in these cases usually consists not of a single altruistic act but of forsaking reproduction for a season and instead playing a large part in caring for nestlings.

The altruist may benefit later by: (a) gaining such valuable experience of the breeding process that his own reproduction, although delayed and therefore presumably shortened, will be more successful (Brown, 1974); (b) developing social bonds which enable the altruist later to find other individuals who will accept him (Emlen, 1980); (c) surviving better against food shortage and predators as a result of participating in group activities (Stallcup & Woolfenden, 1978); (d) being well established to take over a breeding position when this becomes possible (Woolfenden & Fitzpatrick, 1978); or (e) causing a better mate to select him as a result of higher status associated with a propensity to be altruistic (Zahavi, 1977). These possible long-term benefits are not in any way mutually exclusive: an altruist may gain different independent reproductive benefits at different later stages.

In these cases, the form of the benefit to the recipient and of the benefit regained later by the altruist are different. In the case of a nest helper, the recipient receives its benefits in the form of food, whereas the altruist's delayed benefit is in the form of experience, survival, breeding position or status. It is possible that the delayed benefit may even be gained not by the altruist but by the altruist's offspring. Note that the overall *currency* in which the benefits are measured is still reproductive success, but the *form* in which it is offered can vary.

Reciprocity provides another mechanism by which altruism by an individual may result in benefits to him subsequently. Trivers (1971) drew attention to what he called 'reciprocal altruism', and outlined how it might evolve if the benefit to the recipient is greater than the cost to the altruist, and if the recipient subsequently reciprocates. Trivers discussed in detail the problem of cheating, whereby the recipient of the altruistic act fails to reciprocate subsequently. There can be confusion about terminology. 'Reciprocal altruism' may be defined as 'the trading of altruistic acts by individuals at different times' (Wilson, 1975, p. 593); it is the *system* of exchange, it can take place between relatives as well as between non-relatives, and it does *not* refer to the mechanism by which such exchange has evolved. The mechanism whereby it may evolve between non-relatives may be called reciprocity. It is probably best to confine the term reciprocal altruism to the trading of similar altruistic acts, such as food for food, rescue for rescue (Trivers, 1971), or help in fighting for help in fighting (Packer, 1977).

Reciprocity differs in two general ways from the other types of evolutionary causes of delayed benefit altruism. The first (above) is that the form of the repayment is the same as that of the original altruistic act. The second is that the repayment depends on a particular other individual who may die, elope or cheat; by contrast the other types of delayed benefit depend on the altruist's building up a more vague social position for himself within a social network of more other individuals and therefore with possibly greater certainty.

These cases of altruism where there is a delayed benefit to the altruist may be regarded as a form of investment by the altruist. Similarly, a bird or small mammal will expend time and energy storing food during times of food abundance; this food is an investment in the sense that it will be more valuable to the investor at a later date, during food shortage. There is a degree of uncertainty as to whether it will be possible to recover the food, because it may have been discovered by other animals, whose behaviour is difficult to predict. An altruist who helps another individual is likewise making an investment, again with some uncertainty about its recoverability. There may or may not be greater uncertainty than for the solitary food hoarder above – it depends on the type of social system in which the altruist lives.

Compulsion

In some cases altruism may be imposed by the society (including the family) in which an animal lives. The compulsion could take different forms. For example it is possible that helping to rear offspring is the price 'insisted on' by adult babblers (*Turdoides* spp.) in exchange for allowing auxiliaries to be accepted into the group (Gaston, 1977; Zahavi, 1977). It is possible that a dominant male chimpanzee (*Pan troglodytes*) will subsequently be aggressive towards a subordinate if the latter does not 'altruistically' give him a piece of meat. Lionesses (*Panthera leo*) catch prey and relinquish it to males because the latter, being larger, may attack them if they do not (Schaller, 1972; unpublished observation). A subordinate male impala (*Aepyceros melampus*) is forced to be at the edge of the herd where for its own safety it has to be more alert and thus acts 'altruistically' as a lookout, benefiting the rest of the group (P.J. Jarman, personal communication). A dominant *Polistes* paper-wasp female obliges her subordinates to feed her (Wilson, 1975). Human mothers compel their offspring to share their food and possessions – they enforce 'altruism' onto them.

Compulsion by stronger members of the society may be a fairly general cause of altruism by the weaker members. It is worth noting that the distinction between compulsion and delayed benefit as explanations for the evolution of altruistic acts is a blurred one. There is little difference between receiving future benefits and reducing future costs. If babblers 'demand' altruistic behaviour from an auxiliary as the price of entering the group, and if it is in the auxiliary's long-term interests to join the group despite the entry price, the altruistic behaviour will evolve; we cannot say that the mechanism was delayed benefit rather than compulsion. In a sense the entry price has become a feature of the society, and the helping has become a part of growing up. There is no *a priori* reason why we should be more interested in the 'altruistic' genes in the helper than in the 'compulsion' genes in the older members of the society.

One particular form of compulsion is parental manipulation. Alexander's (1974) argument that for genetical reasons parents must always win in evolutionary conflicts with their offspring has been shown to be invalid (Dawkins, 1976). Nonetheless, parents may often be able to manipulate their offspring in practice in such a way as to compel them to be more altruistic than those offspring would otherwise be. Parents are larger and more powerful, at least at an early stage, than their offspring. If a mother is able to partially castrate some of her offspring, they are in effect compelled to be altruistic towards their kin as their only way of reproducing (the problems of 'altruism' by non-reproductive animals is discussed below). In the case of many social insects, offspring are rendered sterile, usually irrevocably, by the type of food they are given early in life. This does not mean that they are defeated in all evolutionary conflicts by their mother; for example Trivers & Hare (1976) showed that workers apparently win the conflict with the queen over the degree of investment in male versus female reproductives.

Nonadaptive

If altruism is imposed by an altruist's unrelated companions, it may be said to be nonadaptive to him. By definition it benefits the recipient, to whom it presumably is adaptive. Intra-specific slave workers of *Myrmecocistus* ants (Hölldobler, 1976), for example, benefit only the members of the colony which captured and enslaved them, and their altruism is clearly adaptive only to the captors. In the less extreme bird cases, the altruist is making the best of a bad job, and the job is made worse by the impositions of the more powerful recipient; it is more difficult to say whether the altruism is adaptive to either the altruist or the recipients.

For altruism to be adaptive, it must occur often enough to be of selective value. Some accidental cases of altruism probably occur so rarely that they are of negligible importance in evolution. For example it may very occasionally happen that newly born herd animals can be muddled up and reared by the wrong parent. The behaviour of rearing the unrelated offspring we would have to label as altruistic, but we would not consider it to be adaptive, any more than we would consider the raising of Romulus and Remus to have been adaptive behaviour by the wolf.

An example of altruistic behaviour, occurring often enough to be of importance in selection, may still be nonadaptive in some circumstances. One set of such circumstances would be if it was being currently selected against (perhaps because of an environmental change) but had not yet had time to disappear. Another would be if the genes responsible were closely linked to genes which had some independent beneficial effect; in this case the linkage if arbitrary will eventually be broken in the course of evolution, but until it is broken the genes responsible, and hence the altruistic behaviour, will persist.

To suggest that some instances of altruism may be nonadaptive is not to suggest that this is often likely to be a useful explanation of altruism, but it is a possibility that should be borne in mind.

Some examples of altruism

I shall take three examples of altruism and consider the various ways in which natural selection may have been responsible for their evolution, mainly in order to emphasise the interaction and joint action of these different ways.

Male baboon coalitions

Packer (1977) described the way in which a male olive baboon (*Papio anubis*) will enlist the help of a second to deprive a third of an oestrous female; while the second is engaged in fighting the third, the first gains access to the female. The males were shown to reciprocate, such that the first would help the second in similar circumstances, and because of the excellent long-term records, they were shown to be unlikely to be close relatives. Reciprocity appears to be the main cause of the evolution of the altruistic behaviour of the second male, who risks injury while his enlistor gains reproductively. However, other factors may also have played a part. For example, the data are scanty as to whether the enlisted male ever gains the female himself – he did not in the six occasions recorded. But if he does only occasionally, this may be enough to compensate for the risks he runs in fighting the third male, in which case we would think twice about labelling his behaviour as altruistic. He would gain an immediate net benefit himself, even if not as great a benefit as his enlistor was likely to gain. Whether we call his behaviour altruistic thus depends on what is the alternative possible behaviour (discussed below).

Baboons enlist one another's help quite often. Obviously if they did so at frequent enough intervals, such that reciprocation occurred within seconds, we should call the behaviour cooperative rather than altruistic. If the first baboon were to pay for the services of the second by means of a cheque, we would still call the second's behaviour cooperative (and astonishing, of course!). But even without visible payment, the obligation imposed on the second may be just as strong, in as complex a society as that of baboons. The time lag until reciprocation of this particular favour may be long, but the two male baboons may have built up so extensive and important a record of cooperative activities, both immediate and spaced, that each individual altruistic act is relatively trivial. Such a cooperative relationship can and does of course develop between relatives, and is probably even more important in those cases; but Packer's observations show that it is possible for it to develop between unrelated individuals. Reciprocity probably allows a greater degree of altruism between kin than would be expected on the basis of their degree of relatedness alone.

Bird alarm calls

Several passerine species on seeing an avian predator, utter an alarm call which warns their companions of the danger; the structure of the call makes it hard for the predator to locate, suggesting that the caller thereby exposes himself to danger, i.e. is being altruistic. Maynard Smith (1965), Trivers (1971) and Harvey & Greenwood (1978) among others have amply explored the mechanism by which this type of altruistic behaviour may have evolved. Almost certainly a number of mechanisms are involved. Close relatives may be protected at least at certain seasons; so too may the caller's mate (Witkin & Ficken, 1979) and descendants at some seasons. Reciprocity is unlikely to be important because cheating by failing to reciprocate would be easily selected for. There are a wide range of possible delayed benefits from calling, involving in various ways discouraging the predator from hunting either the caller or conspecifics nearby. There is a shortage of observations or experimental data, which are needed not in order to distinguish between different hypotheses, but in order to measure the relative importance of the different complementary selective forces in any particular case.

Lion communal suckling

Lionesses allow cubs other than their own to suckle from them (Schaller, 1972; Bertram, 1975), and communal suckling probably results in improved cub survival. It has been shown (Bertram, 1976) that the recipients are probably close relatives of the lioness, and the enhanced survival of kin is probably an important and perhaps sufficient cause of the evolution of such altruistic behaviour. However this does not mean that it is the only cause. Reciprocity may be an important contributing cause – it would be simple for lionesses to retaliate successfully against one of their number who failed to reciprocate. The delayed benefits of allowing others' cubs to suckle are gained by the lioness' offspring, who survive better in the presence of companions, and who if they are male have a much more successful reproductive life if they have male partners (Bygott, Bertram & Hanby, 1979). It should be possible soon to quantify the relative importance of the kin effects and of the delayed benefit effects in the evolution of this example of altruism.

Further problems with altruism
How should we expect a finite quantity of altruism to be allocated?

We know the general conditions under which altruistic behaviour towards a close relative will be selected for: if the ratio of the recipient's gain to the altruist's loss is greater than the reciprocal of the degree of relatedness between them. However, given a choice of relatives who might be aided, the above does not tell us in what proportions a limited amount of aid should be distributed. Altmann (1979) has pointed out the fallacy of assuming that aid should be apportioned according to the degree of relatedness (Dawkins, 1976); rather, all the aid should be given to the closest relative. Obviously a point of diminishing returns is reached, after which increased aid yields a progressively smaller benefit (e.g. offering food to an almost satiated individual). At that point the altruist's inclusive fitness is maximised if he switches to the next closest relative. Other things being equal, this is the optimal strategy.

But other things rarely are equal. The closest relative may not be available (Altmann, 1979), and there may be considerable uncertainty over its relatedness (Bertram, 1976). The altruist should take account too of the recipient's need for assistance (Dawkins, 1976), and of its reproductive value (Hamilton, 1964). In addition the altruist should take account of any delayed benefits to itself from helping that individual (who happens to be a relative), such as whether the latter will reciprocate, or will in some other way assist the altruist or the altruist's offspring. Obviously there is a great deal of uncertainty about many of these factors. However there is likely to be somewhat less uncertainty about most of them if the recipient is an offspring, because offspring are more likely to be available, are less likely to be less closely related than expected, and are more likely to reciprocate. For these reasons it is probably not surprising that aid to offspring is much commoner than aid to others. We will one day be able to compare the optimal with the actual allocation of altruism in a species, but we cannot do so yet.

What are the alternatives to an altruistic act?

We have already encountered, in connection with baboon reciprocation, the problem of determining what is an altruistic act, because it depends on what the alternatives are. If an animal encounters a piece of food, he has in fact several options; to eat it all himself or have only part of it, to give it all to one companion, to divide it among several companions and of course to do so in different proportions, to destroy it, to ignore it, and so on. The payoffs to himself of the different options will range between a large benefit, small benefit, no benefit, small cost and large cost. Is accepting a smaller benefit to be considered to be incurring a cost? Thus, should we consider behaviour to be altruistic if a donor animal helps a recipient by behaving in such a way that the donor benefits only slightly when he might have benefited more?

Must altruistic acts be positive?

Related to the point above is the similar question whether refraining from inflicting a cost or from inflicting a larger cost on another individual is to be considered an instance of being altruistic towards that individual? Is an animal being altruistic if it only wounds instead of killing a rival who might therefore fight him again? Again it depends on what the realistic alternatives are.

Can non-reproductive animals be altruistic?

The ant worker who spends her whole life caring for her siblings, and the worker honeybee (*Apis mellifera*) who dies in defence of her hive, are often quoted as supreme examples of altruism (Ridley & Dawkins, 1980). According to my definition and others' definitions of altruism in biology, an essential feature of altruism is a reduction in the donor's reproductive output. Yet the insect above suffers no reduction in her individual fitness because being sterile she has zero fitness anyway. Is it an example of altruism after all then? One can attempt to escape from the problem in the case of the honeybee by pointing out that a worker *may* occasionally become reproductive if the hive's queen dies, and if the worker dies that option is closed to her; but that option is in fact closed to her anyway, because the queen's replacement is drawn from among the younger inside workers not the older self-sacrificing guards outside the hive. At an earlier stage in the evolution of eusociality, before workers were sterile, their behaviour could certainly have been described as altruistic, but now? The problem is an awkward one, although largely a semantic one.

Conclusion

Only a few years ago altruism was a phenomenon whose evolution and maintenance was difficult to explain. Now, thanks to major theoretical advances and to mental ingenuity we are faced with a multiplicity rather than a dearth of possible explanations as to how a particular piece of altruistic behaviour could be selected for in the course of evolution. Most of them are not competing explanations – for example reciprocity, kin effects and parental manipulation can all act together in enabling the spread of a gene which favoured altruism. Out main task nowadays is to measure and compare the relative importance of each in any particular set of circumstances where an animal performs the previously puzzling behaviour of being altruistic towards a companion.

Summary

1. A new definition of altruism is proposed.
2. 'Altruism in biology is defined as behaviour which is likely to increase the reproductive output of another member of the same $(pR \, ZSZ)$. species who is not a descendant of the actor, and which at least in the short term is likely also to reduce the number of the actor's own descendants'.
3. Previous definitions are not explicit on a number of important points, and in some cases contradict one another.
4. Altruism may be favoured by kin effects, by delayed benefits including reciprocation, and by compulsion.
5. Three types of altruistic behaviour are examined and the interaction of evolutionary causes is emphasized.

It is a pleasure to express my gratitude to all associated with the King's College Research Centre for contributing to a most stimulating time there. I should also like to thank Drs Robin Dunbar and Richard Wrangham for their helpful comments on this paper.

References

Alexander, R.D. (1974). The evolution of social behavior. *Annual Review of Ecology and Systematics*, **5**, 325–83.
Alexander, R.D. (1977). Natural selection and the analysis of human sociality. In *Changing Scenes in the Natural Sciences*, 1776–1976, ed. C.E. Goulden, pp. 283–337. The Academy: Philadelphia.

Altmann, S.A. (1979). Altruistic behaviour: the fallacy of kin deployment. *Animal Behaviour*, **27**, 958–9.

Bertram. B.C.R. (1975). Social factors influencing reproduction in wild lions. *Journal of Zoology*, **177**, 463–82.

Bertram, B.C.R. (1976). Kin selection in lions and in evolution. In *Growing Points in Ethology*, ed. P.P.G. Bateson & R.A. Hinde, pp. 281–301. Cambridge University Press: Cambridge.

Brown, J.L. (1974). Alternate routes to sociality in Jays – with a theory for the evolution of altruism and communal breeding. *American Zoologist*, **14**, 63–80.

Bygott, J.D., Bertram, B.C.R. & Hanby, J.P. (1979). Male lions in large coalitions gain reproductive advantages. *Nature*, **282**, 839–41.

Davies, N.B. & Krebs, J.R. (1978). Introduction: Ecology, natural selection and social behaviour. In *Behavioural Ecology*, ed. J.R. Krebs & N.B. Davies, pp. 1–18. Blackwell: Oxford.

Dawkins, R. (1976). *The Selfish Gene*. Oxford University Press: Oxford and New York.

Dawkins, R. (1979). Twelve misunderstandings of kin selection. *Zeitschrift für Tierpsychologie*, **51**, 184–200.

Emlen, S.T. (1978). The evolution of cooperative breeding in birds. In *Behavioural Ecology*, ed. J.R. Krebs & N.B. Davies, pp. 245–81. Blackwell: Oxford.

Emlen, S.T. (1980). Altruism, kinship and reciprocity in the White-fronted Bee-eater. In *Natural Selection and Social Behavior*, ed. R.D. Alexander & D. Tinkle, pp. 185–92. Chiron Press: Ann Arbor, Michigan.

Gaston, A.J. (1977). Social behaviour within groups of jungle babblers (*Turdoides striatus*). *Animal Behaviour*, **25**, 828–48.

Hamilton, W.D. (1963). The evolution of altruistic behavior. *American Naturalist*, **97**, 354–6.

Hamilton, W.D. (1964). The genetical evolution of social behaviour I and II. *Journal of Theoretical Biology*, **7**, 1–16 and 17–52.

Harvey, P.H. & Greenwood, P.J. (1978). Anti-predator defence strategies: some evolutionary problems. In *Behavioural Ecology*, ed. J.R. Krebs & N.B. Davies, pp. 129–51. Blackwells: Oxford.

Hölldobler, B. (1976). Tournaments and slavery in a desert ant. *Science*, **192**, 912–14.

Lack, D. (1968). *Ecological Adaptations for Breeding in Birds*. Methuen: London.

Lin, N. & Michener, C.D. (1972). Evolution of sociality in insects. *Quarterly Review of Biology*, **47**, 131–59.

Maynard Smith, J. (1964). Group selection and kin selection. *Nature*, **201**, 1145–7.

Maynard Smith, J. (1965). The evolution of alarm calls. *American Naturalist*, **99**, 59–63.

Packer, C. (1977). Reciprocal altruism in *Papio anubis*. *Nature*, **265**, 441–3.

Ridley, M. & Dawkins, R. (1980). The natural selection of altruism. In *Altruism and Helping Behavior*, ed. J.P. Rushton & R.M. Sorrentino, pp. 19–39. Erlbaum: Hillsdale, New Jersey.

Ruse, M. (1979). *Sociobiology: Sense or Nonsense?* Reidel: Dordrecht, Holland.

Schaller, G.B. (1972). *The Serengeti Lion*. Chicago University Press: Chicago & London.

Stallcup, J.A. & Woolfenden, G.B. (1978). Family status and contributions to breeding by Florida Scrub Jays. *Animal Behaviour*, **26**, 1144–56.

Trivers, R.L. (1971). The evolution of reciprocal altruism. *Quarterly Review of Biology*, **46**, 35–57.

Trivers, R.L. & Hare, H. (1976). Haplodiploidy and the evolution of the social insects. *Science*, **191**, 249–63.

West Eberhard, M.J. (1975). The evolution of social behavior by kin selection. *Quarterly Review of Biology*, **50**, 1–33.

Wilson, E.O. (1971). *The Insect Societies*. Belknap Press: Cambridge, Massachusetts.

Wilson, E.O. (1975). *Sociobiology*. Belknap Press: Cambridge, Massachusetts.

Wilson, E.O. (1978). *On Human Nature*. Harvard University Press: Cambridge, Massachusetts.

Witkin, S.R. & Ficken, M.S. (1979). Chickadee alarm calls: does mate investment pay dividends? *Animal Behaviour*, **27**, 1275–6.

Woolfenden, G.E. & Fitzpatrick, J.W. (1978). The inheritance of territory in group-breeding birds. *Bioscience*, **28**, 104–8.

Zahavi, A. (1977). Reliability in communication systems and the evolution of altruism. In *Evolutionary Ecology*, ed. B. Stonehouse & C.M. Perrins, pp. 253–9. Macmillan: London.

13

Mutualism, kinship and social evolution

R.W. WRANGHAM

Introduction

In many animal groups, especially among social insects, birds and mammals, close kin tend to associate. Why? A simple explanation is merely that relatives are born near each other. This is clearly inadequate, however, because even closely related species differ widely in the extent to which females and males breed in their natal groups (Packer, 1979a). A stronger theory is therefore required to explain species differences in the way kin associate and interact.

Two important approaches to the problem come from behavioural ecology and kinship theory. First, behavioural ecology shows that in a variety of species, correlations occur between grouping patterns and environmental factors. It therefore indicates how natural selection can generate groups of different size, sex ratio and degree of cohesion (Crook, 1970; Emlen & Oring, 1977; Clutton-Brock & Harvey, 1978). Second, kinship theory explains the advantages to individuals of interacting in different ways with different classes of kin (Hamilton, 1964; West-Eberhard, 1975). Both approaches are useful but on their own neither has yet succeeded in explaining why social groups tend to be composed of particular combinations of relatives. They seem more likely to do so when appropriately combined, and considerable thought has therefore been given to ways of linking them (Alexander, 1974; West-Eberhard, 1975; Wilson, 1975; Clutton-Brock & Harvey, 1976; Brown, 1978; Vehrencamp, 1979; Chase, 1980).

The classical method of combining them is to treat them in sequence. First, ecological factors are suggested to determine the pattern of aggregation. Second, genetic relationships are considered to determine the ways in which individuals interact, within the ecologically generated groups. This method has the merit of distinguishing different factors influencing social evolution, but it has the concomitant disadvantage that it tends to divorce two processes which may in fact depend intimately on each other for their operation. For instance, ecological factors could favour the aggregation of particular classes of kin, rather than merely leading to undifferentiated groups. If so, behavioural ecology and kinship theory need to be linked more directly.

This paper therefore suggests a new way of combining them. Hamilton (1964) showed that when animals interact their relatedness matters, and both he and subsequent authors have applied this result principally to the evolution of altruism. Here, by contrast, I focus on mutualism. I suggest that mutualism is a useful focus of attention for three reasons. First, where mutualism is favoured by natural selection it can lead to the evolution of preferences for associating and interacting with kin. Second, the ecological factors which lead animals to behave mutualistically can in some circumstances be identified, allowing empirical tests of their importance. Third, mutualistic relationships can generate complex patterns of social organisation within groups. As a result a focus on mutualism may provide organising principles for understanding the evolution of a variety of social relationships, ultimately in terms of ecological adaptation.

Two types of mutualism, differing in the kinds of advantages they confer, are discussed. The paper uses only simple phenotypic considerations, and the underlying assumption is that strategies have evolved which tend to maximise expected inclusive fitness (Hamilton, 1964).

Mutualism and kinship

The nature of mutualism

Mutualistic relationships are defined as those by which two or more individuals gain greater reproductive potential (i.e. expected number of future offspring) than they would by acting alone. Examples include animals hunting together, keeping each other warm, or fighting against a common opponent. Mutualism is found between many forms of life, from different cells to different species, but this paper considers relationships only within species, particularly between individuals of the same sex.

Mutualistic relationships can include two types of mutually beneficial interaction. First, in *mutualistic interactions* all partners gain benefit as a direct result of their joint action (Table 13.1). Second, *altruistic interactions* can have mutualistic effects, if altruists themselves subsequently receive altruism (defined as a phenotypic benefit conferred on the beneficiary at a phenotypic cost to the actor). However, altruism and mutualism are not necessarily linked in this way. In particular, altruistic interactions which do not increase the actor's reproductive potential are by this definition not mutualistic (Table 13.1).

The long-term effects of the two types of interaction are similar, but they depend on different conditions. Mutualistic interactions depend only on two individuals acting together for their immediate joint benefit. They should therefore occur whenever the expected net benefit is sufficiently high. By contrast, the long-term mutualistic effect of an altruistic interaction depends not only on the immediate cost and benefits of the interaction, but also on whether the act is reciprocated. This means that the conditions favouring such interactions include circumstances unrelated to the interaction itself.

Trivers (1971) discussed these conditions and concluded that three were particularly important. First, there should be a large number of opportunities to act altruistically. Second, many of the interactions should be similar, i.e. with roughly equivalent costs and benefits. Third, the same individuals should interact repeatedly. This generally means that group-living is a pre-condition. Mutualistic interactions, by contrast, require no such pre-conditions to be favoured. Their consequences are therefore discussed without assuming the existence of stable groups.

Table 13.1 *Types of interaction classified by their effects on fitness*

Type of interaction	Actor Change in reproductive potential		Recipient Change in inclusive fitness	Identity of recipient
	Short-term	Long-term		
Selfish	− or +	+	−	Any
Altruism, without expectation of reciprocity	−	−	+	Kin
Altruism, with expectation of reciprocity	−	+	+	Any
Mutualism	+	+	+	Any

All interactions are assumed to increase the actor's inclusive fitness in the long-term. Cells show gains (+) or losses (−) to the reproductive potential of the actor, and to the inclusive fitness of the recipient of Ego's act. Differences between altruism and mutualism depend on the effects of the behaviour on Ego's reproductive potential.

Interactions in the lower half of the Table are mutually beneficial for actor and recipient. Those in the upper half are not.

The importance of kin in mutualistic interactions

With respect to the importance of kin as partners, mutualistic interactions vary between two types. In both types interactions lead to a gain in reproductive potential for each mutualist. However, they differ according to their effect on the reproductive potential of non-partners. The key difference is whether or not the advantage gained by acting mutualistically is necessarily gained at the expense of conspecifics.

At one extreme, here called 'non-interference mutualism' (NIM), it is not. For example, two pelicans which cooperate in hunting fish may each catch more than they would by hunting alone. As a result they would achieve an increase in reproductive potential. But this increase is not necessarily gained at the expense of any other individuals. For instance, it would occur if the species consisted of isolated pairs, all of which behaved mutualistically. Provided that others can themselves behave mutualistically, those practising NIM fare better than they would alone but not necessarily better than others. Possible examples include joint action in prey capture (Bertram, 1978), defence against predators (Lin & Michener, 1972) and defence of food sources against other species (Robertson, Sweatman, Fletcher & Cleland, 1978).

In 'interference mutualism' (IM) by contrast, the benefit of cooperation is necessarily achieved at the direct expense of conspecifics. The simplest case consists of two animals cooperating to exclude a third from access to a desired resource. Consider, for example, three hyaenas finding a dead gazelle. Any two who jointly prevent the third from eating will each be able to get more food than if all eat together. In such a case the benefit of cooperation is solely the result of excluding a conspecific, with the consequence that some individuals fare better than others even if all behave mutualistically. Examples include cooperative defence of nest sites (Gamboa, 1978), of food sources (Wrangham, 1980), of territories (Emlen, 1978) and of mates (Bygott, Bertram & Hanby, 1979).

Many cases of mutualism can be imagined which would fall between the two extremes of NIM and IM. Suppose that a lake holds three pelicans, that the optimal group size for hunting fish is two, and that it therefore pays a hunting pair to exclude the third. This could be viewed as NIM, because the advantage of cooperation does not in principle depend on excluding a conspecific. Yet it would also be IM, because the two who cooperate necessarily impose a cost on the third. NIM and IM are blended in this way wherever competition occurs for membership of a group of non-interference mutualists. Nevertheless they are considered separately, in order to distinguish their effects.

The different effects of NIM and IM occur as a result of the way in which mutualism between two or more individuals affects other individuals. Consider three individuals, i, j and k, in a situation where mutualism between two (and only two) individuals is favoured. j and k are assumed to be equally willing to serve as i's partner, and differ only in that j is more closely related to i than is k. Let the benefit of acting mutualistically be B_M. If i can choose either j or k as a partner, which choice maximises i's inclusive fitness?

First, in extreme NIM all individuals can gain the same benefit. Hence, whether i chooses j or k as a partner the gain to i's inclusive fitness is

$$B_M(1 + b_{ij} + b_{ik})$$

where b is the coefficient of relatedness (Hamilton, 1972). Thus partner choice is immaterial, and there is no expected bias for interacting with kin.

Second, in IM the cooperators exclude the third individual from the desired resources. The reproductive potential of the excluded individual therefore changes by B_E, where B_E is less than B_M and may be less than zero. Accordingly, i's inclusive fitness rises by

$$B_M(1 + b_{ij}) + B_E b_{ik} \quad \text{(if i partners j)}$$

or by

$$B_M(1 + b_{ik}) + B_E b_{ij} \quad \text{(if i partners k).}$$

Since $b_{ij} > b_{ik}$, it pays i to partner j in preference to k; thus, the closer relative is the preferred partner.

Other things being equal, therefore, NIM neither favours nor disfavours kin as partners, whereas IM favours kin partnerships. The important point is that interactions between kin can be favoured purely as a result of mutualism, even in the absence of altruism (cf. West-Eberhard, 1978). A second issue is that in species where mutualism is important, differences in the tendency for kin to associate may be related partly to differences in the importance of NIM and IM.

Because other things are not always equal, caution is necessary in applying these conclusions. In particular, the difference in the effects of NIM and IM may be reduced when potential partners differ in other ways than their relatedness. For example, potential partners may differ with respect to their competitive ability, or in the effect of a given amount of resource on their reproductive potential. These and other such differences could lead either to kin being preferred in NIM (e.g. if familiar individuals cooperate more effectively than unfamiliar individuals), or to a more distant relative being preferred in IM (e.g. if it has greater competitive ability than a closer relative). Phenotypic effects like these weaken the prediction that systematic kin association is associated with IM rather than NIM. To the extent that they occur systematically, therefore, the expected relationship will be confounded. It is assumed here that such effects are minor, but it is recognised that they must ultimately be taken into account and may be of major importance in certain species.

Group stability
Partner preferences have been discussed so far on the assumption that partner choices are made at the time that the interaction occurs. However, if mutualistic interactions occur repeatedly individuals may benefit by developing relationships, i.e. a consistent choice of partner across many interactions. Such relationships are favoured if there is a risk of failing to find an appropriate partner when needed. As a result, they may influence the way in which individuals associate.

The risk is particularly severe in the case of IM. In this case partnerships are expected to form along kin lines, and individuals travelling with conspecifics but without close kin are liable to find themselves without an ally. For example, suppose that three individuals encounter a resource where IM is favoured. Other things being equal, the two who are most closely related should cooperate at the expense of the third. To minimise the risk of being excluded in this way, individuals should associate with their closest possible relative at all times.

A result of partner preferences, therefore, is that individuals should travel in relatively stable groups. Because partner preferences are expected to be more systematic in IM than in NIM, groups are expected to be more stable where IM is more important (Fig. 13.1). In the simplest case, groups are pairs. If resource distribution favours IM in larger groups, however, stable groups of considerable size may develop. Relationships between these groups would normally be aggressive, unlike those between NIM groups. Thus NIM and IM groups are expected to differ not only in composition, but also in stability and inter-group relationships.

Sex-specific 'key strategies' and intra-sexual relationships
Fig. 13.1 suggests that a resource distribution favouring IM leads to stable groups of close kin. Yet this is only one of many ecological pressures. To understand the effects of any particular pressure we need to evaluate its contribution to social evolution compared to those of other influences.

This can be done by finding out whether IM (for example) is the optimal strategy for acquiring the 'key resource'. The key resource is whichever resource is most cost-effective in raising the reproductive success of breeding animals. Since, by definition, animals whose strategies are directed to competing for this resource have the highest reproductive success, selection tends to favour those 'key strategies' (Wrangham, 1979, 1980). If IM is the key strategy, it can be said to be responsible for kin-groups. If not, kin-groups are adaptive for other reasons.

In the case of breeding males, theory and data show that in general, effort put into acquiring mates has greater effects on fitness than effort put into acquiring food, water, safety from predators or other resources (Williams, 1966; Trivers, 1972). Though in many species breeding males have to eat, increased access to food gives less benefit than increased access to mates once males are in sufficiently good condition to breed. Unless the distri-

Fig. 13.1. Grouping patterns in relation to two types of mutualism.

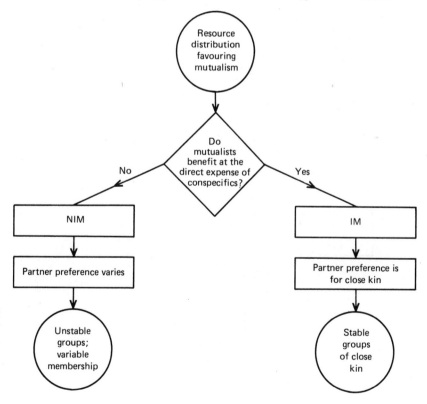

bution of females make male–male competition for females uneconomic, the foraging strategies of breeding males are therefore adapted to mating strategies, and not vice-versa.

The reproductive success of breeding females, on the other hand, is not normally limited by the availability of mates. Instead, breeding rate is constrained by environmental resources. If such resources can be ranked in terms of cost-effectiveness, a key resource can be identified.

The concept of a key resource for females is helpful because it draws attention to the difference in the ways each sex is affected by environmental pressures. The classical view of the relationship between ecology and social evolution acknowledges the uniqueness of male strategies, but considers

Fig. 13.2. Sexual selection view of social evolution.

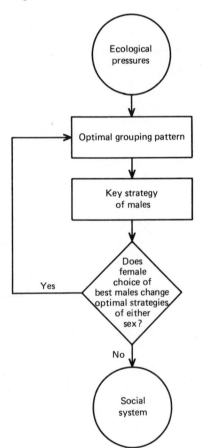

both sexes equally influenced by the environment (Fig. 13.2). More recent ideas, by contrast, suggest that males are influenced by environmental resources only to the extent that female strategies are affected (Fig. 13.3) (Emlen & Oring, 1977; Bradbury & Vehrencamp, 1977; Wrangham, 1979; Wittenberger, 1980). Thus female strategies are considered to be directly influenced by the distribution of environmental resources in a way which male strategies are not. Following Fig. 13.3, any consideration of the way environments shape social systems must begin by analysing ecological effects on females.

Fig. 13.3. Female-focus view of social evolution.

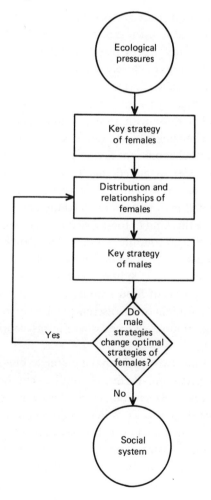

Mutualism and social evolution

The significance of the principles discussed above depends on whether they can be used to provide testable explanations of the species distribution of grouping types. Previous classifications of social groups tend to turn on the way males compete for females, and therefore cannot easily be used here. Rather than discuss mutualism in relation to different types of mating system, therefore, I briefly suggest how its importance might be recognised in three major classes of relationship, i.e. those within each sex and between the sexes. An implication of this discussion is that groups could usefully be classified according to these relationships.

Intra-sexual mutualism

Females. If social evolution proceeds as suggested, a female key resource inducing NIM should lead to open groups composed of females who may or may not be close relatives. Key resources favouring IM, by contrast, should lead to closed groups of closely related females.

By turning them on their head these expectations have been tested for primates; species with female kin-groups were expected to have female key resources which induce IM, while those with groups of unrelated females were not (Wrangham, 1980). The female key resource was assumed to be food, and a model of the ecological conditions favouring IM was tested in 33 species of primates. The model suggested that two conditions were necessary for stable female kin-groups to evolve. First, they are favoured if high-quality foods are distributed in discrete patches containing a limited number of feeding sites, because this kind of food distribution favours IM. This is a necessary but not a sufficient condition; it takes no account of the fact that during periods of food scarcity, food patches are likely to shrink with the result that groups are expected to split up. The second condition, accordingly, was that during periods of food scarcity the species should switch from eating high-quality foods in small, discrete patches, to selecting lower-quality items in large continuous patches where intra-group competition has less importance.

The food distribution of all but two species having female kin-groups was found to conform to expectation. Preferred foods occur in finite patches (principally fruiting trees) at which competition between groups is observed. When food is scarce these species switch to diets composed of abundant, lower-quality items, distributed in such a way that IM appears to be relatively unimportant. Food distribution could not be described in quantitative terms, so the fit to expectation was testable only broadly. However, in a second test the model was given further support by data from the only four species whose social groups are composed of females who are only distantly related to each other. The food distribution of these species differ markedly from those with female kin-groups, as expected. In three cases the species do not eat ripe fruit, and foods are therefore distributed in a way which does not favour IM. In the fourth, ripe fruit are preferred but no major alternative foods are eaten, so groups are forced to disperse during periods of food scarcity.

The primate evidence thus suggests that in many cases breeding females who live in groups of female relatives do so specifically because of the advantages gained in competing mutualistically for access to key resources. This is supported by the fact that kin-groups occur even in species having high levels of intra-group competition over food. Such competition might have been expected to cause relatives to live in different groups, to avoid imposing costs on kin. In fact, however, spatial clumping of relatives occurs even within groups (Kurland, 1977). The implication is that the disadvantages of competition with close relatives are an inevitable outcome of the key strategy of cooperating with them, both within and between groups. In support of this idea, mutualistic interactions by female relatives competing for food or dominance are frequently observed in species with female kin-groups (Chapais & Schulman, 1980; Wrangham, 1981).

Groups of unrelated females were not expected to be found where female key resources induce IM, and none such are known in primates. Instead, they should occur either where the key resource induces NIM, or where group-living is an incidental effect of other pressures. There are no clear cases of NIM causing female grouping in primates. Possibly they occur in species with unstable groups such as some ungulates or ostriches (*Struthio camelus*), for which defence against predators may be a critical factor favouring NIM (Bertram, 1980). Group-living as an incidental effect (of intersexual mutualism) is discussed below.

Males. In many species social groups tend to include only one adult male, but at least two types of group are found in which two or more males live together.

First, a comparatively rare system is the occurrence of closed male kin-groups. As with female kin-groups, these suggest that the key resource induces IM, but here the key resource is expected to be access to females rather than an environmental resource. In a variety of species having male kin-groups males do indeed cooperate with relatives in competition for access to females (e.g. hamadryas baboons *Papio hamadryas*, Kummer (1968), Abbeglen (1976); lions *Panthera leo*, Bygott *et al.* (1979); turkeys

Meleagris gallapavo, Watts & Stokes (1971). However no models have been proposed to explain why IM might pay in these species as opposed to others. Unlike female primates, therefore, there is no independent evidence that these kin-groups arise in response to resource distribution. Instead, it is possible that kin-groups were favoured for other reasons, and that IM between relatives is an incidental effect. Models of the way female distribution influences male strategies are therefore needed, to test the hypothesis that male kin-groups arise because IM is favoured in competition for access to fertile females.

Second, breeding groups may include several unrelated adult males. Here the lack of kinship means that the key resource is not expected to favour IM. Instead, it is expected either to lead to NIM between males, or (more probably) to favour inter-sexual mutualism in such a way as to induce tolerance between males (Wrangham, 1980). In some species males do in fact compete mutualistically for access to oestrous females, though IM appears not to be necessary for successful competition because the most successful males often compete alone (baboons *Papio anubis* and *P. cynocephalus*, Packer (1977, 1979*b*), Hausfater (1975). Nevertheless the fact that IM occurs means that its possible influence on the evolution of such groups should be examined. Where the distribution of females appears to favour IM among males, an important problem will be to explain why males do not associate with kin.

Inter-sexual mutualism

Inter-sexual mutualism occurs wherever members of each sex gain mutual advantage from the behaviour of one or more members of the opposite sex. It is discussed here in order to illustrate how it can lead to group-living even where intra-sexual mutualism is not important. As before, two types of mutualism can be distinguished.

First, NIM is defined as before, and has similar effects. Systematic partner preferences are not generally expected because there are no necessary costs on conspecifics.

Second, IM between sexes is again defined as incurring a cost on others, but its effects on partner choice can differ from those produced by IM within sexes. This occurs where the benefit of mutualism lies in having a mating partner. If so, the normal advantage gained by favouring kin is offset by a potential loss of fitness as a result of inbreeding (Ralls, Brugger & Ballov, 1979).

Even if kin are not preferred partners, however, IM between the sexes can favour other partner preferences, especially by females, and can thereby lead to stable groups. The classic example concerns polygynous birds, in which females benefit by pairing with already-mated males in good habitat rather than with unmated males in poor habitat (Verner & Willson, 1966; Orians, 1969). Differences in habitat quality have been the principal focus of attention in application of the Orians-Verner model ('resource defence polygyny', Emlen & Oring 1977), but other characteristics of males can have similar effects, though less easily quantifiable.

For example, where the distribution of environmental resources makes inter-individual competition uneconomic, there need be little disadvantage to living in groups. If so, male success in mate-guarding may be critical for females as well as for males. In mountain gorillas *Pan gorilla berengei* several unrelated females travel with a single breeding male who defends them from other males; females cooperate by following him. Male courtship is aggressive and imposes high costs on females. Consequently females prefer males who are the most effective protectors from the courtship of other males (Harcourt, 1978). Since there is little feeding competition and no ecological reasons have been found to account for gorilla groups, female–male mutualism appears to be directly responsible (Wrangham, 1979). It may similarly be important in the evolution of groups of other species with stable groups of unrelated females (e.g. plains zebra *Equus burchelli*, Klingel (1975); red colobus, *Colobus badius*, Marsh (1979).

Female choice can thus lead to groups, but the type of group is different from those developed through IM among females. First, females do not form alliances with other females, so there is no bias in favour of relatives. Second, group membership is stable only so far as the female–male bond is stable; if the male's superiority over other males wanes, females are expected to leave, and they do (Harcourt, 1978; Marsh, 1979).

'Female-choice groups' differ also from those arising from NIM. They are expected to be more closed and more stable, with more highly differentiated relationships between females and males, but with equally bland relationships among females. There is good evidence of a trend in this direction in primates (Harcourt, 1979; Wrangham, 1980). This suggests that female-choice groups can be recognised partly through the types of social relationship found within them, and therefore that appropriate models of the ecological conditions responsible for them can be developed and tested.

Altruism within IM groups

Interference mutualists are bonded by the need to compete against others; but if competition is important in establishing relationships, it cannot normally be avoided within them also. Since mutualists have particular partner preferences, competitive strategies within bonds must take into account not only immediate costs and benefits, but also the future of the relationship. This has two implications for the evolution of altruism.

First, within alliances competitive strategies should be more inhibited than those between unallied individuals, in order to allow the alliance to be maintained; such inhibition can be regarded as passive altruism. For example winners should refrain from killing defeated rivals. This is not necessarily true of competition between lone individuals, or between those in different alliances. Male chimpanzees *Pan troglodytes* have violent aggressive interactions within alliances ('communities') but do not inflict serious bodily injury. Aggression between males of different communities, however, can lead to serious injuries and deaths (Bygott, 1979; Goodall, 1979). Conventions in animal fighting are normally analysed without regard to the significance of long-term bonds (e.g. Maynard Smith & Parker, 1976), but this suggests they should be taken into account.

Second, the need to obtain the best possible ally can favour active short-term altruism. This occurs if there is competition between two individuals for the mutualistic support of a third. Suppose, for instance, that two individuals are distantly related to each other but are closely and equally related to a third, who is their preferred partner. Other things being equal, if one of the two is more altruistic than the other, it should be chosen as an ally by the preferred partner. Consequently, competition to receive support from a preferred potential partner could lead to competition to provide altruism, purely as a result of the need for the better ally.

Primates appear to offer examples of this process. Alliances within primate kin-groups are commonly formed between close kin (Cheney, 1977; Kurland, 1977; Massey, 1977; de Waal, 1978; Lee & Oliver, 1979). However, kinship is not the only factor affecting alliance formation. Individuals vary also in dominance rank, and those of high rank are preferred allies (e.g. Kaplan, 1978; Fairbanks, 1980). One way in which subordinate animals compete for dominant partners is to groom them. Field data show not only that subordinates tend to groom dominant individuals more than vice-versa, but also that subordinates compete for the opportunity to groom dominants; furthermore, high rates of alliance formation are correlated with high rates of grooming (Seyfarth, 1977, 1980). The implication is that the pattern of grooming is explicable partly because more effective alliances are obtained by more generous groomers (Seyfarth, *loc. cit.*).

This is of interest because it means that altruism can evolve as a consequence of interference mutualism, without being dependent on kin selection or the expectation of reciprocal altruism. (Grooming is assumed to be an altruistic act since it incurs a finite cost to the groomer, without any immediate benefit; and the fact that dominant animals allow themselves to be groomed implies that they receive a benefit.) It is not at first obvious that this is so, both because grooming tends to be given to kin, and because it is associated with reciprocal benefits. However, the tendency for altruism to be given to kin may be only an incidental effect of the fact that in general, kin are preferred mutualistic allies, as argued above. If so, altruism given to kin within IM groups need not follow Hamilton's rules (Hamilton, 1964). Again, although an altruist expects to receive a reciprocal benefit (i.e. mutualistic support), the benefit is not necessarily altruistic. In particular, support in an alliance is not altruistic if it is provided by an individual which itself benefits directly from the alliance. Reciprocal altruism is therefore not necessarily the appropriate way to describe the altruism observed within IM groups.

This suggests that IM can lead not only to the evolution of relatively closed, stable groups, but also to complex patterns of differentiated relationships within such groups (see Caplow, (1968) for discussion and examples). If so, a focus on mutualism may be able to unite two recent advances in primate sociobiology, namely the appreciation of the importance of alliances (Caplow, 1968), and the development of models which generate complex social networks from simple rules (e.g. Seyfarth, Cheney & Hinde, 1978). In the past the ultimate origins of complexity have been explained principally in terms of sexual selection, kin selection and reciprocal altruism. Interference mutualism appears to provide additional explanatory power, not only in primates but also in other species having closed, stable and mutually protective kin-groups.

Discussion

This paper proposes that two major types of mutualistic social grouping can in principle be identified. First, NIM groups are those in which individuals benefit from each other's presence but do not, as a result, necessarily impose costs on others. Herds of some ungulates (e.g. wildebeest *Connochaetes taurinus*) may provide examples of NIM groups if by grouping, individuals indeed obtain mutual benefits, for example in escaping from predators. Second, in IM groups individuals benefit from each other's presence and necessarily impose costs on others (e.g. in primate kin-groups). IM groups include female-choice groups as a special case, in which individuals of each sex gain complementary benefits and where relationships within sexes are not necessarily mutualistic (e.g. mountain gorillas).

The value of classifying groups in this way is that it suggests that different types of group are favoured by different sets of ecological conditions, and have different consequences for group structure. Consequently, the adaptive significance of each grouping type should be analysed by different methods.

Methods for examining the importance of IM have already been proposed for some species (e.g. Wittenberger, 1980; Wrangham, 1980). To develop satisfactory theories of social evolution in groups, however, we need to understand not only the influence of particular pressures on grouping patterns, but also whether or not other pressures have effects. This will ultimately allow the combined influence of different pressures to be understood. With respect to mutualism several gaps therefore need to be filled.

First, we need more explicit models of the causes and consequences of NIM, so that its role in social evolution can be clearly distinguished from that of IM and of selfish behaviour. For instance, the influence of NIM was suggested here to be limited to a pressure for individuals to associate. It is possible, however, that more sophisticated predictions could be generated when factors such as the need for partners with particular abilities are taken into account. If so, it will become easier to recognise species in which NIM is important, and to model the factors responsible for their social evolution.

Second, we need further models of the ways in which IM can favour sociality in different species, especially among males. These will not be easy to develop because male groups appear not only to arise in response to female distribution but also, frequently, to change it (Fig. 13.3). An ESS model is therefore required. A second problem, for both females and males, is to understand the role of factors other than kinship. An obvious candidate for attention is variation in individual competitive ability (Caplow, 1968).

Third, although female-choice groups have been modelled in species where males control access to resources (Orians, 1969; Wittenberger, 1980), they have not been analysed in detail in other cases, such as where the male role is limited to protecting females from male harassment. The same problem applies here as to IM groups of males; male behaviour can affect female behaviour, and can thereby alter the nature of the optimal strategy for males. Again, therefore, ESS models are required.

By pursuing the different effects of NIM and IM it should ultimately be possible to combine them in a unified analysis of a given social system. At present the easiest research strategy is often to focus on single pressures. However, although a tight focus is helpful in the first analysis it is clearly inadequate for understanding the richness of social behaviour. As a simple example, lions (*Panthera leo*) are often suggested to form groups because they can thereby hunt more effectively (Bertram, 1978), i.e. they are considered to form NIM groups. Nevertheless the fact that females often form closed kin-groups which compete over carcasses (Schaller, 1972), while males tend to have kin-groups which compete for access to females (Bygott *et al.*, 1979), suggests that IM is just as important as NIM for both sexes. Since lions commonly hunt in small parties within their larger social units, both NIM and IM are probably necessary to explain the patterns of social behaviour. Thus in this and many other cases a broad perspective is necessary.

In this respect an intriguing feature of mutualism is the way it has affected the evolution of human behaviour. A variety of mutualistic relationships appear to be important. For instance, NIM is clearly a major influence on diverse human activities including farming, hunting and tool-making, and is often suggested to be responsible for the occurrence of groups. Whether or not the latter is true, there can be no doubt of the importance of NIM in shaping intra-group relationships.

At the same time IM may well have been a critical factor influencing the development of inter-group warfare, and is perhaps responsible for the origin of human groups. The evolution of war is sometimes explained in terms of group selection (Alexander, 1974; Hamilton, 1975). However, this is implausible because group selection requires unusual and improbable conditions to be effective (Maynard Smith, 1976). Individual selection, by contrast, could lead easily to warfare if the distribution of resources favours IM, and increasingly large groups could be favoured purely as a result of the ability of large groups to dominate small groups.

Again, different types of group may be generated by the different ways in which the resource distribution favours mutualism. In many human groups males tend both to be more closely bonded and (between alliances) more aggressive than females (Tiger, 1969; Chagnon, 1979); and kin-groups tend to be based more on male than female kin relations (Murdock, 1957). However this is not universal, and specific correlations between ecology and grouping type will allow the significance of such trends to be tested. For instance, pastoral societies are almost exclusively patrilineal (Goody, 1976). A model could therefore be developed to test the hypothesis that an economy based on animal production generates a key resource favouring IM among males. On the other hand where females tend to form closed kin-groups which compete with each other (e.g. Richards, 1939) IM among females may be important. To the extent that such proposals are testable they offer intriguing possibilites for understanding the ultimate causes of variation in the structure, size and cohesion of human groups. Just as IM can generate complex patterns of altruistic and competitive relationships in monkeys, it may have far-reaching effects on the development of human social relationships.

Summary

1. It is useful to distinguish two types of mutualism. Non-interference mutualism (NIM) does not necessarily reduce the fitness of conspecifics, whereas interference mutualism (IM) does. The distinction is useful because kin are more likely to be favoured as partners in IM than in NIM.
2. Consequently, a resource distribution which favours IM is expected to lead to kin-groups. This hypothesis can be tested by identifying key resources and determining whether they favour IM within sexes. Data from primates show that in many species female kin-groups are indeed associated with a resource distribution favouring IM among females. Similar tests are possible in other groups.
3. Mutualism between sexes can favour group-living even where access to environmental resources is not controlled by either females or males. This occurs where male success in mate-guarding is critical for the reproductive success of both sexes.
4. In groups which arise as a consequence of a resource distribution favouring IM, complex social relationships can develop purely as a result of mutualism. In particular, altruism can be favoured directly by mutualism, without relying on kin selection or the benefit of reciprocal altruism.

I am grateful to Brian Bertram, Napoleon Chagnon, Robin Dunbar, Paul Harvey, Sarah Hrdy, John Maynard Smith and Dan Rubenstein for comments on an earlier draft.

References

Abbeglen, J.J. (1976). *On Socialisation in Hamadryas Baboons*. Ph.D. thesis, Zurich University.

Alexander, R.D. (1974). The evolution of social behaviour. *Annual Review of Ecology and Systematics*, **5**, 325–83.

Bertram, B.C.R. (1978). Living in groups. In *Behavioural Ecology*, ed. J.R. Krebs & N.B. Davies, pp. 64–96. Blackwells Scientific Publications: Oxford.

Bertram, B.C.R. (1980). Vigilance and group size in ostriches. *Animal Behaviour*, **28**, 278–86.

Bradbury, J.W. & Vehrencamp, S.L. (1977). Social organisation and foraging in emballonurid bats. *Behavioural Ecology and Sociobiology*, **2**, 1–17.

Brown, J.L. (1978). Avian communal breeding systems. *Annual Review of Ecology and Systematics*, **9**, 123–55.

Bygott, J.D. (1979). Agonistic behaviour, dominance, and social structure in wild chimpanzees of the Gombe National Park. In *The Great Apes*, ed. D.A. Hamburg & E.R. McCown, pp. 405–27. Benjamin/Cummings: Menlo Park.

Bygott, J.D., Bertram, B.C.R. & Hanby, J.P. (1979). Male lions in large coalitions gain reproductive advantage. *Nature*, **282**, 839–41.

Caplow, T. (1968). *Two Against One*. Prentice–Hall: New Jersey.

Chagnon, N.A. (1979). Mate competition, favoring close kin, and village fissioning among the Yanomamo Indians. In *Evolutionary Biology and Human Social Behavior: An Anthropological Perspective*, ed. N.A. Chagnon & W. Irons, pp. 86–132. Duxbury Press: North Scituate, Mass.

Chapais, B. & Schulman, S.R. (1980). An evolutionary model of female dominance relations in primates. *Journal of Theoretical Biology*, **82**, 47–89.

Chase, I.D. (1980). Cooperative and noncooperative behavior in animals. *American Naturalist*, **115**, 827–57.

Cheney, D.L. (1977). The acquisition of rank and the development of reciprocal alliances among free-ranging immature baboons. *Behavioural Ecology and Sociobiology*, **2**, 303–18.

Clutton-Brock, T.H. & Harvey, P.H. (1976). Evolutionary rules and primate societies. In *Growing Points in Ethology*, ed. P.P.G. Bateson & R.A. Hinde, pp. 195–237. Cambridge University Press: Cambridge.

Clutton-Brock, T.H. & Harvey, P.H. (1978). Mammals, resources and reproductive strategies. *Nature*, **273**, 191–5.

Crook, J.H. (1970). The socio-ecology of primates. In *Social Behaviour in Birds and Mammals*, ed. J.H. Crook, pp. 103–66. Academic Press: London.

Emlen, S.T. (1978). The evolution of cooperative breeding in birds. In *Behavioural Ecology*, ed. J.R. Krebs & N.B. Davies, pp. 245–81. Blackwells Scientific Publications: Oxford.

Emlen, S.T. & Oring, L.W. (1977). Ecology, sexual selection and the evolution of mating systems. *Science*, **197**, 215–23.

Fairbanks, L.A. (1980). Relationships among adult females in captive vervet monkeys: testing a model of rank-related attractiveness. *Animal Behaviour*, **28**, 853–9.

Gamboa, G.J. (1978). Intraspecific defense: advantage of social cooperation among paper wasp foundresses. *Science*, **199**, 1463–5.

Goodall, J. (1979). Life and death at Gombe. *National Geographic Magazine*, **155**(5), 592–621.

Goody, J. (1976). *Production and Reproduction*. Cambridge University Press: Cambridge.

Hamilton, W.D. (1964). The genetical evolution of social behaviour. *Journal of Theoretical Biology*, **7**, 1–52.

Hamilton, W.D. (1972). Altruism and related phenomena, mainly in social insects. *Annual Review of Ecology and Systematics*, **3**, 193–232.

Hamilton, W.D. (1975). Innate social aptitudes of man: an approach from evolutionary genetics. In *Biosocial Anthropology*, ed. R. Fox, pp. 133–55. Wiley: New York.

Harcourt, A.H. (1978). Strategies of emigration and transfer by primates, with particular reference to gorillas. *Zeitschrift für Tierpsychologie*, **48**, 401–20.

Harcourt, A.H. (1979). Social relationships between adult male and female mountain gorillas in the wild. *Animal Behaviour*, **27**, 325–42.

Hausfater, G. (1975). Dominance and reproduction in baboons (*Papio cynocephalus*): a quantitative analysis. *Contributions to Primatology*, **7**. S. Karger: Basel.

Kaplan, J.R. (1978). Fight interference and altruism in rhesus monkeys. *American Journal of Physical Anthropology*, **49**, 241–50.

Klingel, H. (1975). Social organisation and reproduction in equids. *Journal of Reproduction and Fertility*, **23**, 7–11.

Kummer, H. (1968). *Social Organisation of Hamadryas Baboons*. University of Chicago Press: Chicago.

Kurland, J.A. (1977). Kin selection in the Japanese monkey. *Contributions to Primatology*, **12**, S. Karger: Basel.

Lee, P.C. & Oliver, J.I. (1979). Competition, dominance and the acquisition of rank in juvenile yellow baboons (*Papio cynocephalus*). *Animal Behaviour*, **27**, 576–85.

Lin, N. & Michener, C.D. (1972). Evolution of sociality in insects. *Quarterly Review of Biology*, **47**, 131–59.

Marsh, C.W. (1979). Female transference and mate choice among Tana River red colobus. *Nature*, **281**, 568–9.

Massey, A. (1977). Agonistic aids and kinship in a group of pigtail macaques. *Behavioural Ecology and Sociobiology*, **2**, 31–40.

Maynard Smith, J. (1976). Group selection. *Quarterly Review of Biology*, **51**, 277–83.

Maynard Smith, J. & Parker, G.A. (1976). The logic of asymmetric contests. *Animal Behaviour*, **24**, 159–75.

Murdock, G.P. (1957). World ethnographic sample. *American Anthropologist*, **59**, 664–87.

Orians, G.H. (1969). On the evolution of mating systems in birds and mammals. *American Naturalist*, **103**, 589–603.

Packer, C. (1977). Reciprocal altruism in *Papio anubis*. *Nature*, **265**, 441–3.

Packer, C. (1979*a*). Inter-troop transfer and inbreeding avoidance in *Papio anubis*. *Animal Behaviour*, **27**, 1–36.

Packer, C. (1979*b*). Male dominance and reproductive activity in *Papio anubis*. *Animal Behaviour*, **27**, 37–45.

Ralls, K., Brugger, K. & Ballou, J. (1979). Inbreeding and juvenile mortality in small populations of ungulates. *Science*, **206**, 1101–3.

Richards, A.I. (1939). *Land, Labour and Diet in Northern Rhodesia*. Oxford University Press: Oxford.

Robertson, D.R., Sweatman, H.P.A., Fletcher, E.A. & Cleland, M.G. (1976). Schooling as a mechanism for circumventing the territoriality of competitors. *Ecology*, **57**, 1208–20.

Schaller, G.B. (1972). *The Serengeti Lion*. Chicago University Press: Chicago.

Seyfarth, R.M. (1977). A model of social grooming among adult female monkeys. *Journal of Theoretical Biology*, **65**, 671–98.

Seyfarth, R.M. (1980). The distribution of grooming and related behaviours among adult female vervet monkeys. *Animal Behaviour*, **28**, 798–813.

Seyfarth, R.M., Cheney, D.L. & Hinde, R.A. (1978). Some principles relating social interactions and social structure among primates. In *Recent Advances in Primatology: Volume I, Behaviour*, ed. D.J. Chivers & J. Herbert, pp. 39–51. Academic Press: London.

Tiger, L. (1969). *Men in Groups*. Nelson: London.

Trivers, R.L. (1971). The evolution of reciprocal altruism. *Quarterly Review of Biology*, **46**, 35–57.

Trivers, R.L. (1972). Parental investment and sexual selection. In *Sexual Selection and the Descent of Man*, ed. B. Campbell, pp. 136–79. Aldine: Chicago.

Vehrencamp, S.L. (1979). The roles of individual, kin and group selection in the evolution of sociality. In *Handbook of Neurobiology, Vol. 3: Social Behavior and Communication*, ed. P. Marler & J.G. Vandenburgh, pp. 351–94. Plenum Press: New York.

Verner, J. & Willson, M.F. (1966). The influence of habitats on mating systems of North American passerine birds. *Ecology*, **47**, 143–7.

de Waal, F.B.M. (1978). Exploitative and familiarity-dependent support strategies in a colony of semi-free-living chimpanzees. *Behaviour*, **66**, 268–312.

Watts, C.R. & Stokes, A.W. (1971). The social order of turkeys. *Scientific American*, **224**, 112–18.

West-Eberhard, M.J. (1975). The evolution of social behaviour by kin selection. *Quarterly Review of Biology*, **50**, 1–34.

West-Eberhard, M.J. (1978). Temporary queens in *Metapolybia* wasps: non-reproductive helpers without altruism? *Science*, **200**, 441–3.

Williams, G.C. (1966). *Adaptation and Natural Selection*. Princeton University Press: Princeton.

Wilson, E.O. (1975). *Sociobiology: the New Synthesis*. Harvard University Press.

Wittenberger, J.F. (1980). Group size and polygamy in social mammals. *American Naturalist*, **115**, 197–222.

Wrangham, R.W. (1979). On the evolution of ape social systems. *Social Science Information*, **18**, 335–68.

Wrangham, R.W. (1980). An ecological model of female-bonded primate groups. *Behaviour*, **75**, 262–300.

Wrangham, R.W. (1981). Drinking competition in vervet monkeys. *Animal Behaviour*, **29**, 904–10.

14

Sociodemographic attributes of nepotism in tribal populations: man the rule-breaker

NAPOLEON A. CHAGNON

Introduction

Let me begin by drawing attention to the fact that human sociality evolved in a context of small groups within which individuals were highly dependent on their neighbours for a number of critically important forms of support: acquiring food resources and cooperatively allocating them, protection from conspecifics both within and outside the group and from predators, and finding and keeping mates. While my comments are germane to all three forms of support, I want to emphasise in this paper the significance of cooperation and aid found among humans in finding and keeping mates, particularly during the long phase of our evolution when we lived as hunter/gatherers and as tribesmen.

The main thrust of this paper is to draw attention to the importance of broad features of tribal demography, such as mortality patterns, age/sex distributions, age difference between the sexes at birth of first child, and the longer reproductive life span of males, and to show how these relate to:

(a) ontogenetic changes during the life cycle of every individual, such changes being defined both physiologically and culturally;

(b) the high degree to which individuals in tribal societies must derive support from neighbours other than parents; and

(c) strategies for manipulating neighbours for selfish inclusive fitness interests.

I suggest that given the high degree of inter-individual dependence in such things as finding mates, the mortality patterns in tribal societies, and the chronic discrepancy between absolute age and generation classification, tribesmen probably *have always had to manipulate kinship information.* This is not to imply that local groups (bands, small communities) are invariably comprised of relatives or that manipulations are confined only to those individuals who are known kin. I do believe, however, that the composition of local groups historically and in the ethnographic present is heavily dominated by related individuals. While dyadic interactions in such groups can readily be analysed as a kind of reciprocity (West-Eberhard, 1975; Trivers, 1971), I will emphasise the kin selection aspects (Hamilton, 1964) of the interactions in this paper and the implications for nepotistic behaviour (Alexander, 1979).

This chapter appears in a book whose other contributors are all biologists in the broad sense of the term. As the only social scientist and only contributor who is dealing specifically with the application of sociobiological theory to human behaviour, the contemporary climate among social science experts who claim expertise in the interpretation of human behaviour affects my freedom of expression more than it does the positions developed by others in this volume. Even biologists seem uneasy or reluctant to extend the theory to humans. At the final conference of the group that presents this book, Professor John Maynard Smith asked, quite seriously, at the end of my comments: 'Why are anthropologists interested in this theory for "chaps" [humans]?' The question implies two kinds of answers. Either he thinks that it does not apply to man, in which case he would like to know why anthropologists are trying to apply it, or, he thinks that it does not apply to *any* social behaviour in any species, leaving himself in the unenviable position of having to explain why he goes about making theory that does not apply to real behaviour. Whatever the answer is to Maynard Smith's question, let me simply acknowledge the obvious: applying the theory to human social behaviour is greeted with less enthusiasm than it is when applied to the behaviour of other animals. With this in mind, I will rely extensively on the behavioural and reproductive data I have collected among the Yąnomamö Indians of southern Venezuela, a large tribe of Tropical Forest cultivators whose communities range in size from about 40 individuals to about 300, a tribe consisting of some 12 000 individuals.

Sociodemographic limitations to parental investment

Social anthropologists often conceive of the organization of band and tribal society as nested hierarchies beginning with the 'nuclear family' and building up into larger, more extensive units such as extended families, clans, lineages, etc. In speaking of the general composition of band societies, Elman Service offered the following generalization: 'Hence, husband–father, wife–mother, offspring, and perhaps an aged dependent make up the most cohesive unit in band society' (1971, page 57). How frequent is this cohesive unit in specific band (or tribal) societies? If it is commonplace or near-universal as a 'building block' in primitive social organization, then we would be led to assume that investments by parents in the well being of offspring are equally commonplace, and statistically common enough to direct our attention in the field to studying the quality and quantity of parental investment in 'typical' nuclear families. However, I rather suspect that the nuclear family so defined is not only rare in real primitive societies, but that it is relatively insignificant as a source of investment to individuals beyond the period of late juvenile development when aid from neighbours, especially for males in the context of acquiring mates, becomes critically important.

Consider the following statistics on the Yąnomamö Indians. Fig. 14.1 shows, for a large number of individuals ($N = 1326$), the proportion of cases in which any given person (males and females) has a coresident grandparent ('... an aged dependent ...') and the monogamously married couple that produced the individual, arranged by five-year age intervals.

Fig. 14.1. Percentage of individuals of both sexes who live in a household consisting of monogamously married parents plus one grandparent, arranged by 5-yr age intervals (c.f. Fig. 10.6).

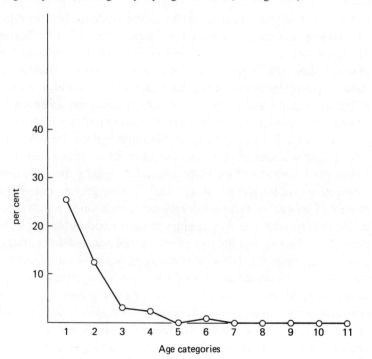

When they are between the ages of birth and four years, only about 25% of individuals in this population fit the description 'most cohesive unit' in band society, i.e., live in a household containing both living parents married (monogamously) to each other, and one grandparent. The fraction drops to about 12% in the age category five-to-nine years, and approaches zero by the time the age category 10–14 years is reached! As we shall see in a moment, the rarity of the 'nuclear family' defined in this fashion is largely due to the restriction of including an 'aged dependent,' a grandparent in this case, and partly due to the restriction that the parents can only be married monogamously. It is caused also by the divorce of parents after the birth of children, and by the relatively high incidence of mortality among adults, especially males. Still, the data draw attention to the statistical rarity of the social building block that many anthropologists assume to be relatively common in band and tribal society. From the vantage of sociobiological theory in general and investment theory in particular, a major question emerges: whence comes the investment that individuals need in a society where cooperation and mutual interdependence are crucial in acquiring and sharing material resources, for mutual defence and protection and, most important for young males, finding and keeping wives?

That a high degree of aid for males appears to come from non-parental kin in this society can be illustrated statistically. Apart from indicating that males who are successful at acquiring wives appear to have more kin in an absolute sense, the following data also indicate that the *kinds* of kin they have is equally significant. What this in fact says is that cultural definitions of kin are crucial variables in understanding human investment and nepotism patterns: having large numbers of the 'right kind' of kin where 'kind' is culturally defined. It must be kept in mind that in this society, and in many other primitive societies, marriages are arranged for young people by adult siblings and members of the older generation, usually the parents and the close relatives of the parents of both the bride and groom. Indeed, the very essence of politics in such societies is intimately bound up with the machinations of the adults as they attempt to acquire desirable mates for their dependent offspring and siblings' offspring, and much of the conflict in such societies emanates from these machinations. Since the offspring for whom the marriages are arranged are often very young – as young as five years old for females and mid-teens for males – the manipulations of the *parents* are central to understanding tribal fitness-maximizing strategies. Parents gain allies with families that are more or less powerful in local group activities, and the alliances entail obligations to continue ceding marriageable daughters over the generations. In a word, because humans arrange marriages for their offspring and other dependent relatives (many of whom are more important than others because of cultural definitions of 'importance' in local cultures), understanding strategies of mating among humans necessarily requires an understanding of both the individual's strategies as well as those of his elder kin.

This situation resembles, in a formal sense, 'parent/offspring conflict' (Trivers, 1974) in that it deals with the nature of investment patterns of elder and younger kin (often, though not invariably, separated by a generation). However, it often differs from parent/offspring conflict because the interests of the elder generation and the younger generation overlap extensively, particularly in the case of young males who strive to find a mate in a situation where mates are scarce, a condition brought about largely because some particularly successful males acquire multiple wives (Chagnon, Flinn & Melancon, 1979). If humans have been mildly polygynous throughout their history (Alexander, 1979) and if the marital success of males has been contingent on aid from parental and non-parental elder kin, young males have probably always been dependent on older males for support in acquiring mates, and older males have always been in a position to tender such aid, which benefits them as well as their young males dependants, in inclusive fitness terms.

Fig. 14.2 gives the distribution of patrilateral kin for all males aged 25 years or older among 529 living Yąnomamö who comprise the 'Shamatari'

Fig. 14.2. Average number of patrilateral relatives for men aged 25 or older who are (a) polygynous ($N = 36$), (b) monogamous ($N = 42$) or (c) single ($N = 9$).

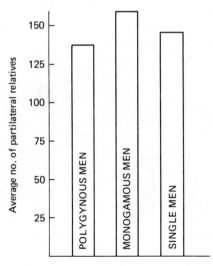

population bloc, a cluster of some half-dozen villages that have all derived through fissioning from a common village (Chagnon, 1974). The males have been segregated according to whether they were (1) polygynous, (2) monogamous or (3) single at the time of the last census (1975) of their villages. Thirty-six males were polygynous, 42 were monogamous and 9 were single in 1975. Every male in each category was examined to determine how many living kin he presently had who were related to him through patrilateral connexions, and an average was taken for males in each of the three matrimonial categories. The results show that males of the three matrimonial classes have roughly the same average number of patrilateral relatives (of all generations), suggesting that the number of this (culturally defined) kind of kin is not a critical variable in explaining marriage differences among them. The same kind of analysis was performed to determine the number of *matrilateral* kin that the males of the three matrimonial classes had. Fig. 14.3 gives this distribution. The statistics in Fig. 14.3 indicate that males who are single are 'handicapped' compared to monogamous or polygynous males in that they have fewer matrilateral kin than the matrimonially successful males of their own age. This is probably due to the *cultural* prescription, in this society, that males are obliged to find mates among their patrilateral *or* matrilateral cross-cousins (Chagnon, 1977) and having supportive kin in *both* social/

Fig. 14.3. Average number of matrilateral relatives for men aged 25 or older who are (a) polygynous ($N = 36$), (b) monogamous ($N = 42$) or (c) single ($N = 9$).

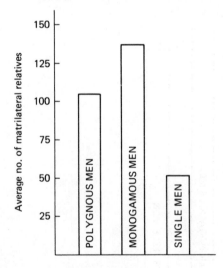

genealogical categories is crucial. Females who marry into local groups, either by amicable arrangements or through abductions, confer on their sons a disadvantage: the matrilateral relatives of those sons are living elsewhere, in distant villages, and are unlikely to tender aid to them, and their matrimonial fates largely depend on locating available patrilateral cross-cousins.

Finally, the culturally defined kinship axis 'laterality' is only one of several important cultural aspects of kinship. In this society, and many other tribal societies with identical marriage prescriptions (Murdock, 1949, 1957), the relative numbers of *ascending generation* kin or *own generation* kin are likewise important to males who strive to locate mates. Figs. 14.4 and 14.5 show the distributions, respectively, of *ascending* generation and *own* generation kin for the three matrimonial classes under consideration. Bearing in mind that marriages are arranged by the older patrilineal kin (siblings and men of father's generation), the more support a male has from such kin the greater is the likelihood that he will find a mate. Given the mortality patterns (Chagnon, 1974; Melancon, 1981) in this population, and with increasing age, a male must rely more and more heavily on his own-generation kin for support in his quest not only to find a mate, but to keep her as well (Fig. 14.5). This is also implied in the statistics on the distribution of the 'nuclear family' (as in Fig. 14.1) without the restriction of including an 'aged dependent'. Technically, the several curves in Fig. 14.6 refer to the potential sources of parental investment that individuals in the 11 age categories can draw on as they mature. The important features of the data in Fig. 14.6 are:

(a) An individual is more likely to have his or her mother alive and coresident for a significant fraction of infancy and adolescence than he or she is likely to have a father alive and coresident (cf. Figs. 14.2 and 14.3 for relatives of father and mother of married and unmarried men age 25 or older).

(b) At a relatively young age many individuals do not have both parents alive and coresident, e.g., by age 10–14 (curve C) some 60% do not have married coresident parents, and by ages 15–19 more than 75% do not. For males, this is a serious handicap if parental aid in finding mates is important.

(c) Individuals must expect to 'share' their potential parental aid with half-siblings in a large fraction of cases. Curve D gives the distribution of cases in which individuals live in monogamous households, showing that at ages between nought and four years only 50% of the individuals enjoy that security. Thus, while over 85%

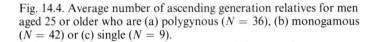

Fig. 14.4. Average number of ascending generation relatives for men aged 25 or older who are (a) polygynous ($N = 36$), (b) monogamous ($N = 42$) or (c) single ($N = 9$).

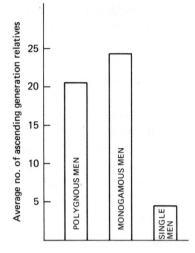

Fig. 14.5. Average number of own generation relatives for men aged 25 or older who are (a) polygynous ($N = 36$), (b) monogamous ($N = 42$) or (c) single ($N = 9$).

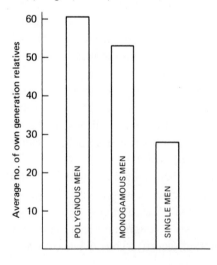

of individuals between nought and four years old have coresident married parents (curve C), a large proportion of these cases entail an extra spouse of one of the parents (usually the father).

Of all the features of these data, perhaps the most important is that individuals of both sexes have a relatively low probability of deriving aid from both of their natural parents by the time they are teenagers or young adults, just entering the matrimonial phase of their lives. The loss of a father (either by death or migration) restricts the amount of support that a young individual, particularly a young man, can expect from patri-kin and

Fig. 14.6. Percentage of individuals of both sexes, arranged by 5-yr age intervals, where (A) the mother is alive and coresident, (B) the father is alive and coresident, (C) both parents are alive, coresident and married either monogamously or polygamously, (D) both parents are alive, coresident and married only to each other and (E) both parents are alive, coresident, married monogamously and have at least one grand-parent alive and coresident. $N = 1326$. Curve E presents data from Fig. 14.1.

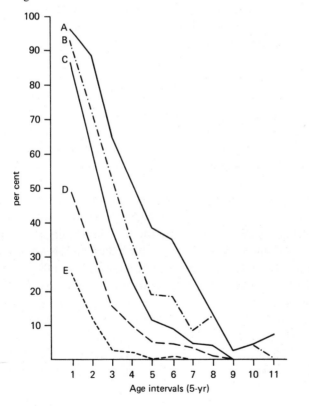

the loss of a mother restricts potential aid from relatives on her side of the family. Irons (1981) has drawn attention to the significance of the 'pooling' of resources, including marriageable females, among clusters of closely related males, as an efficient means for obtaining mates in a milieu of competition for mates, and he shows why such cooperative male coalitions are exogamic.

In short, the sociodemographic properties of a tribal population such as this one suggest that males in particular must solicit aid and support from neighbours other than parents in order to acquire mates.

Ontogeny: cultural and natural

Among humans, ontogenetic changes are given cultural attributes that often correspond to obvious physiological changes, such as puberty, but many of the cultural attributes are arbitrary and not predictable from the simple facts of physiology. At various stages in the individual's life cycle, he or she will have specific social and 'reproductive' values to individuals around him or her, values that emerge, endure for a time and then change by either diminishing or transforming with increasing age. Similarly, the neighbours with whom the individual must interact also go through the same kinds of social and reproductive transformations from Ego's perspective, and Ego must adjust his social behaviour when this occurs. I suggest that historically one of the most critical forces or 'environmental' factors to which the human individual had to adapt was the constantly changing ontogenetic attributes of the network of coresident neighbours – relatives and non-relatives – with whom Ego interacted socially during the life cycle. While we cannot study this directly, contemporary tribal societies can serve as an approximation to the general conditions to which I refer.

From the perspective of any given Ego striving to survive and reproduce, all neighbours can be conveniently thought of as falling into two broad categories: *social allies*, who are useful to Ego in acquiring material resources, aid in conflicts and finding suitable mates, and *social competitors* whose own survival and reproductive interests are in conflict with Ego's (see Irons, 1979, for a discussion of 'primary social allies and competitors'). In most human societies, Ego's relationships with some neighbours might be neutral or 'mutualistic' (see Wrangham, this volume) at one point in time, but antagonistic and competitive with the same neighbours at other points in time. These differences are not always reducible to changes in the social contexts, but are probably due to ontogenetic changes in the individuals involved. Thus, 12-year-old boys might hunt cooperatively and share in each other's catch, but at the age of 20 might have to oppose each other violently in club-fights because culturally imposed kinship classifications require it.

Given ontogenetic changes and some cultural definitions of social value based on them, individuals must be presumed to develop facultative strategies that are sensitive to changes in the social and reproductive utilities of neighbours, as well as changes in their own status vis-a-vis those neighbours. Thus, individual strategies for reproductive success should be viewed as chronically adjusting responses to chronically changing neighbours: neighbours grow, mature and transform in their social and reproductive utility to Ego, a process that is rooted not only in the biology of ontogeny, but also in the culturally prescribed meanings that humans impose on the individual's 'ideal' relationships to neighbours. In such a milieu, one would expect natural selection to favour highly flexible, facultative responses to the ever-changing social environment.

The individual's initial fund to kin: earned and unearned support

Neighbours can be viewed in this perspective as reproductively useful sources of investment. There is not an abundance of literature in anthropology that describes the genealogical structure of local groups in statistical terms, but the general position in qualitative terms is that in most tribal communities the individual is surrounded by kinsmen, a term that vaguely implies that some people are biological relatives and others are 'fictively' related by extensions of kinship terms. My comments here refer to the kinship structure of Yąnomamö communities where demonstrable genealogical connexions between individuals is defined as kinship. In these communities, very large fractions of the local group are genealogically related to most members of the group (Chagnon, 1979a). There are, however, 'inequalities' among individuals in that a few individuals in most communities will have almost no kin there, and some individuals in the community will have only a modest fraction of relatives compared to the 'in-group' that amounts to the kinship core of the community. Fig. 14.7 gives a graphic view of the distribution of kinship in one Yąnomamö village (from Chagnon, 1979a). It is not known how comparable this population is to other tribal societies insofar as the amount of relatedness within local communities is concerned, but I would suspect that it would be comparable to groups practising bilateral cross-cousin marriage; the latter is a matrimonial system commonly found in the primitive world, and a system that some anthropologists suggest as a good candidate for the organization of societies of early hunter/gatherers (Service, 1971; Fox, 1967).

Reproductive inequalities based on differential numbers of potential supporters begins at birth for each individual. Each has an initial 'fund' of kinsmen on whom he can rely. Initial investments received by children of both sexes derives largely from parents, but as the data in Fig. 14.6 have shown, there is an expectable early limit on purely parental investment for most individuals. Except for full siblings, the network of kin for each individual differs in both quantitative and qualitative aspects. Some individuals will have comparatively large numbers of kin who can aid them whereas others will have comparatively few. Figs. 14.2, 14.3, 14.4 and 14.5 show this for adult males. Individuals with comparatively few kin might, however, have more kin of the 'right' kind. The differences between individuals in their networks of kin at the time of birth must be attributable to the reproductive accomplishments of their immediate ascendants: these differences are relatively insensitive to large changes that might occur through the strivings of individuals. The most dramatic change an individual can affect in this regard is to elect to remain coresident with or separate from neighbours, thereby altering the patterns of nepotism at the local level. In addition, individuals can affect the kinds of relationships they have with some neighbours by manipulating kinship classifications, such as arbitrarily reclassifying a parallel cousin (a prohibited marriage partner) into a cross-cousin (a prescribed marriage partner). I will explore these two phenomena in a later section of the paper. Here, I wish to draw attention to

Fig. 14.7. Kinship relatedness in a typical Yąnomamö village, 16(N = 116), showing the percentage of relatives each individual has in the village arranged by quartiles: (A) individuals related to 25% or fewer of village residents, (B) individuals related to 26–50% of village residents, (C) individuals related to 51–75% of village residents, and (D) individuals who are related to more than 76% of village residents (from Chagnon, 1979a, p. 129).

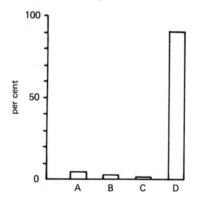

differences in the variation in reproductive success of males and females, and how they set into motion the inequalities in the initial fund of kin support that individuals can draw on during their life cycles.

Due to the success of a few males acquiring multiple wives, variation in reproductive success is higher among Yąnomamö males than it is among females (Chagnon, 1974; 1979*b*; Chagnon *et al*, 1979; Melancon, 1981). Quite predictably, the offspring of such males, particularly the sons, enter society with relatively more kin than the offspring of less-successful fathers. The initial advantage of these sons translates, in turn, to advantages for their own sons, who are surrounded by large numbers of individuals who are cousins of various kinds or siblings and half-siblings. High reproductive success among males thus begets high success among sons and grandsons (MacCluer, Neel & Chagnon, 1971; Chagnon, 1974; 1979*a*; *b*; 1980).

This variability in male reproductive success sets into motion a pattern of local population variability in which some individuals have many more kin of various categories than others do, i.e., they have a different 'fund of kinsmen' to draw on for nepotistic support. We may characterize this initial fund of kinship support, the 'unearned' component of the individual's kinship network, to emphasise the fact that the newborn individual has no control over the magnitude or composition of his kinship network. An individual can, however, affect the structure and size of the group of neighbours he lives with, which in effect structures nepotism at its most effective level in human societies: the local community. This is accomplished by the politics of individual alliance efforts and choices during local group fissioning on the one hand, and by reclassifying some kinds of kin as different kinds of kin on the other. The reclassification essentially moves these kin from a category of one type of social value, say 'negative,' to a category of 'positive' social value – marriageable for example. I will give examples of these below.

I would like to suggest at this juncture that the application of inclusive fitness theory in general and kin selection theory in particular with regard to tribesmen should focus primarily on the social interactions that take place at the local level. In effect, this means the activities among individuals in small, coresident communities such as bands or villages. This is because most of the interactions between individuals in fact take place at the local level, and individual strategies are geared to that level. While theoretically an individual can affect the reproductive success of individuals in distant communities, in fact individual strategies have probably been evolved to affect immediate neighbours. There are, of course, tribal situations in which groups periodically or chronically come into contact with each other, and the interactions can affect the inclusive fitness of individuals in both groups. These, I suggest, should be treated as a special case of the more general pattern of inclusive fitness strategies being designed for local level contingencies.

Through manipulations of local neighbours, an individual can improve his or her comparative fund of nepotistic support and, presumably, comparative inclusive fitness beyond what the initial 'luck of the draw' was regarding genealogical kin. These improvements – comparative increases in potential nepotistic support – can be viewed as 'earned' components in the individual's kinship network. By extension, the individual will have both an earned and an unearned dimension to his or her inclusive fitness characteristics. This is true because individuals will have many reproducing kin in other, non-local, communities whose reproductive accomplishments contribute to the number of genes Ego has represented in future gene pools, but Ego may or may not have been effectively involved ('favouring' or 'disfavouring' them) in affecting that reproductive success. Therefore, their contribution to Ego's fitness must be distinguished from contributions made to Ego's inclusive fitness that entailed Ego's effects on others. I suggest that the contributions to any individual's genetic representation made by individuals who have not been measurably affected by Ego's actions be designated as the 'unearned' component of inclusive fitness. Hamilton's definition of inclusive fitness (1964) refers to that portion of an individual's genetic representation in the population that is due to effects the individual had on the reproductive accomplishments of genetic relatives. These effects are, in practice, extremely difficult to measure. I am suggesting that for some highly social species, humans included, it might be in practice more useful to consider the total genetic representation an individual has in the population that is embodied among all detectable kin within a defined (bounded) region as the 'potential fund of kin' he can affect because of the *possibility* of interacting with them. One can then measure interactions in local communities among individuals, particularly interactions that change the composition and size of local communities, and assess the degree to which the interactions result in a new composition more favourable to the individual whose actions help bring it about. One important dimension of the composition of a group, in studies of humans whose mating practices are in some measure restricted by kinship classifications, is the relative number of mate competitors compared to potential mates in the local group, provided that a significant fraction of the mating takes place within the group.

In practical terms, using inclusive fitness characterizations makes the most sense in that maximal, bounded group within which an individual effectively operates as a social organism, because it is within such a bounded group that individuals can demonstrably affect their inclusive fitness by their influences on their neighbours. This appears to be true for most extant primitive societies and probably has been true throughout human evolution. With the development of agriculture, the Industrial Revolution and communications technology, of course, the bounds have increased dramatically. The problems that result from these changes are beyond the scope of this paper; I believe, however, that they are problems of measurement and that they are tractable.

Applying inclusive fitness theory to tribal societies appears, by comparison to large, national populations, to be relatively simple. Without some procedure to bound the population, however, the problems are still enormous. For example, individuals in tribal societies have many kin in remote villages or bands. In some cases, these kin are living at such a great distance because of conflicts and confrontations within a larger group that fissioned to produce two new communities. For instance, the headman of one of the groups might have expelled the others and driven them away, including some close relatives. That is to say, Ego (the headman) actively disfavoured them and drove them away to reproduce elsewhere. Hence, their reproductive accomplishments after the exodus are the result, in part, of Ego 'disfavouring' them, and one should conclude that some fraction of their reproductive accomplishments should be not only not positively included in Ego's inclusive fitness, but should be subtracted from it! I suspect that the only practical solution to problems of this genre would be to focus on relative changes at the local level of the individual's comparative reproductive success and/or local inclusive fitness as a consequence of observable and measurable influences on immediate neighbours.

Social strategies and two kinds of manipulations by males
Individual choices during fissioning of local communities
Band and tribal societies rarely become larger than a few hundred chronically coresident individuals. The Yąnomamö Indians are typical in this regard: most villages fission when they reach a population of about 125 to 150 individuals, but a few manage to grow larger – upwards of 400 individuals (Chagnon, 1974; 1979a). Fissions are the consequence of internal fighting among adult males, ultimately over sexual infidelity and the possession of females. It is the adult males who decide on fissions and who align the group in such a way that when they depart to create a new village, they will create a village that has a composition congenial to their own

political and social interests. Emically (from the 'native' point of view) this would be a village composed of individuals who are likely to cooperate economically, to lend unflinching support to the village elders in confrontations with other groups, and to be reluctant to disrupt local tranquility by engaging in sexual trysts with the wives of other men. Etically (from the scientific observer's point of view), a village fission keeps clusters of closely related individuals together and separates them from other clusters of individuals, the latter on average being less related to the first cluster than they are among themselves (Chagnon, 1974; 1975; 1979a). In addition, adult males separate from other adult males who are primary social competitors for females – usually distant parallel cousins and remote relatives of various categories. Conversely, they surround themselves with primary social allies – adult males who are siblings, half-siblings and cross-cousins (Chagnon, 1981). The formal characteristics of villages before and after fission, in anthropological terms, entail a transition from villages with a relatively heterogeneous lineage composition to new villages with a more conspicuous dual organization. That is to say, a prefission large village will be characterized by several lineages (groups of individuals related through male kinship and descent ties in this case) of varying size. Table 14.1 summarizes the composition of four villages that fissioned in the early

Table 14.1. *Increase in the percentage of adult males who belong to the two largest lineages in the village after four villages fissioned*

Village	Duality (%)	Increase in duality (%)	No. of adult males in village	Village size
Prefission: 14 + 99	56		45	157
Postfission $\frac{14}{99}$	58	+2	26	120
	56	0	9	37
Prefission: 1 + 8	52		56	222
Postfission $\frac{1}{8}$	61	+9	23	100
	48	−4	33	122
Prefission: 16 + 49	64		50	193
Postfission $\frac{16}{49}$	86	+22	29	116
	76	+12	21	77
Prefission: 18 + 19	75		53	225
Postfission $\frac{18}{19}$	67	−8	33	147
	90	+15	20	78

Five villages resulting from the fissions were more 'dual' (more adult males belonged to the two largest lineages in the village); two were less dual and one remained the same.

1970s, showing the resulting composition of the eight new villages that were formed and the tendency for most of them to be more 'dual' after the fission: five of the eight newly formed villages were more strongly dominated by two lineages. The figures are for adult males (aged 17 years or older) in the populations.

An interesting phenomenon after a fission is the conspicuous attempt on the part of some adult males to persuade allies who have elected to move away to return 'home' to the other village and bring their sisters and daughters with them. These efforts can be costly, such as clearing and planting a garden for the returnees. The process of village fissioning and the relationship of lineage structure to a male's long-term fitness interests can be shown more easily in a schematic representation of village fissioning, as in Fig. 14.8. Fig. 14.8 shows a hypothetical village in which there are 100 adult males divided into four patrilineal descent groups A, B, C and D. Each descent group would have one or more male leaders. Prior to fission, the leader or 'headman' of lineage C would have some authority over about 20% of the adult males of the village. Females from lineage C would be eligible mates for many of the males in lineages A, B and D, as well as eligible sexual partners for these males. The composition of the village prior to fission is 'heterogeneous' in the sense that it has four lineages in it. The advantage for the leader of lineage C to fission can best be seen in the second half of the Figure: although he is now in a much smaller village, his authority extends over *half* of the adult males in the village. In addition, the adult males who comprise the remaining 50% of the village are 'in-laws' to whom men of lineage C give their sisters and daughters and from whom their own wives are taken. The leader of lineage C, as well as the other males in that lineage, are now, after fission, in a village that is more congenial to their social and reproductive interests. It should be clear why males would agitate for a village fission – one of the more dramatic ways an individual male can manipulate his genealogical fund of power to his own reproductive advantage. While the headman of lineage C still has the same number of kin who will contribute to his inclusive fitness, he has established an improved milieu at the local level that is freer from competition and has increased his ability to affect the reproductive success of dependent kin and allies – he is better able to control and manipulate them in the relative absence of competing influences.

The genealogical dimensions of this process entails the accumulation of potential allies (siblings, first cross-cousins) and the simultaneous expulsion of potential competitors (distant parallel cousins, distant male kin of all categories) from the village. Fig. 14.9 shows the life cycle experience of males in one typical village with regard to potential allies and competitors. As a male grows older, he surrounds himself increasingly with siblings and cross-cousins, and simultaneously 'gets rid of' parallel cousins and other distant kin. Thus, between the ages of 0 and 14, a male will have only about 35% of his own-village male relatives falling into the 'allies' category, but after age 45 or so, some 80% of his own-village (male) relatives of his own generation will be siblings and cross-cousins. In terms of reproductive advantage, a fission leads to the reassortment of marriageable females in such a way that men in some villages have more female cross-cousins (eligible mates) than men in other villages created by a fission: some win and some lose. Fig. 14.10 shows the distribution of female cross-cousins for

Fig. 14.8. Schematic representation of fissioning in a Yąnomamö village showing the distribution of lineages before and after fission. Note the comparative increase of lineage C's influence in village composition and, by extension, reproductive advantages of the males in lineage C after fission.

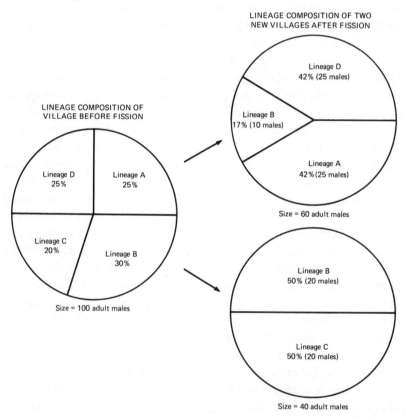

Fig. 14.9. Percent distribution by age category of 'social allies' (A) and 'social competitors' (C) in one Yąnomamö village (see text for definitions) for kin in Ego's own generation.

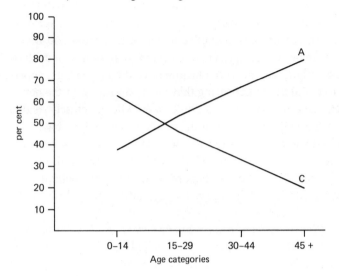

Fig. 14.10. Percent availability of mates (female cross-cousins) for males of different ages before and after the fission of a village into three villages (nos. 09, 16 and 49). Solid line, before fission.

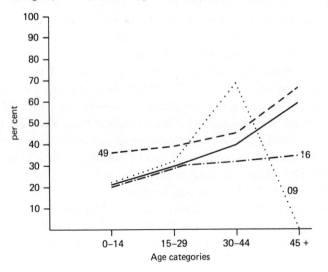

men of four age categories after a particular village fissioned, in this case, into three new villages. Note that the males of village 49 emerged with larger-than-average numbers of female cross-cousins than did the males of villages 16 and 09. In particular, the younger males of village 49 will have relatively large numbers of eligible mates (female cross-cousins).

Thus, a major advantage a male can gain by agitating for a village fission is that he might emerge as the headman of the new village, depending on how successful he is at ensuring that the composition of the new village is characterized by a majority of adult males who are closely related to him through the male line. In a large village a man might have a relatively subordinate status compared to the village headman – even though he might be the most prominent of his own lineage – but in the newly created village he might in fact be the headman and enjoy the perequisites that are associated with headmanship: polygyny and greater political authority.

Manipulation of neighbours by redefining their kinship identities

Individuals manipulate their neighbours by placing them into or removing them from culturally defined kinship categories in such a way as to make them more 'useful' reproductively, economically or politically, or to render them less effective as competitors. The more remote the relationship between individuals genealogically defined, the greater is the ease with which this kind of manipulation can take place without provoking village-wide outrage and reaction. Thus, a man is not likely to be able to redefine his actual daughter as 'wife' and marry her with impunity, but he is likely to redefine a distant female relative that he must call daughter because of remote genealogical ties to her, reclassifying her as 'wife'.

This is perhaps one of the thorniest issues making discourse between anthropologists and biologists difficult, since two distinct notions of 'kinship' are involved. Both are relevant to predicting and understanding human social behaviour (Fox, 1979). From the vantage of social anthropology, the kinship category one is placed in vis-a-vis some other individual prescribes a set of social and behavioural expectations. These are usually defined and identified by the anthropologist via native verbal or ideological expressions, such as 'brothers ought to be friendly to each other, share items willingly and defend each other in fights,' or 'the term for "wife" is the same term you use for your mother's brother's daughter, and you should marry only a woman who is called by that term.' Unfortunately, we social anthropologists rarely document 'brotherhood' or 'wifeship' in micro-behavioural terms such that 'brother' can also be defined in behavioural as well as genealogical or taxonomic ways. We do know that not all 'brothers' have the same biological parents, and this fact is usually taken to be the basis of the argument that you cannot reduce human kinship (which usually means systems of classification, not systems of behaviour) to biological relationships without doing considerable violence to the 'meaning' of kinship. Lamentably, only individual cases and anecdotes are recited to justify this general argument – that genealogy and classification do not mesh (see Sahlins, 1976, pp. 51–2). While it is undoubtedly true that kinship categories affect the behaviour of individuals (Fox, 1979), it is nevertheless true that we have precious little quantitative data that show this for classification and behaviour in real societies (see Chagnon, 1981, for some data).

The fact that human kinship classification deviates so markedly from a purely genealogical paradigm based on the facts of procreation is built into human reproduction practices and the biological facts of ontogeny. In most human societies, the age at which females marry and reproduce is usually significantly lower than that for males. Among the Yąnomamö, the average age of a mother giving birth is 26.8 years, and of the father at that time, 35.4 years. The population is growing, and the generation length for females is 26.3 years and for males 34.6 years. In addition, the effective reproductive life span of females is much shorter than that of males. The net result is that there will be more generations of descendants through females than through males, with the inevitable consequence that kinship classifications will always be discrepant with the biological pedigree based on the reproductive acts of parents. Individuals will therefore always have to 'adjust' the classification system to keep generations more-or-less in harmony with the specifications of the culturally defined kinship taxons. Fig. 14.11 (p. 312) illustrates this by showing the descendants of one Yąnomamö lineage 'founder' through the male and the female lines, i.e., it compares the number of descendants he has through males and descendants through females over four generations. The founder had roughly the same number of sons and daughters (20 and 23 respectively). In the second generation, he has more grandsons through his sons than granddaughters through his daughters, owing to the fact that some of his sons were highly successful because they had many social allies and sisters to cede in marriage. By the third generation, his greatgranddaughters via the female line are more numerous than his greatgrandsons via the male line: the shorter generation length and earlier age at marriage of females is beginning to show up here. Finally, in the fourth descending generation, his descendants (both male and female descendants are given for this generation) through males number only nine, but his descendants through females number 59, about six times as many. One predictable consequence of the fact that the generation length is shorter for females than for males is that with some inbreeding, individuals will be related to their spouses in complex ways. Some of these genealogical relationships are consistent with the cultural specifications of prescriptive marriage – for example, men 'should' marry cross-cousins, and many of them do – but some will be at odds with these specifications: spouses will be linked through relationships such that they are in different genealogical generations. By Yąnomamö definition, any marriage *between* generations constitutes incest, and therefore any generation-discrepant (genealogical) link between spouses amounts to violation of the incest prohibitions. Fig. 14.12 shows the genealogy of a typical Yąnomamö marriage that entails generation-aberrant relationships between spouses. The man, Ego 734, married a woman (403) to whom he was related in three different ways. The closest genealogical connection – MFSD – is a legitimate relationship by cultural rules, since he married his half-matrilateral cross-cousin, i.e., his mother's (half) brother's daughter. The remaining two genealogical connections (FFSDD and MFFSDDD) between the spouses are generation-aberrant and are therefore incestuous. In this particular marriage, and others similar to it, the important connection would be the closest one – which is, in this case, the only 'legitimate' connection between the spouses. In many cases, however, all connections might be equally close or remote and therefore there is ambiguity. In such

Fig. 14.11. Descendants of a successful Yąnomamö male through sons and daughters, showing the effects of shorter generation length through daughters.

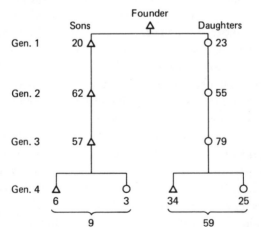

cases, 'interested' males will emphasise the connections that are legitimate and ignore the ones that are incestuous in order to place the female in question into a marriageable relationship. Other males, of course, would be doing the same and thus there would be conflict.

An exhaustive examination of all marriages among all living individuals in two multi-village Yąnomamö populations (approximately 1300 living individuals divided among 13 villages) showed that about 60% of the 817 marriages were consanguineous, i.e., the spouses were demonstrably related in some known genealogical way. Of these 485 marriages in which the spouses were related, 274 of them (56%) contained at least one incestuous link, the overwhelming fraction of which was generation-aberrant incest links (232 of 274, or 85%). Of these, some 40% (88 of the 232) entailed marriages in which there were 'legitimate' genealogical links connecting the spouses, i.e., marriages in which there was room to manipulate genealogical information to selfish ends.

But these do not even begin to cover the full extent to which manipulations actually occur, many of which involve manipulating just the kinship classifications, i.e., what people 'call' each other: these are not all counted in the above statistics on genealogically detectable incest, and it would be very difficult to detect even a fraction of those that entail only manipulations of

Fig. 14.12. Pedigree of a typical Yąnomamö marriage showing the multiple relationships between a male and his spouse. Ego's wife is related to him as (A) MFSD, (B) FFSDD and (C) MFFSDDD where M = mother, F = father, S = son and D = daughter. Only the first genealogical link conforms to the marriage rule; the two additional links are generation-aberrant and, by Yąnomamö definition, incestuous.

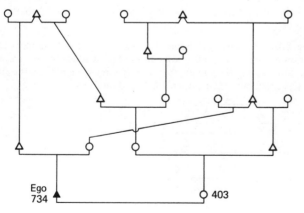

kinship *classifications*. The genealogical approach, in short, just identifies a portion of the incest and reveals, therefore, only a fraction of the manipulations that take place.

The way such manipulations work can best be seen in an example. Fig. 14.13 shows the marriage of Ego to a woman who is technically in a generation superior to his own and to whom he cannot trace a single legitimate genealogical link to make a case that the marriage is in fact 'legitimate' by some kinship tie. By Yąnomamö definition, this would be a definitely incestuous marriage. It came about when the individual labelled A in the diagram 'changed' his kinship terminology with respect to the woman labelled B in the diagram. Technically, he would have to call her (and did so before the manipulation) by a term used for 'brother's daughter.' However, he began calling her by a term meaning 'sister', thereby making her move up one whole generation. Since a man can, by the rules of marriage, marry a woman who is the daughter of a 'father's sister', the kinship manipulation made a whole new category of women available to the sons of A, one of whom is shown in Fig. 14.13 as married to the daughter of B. This incident provoked considerable anger and resentment among many of the adult males of the village, since the manipulation enabled A's son to marry a woman who was eligible to them as a marriage partner and hitherto ineligible to him. In fact, the manipulation ultimately led to a fission of the group with A and his sons forming the core of the group that pulled away from the larger village. Many people in the original village refused to change their kinship classification of the woman and contemptuously referred to the marriage as a blatant case of incest.

This is only one of several hundred cases of 'incest,' i.e., of individuals manipulating categories of kinship in order to define others as more useful reproductively than those which their given reciprocal kinship classifi-

Fig. 14.13. Pedigree of an incestuous marriage resulting from manipulation of kinship classifications: individual A redefined B as a sister, thereby making his son eligible to marry her daughter by the rule that males can marry their father's sister's daughters.

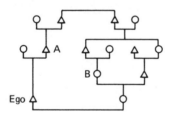

cations prescribed. But it is instructive in that it illustrates how individuals increase reproductive potentials through manipulations, and through these increase their 'earned' inclusive fitness. The given (cultural) kinship classifications are learned through the juvenile period and enculturated into the young people as they grow up. One might view this process as a social means to acquire a knowledge of the rules of kinship classification in order to *break* them efficiently, i.e., calculating the probable risks for so doing and the size of one's support group which will defend the legitimacy of the fabrication. For the demographic and social reasons discussed above, it would appear that classification systems and genealogical relationships are always out of synchrony with each other, and in small tribal communities where life is organized by kinship, chronic manipulations of kinship classification must occur. From this vantage, humans are not so much to be heralded as rule *makers* as they are to be appreciated as rule *breakers*. In the case of kinship classifications and manipulations, it seems likely that the overall patterns of the manipulations have a general tendency to benefit the inclusive fitness interests of the manipulators, a special case of the more general proposition suggested by Alexander (1979): that rules are the outcome of the inclusive fitness maximization efforts of members of our species, and that breaches of them should be viewed in this context.

Insofar as incest is concerned, defined as generation-aberrant marriage in this case, the manipulations appear to take place when individuals are related in multiple ways and the manipulated relationships are relatively remote, such as half-cousins or second-cousins. This is germane to kin-selection studies of humans in the sense that simple closeness of kinship as a predictor of behaviour must be tempered by a consideration of cultural prescriptions and the structure of the genealogical relationships whose combined magnitude, measured by the coefficient of relatedness, expresses that closeness. Previous studies have indicated that closeness of relatedness between individuals in such things as fights (Chagnon & Bugos, 1979) and village fissioning (Chagnon, 1975, 1981) is a reasonably good predictor of behaviour when the relationships are close ones. The data on incest and kinship manipulations suggest that for more remote degrees of relationship, such as second-cousins, the statistic 'r' might not be a very reliable predictor by itself. I suggest that in communities with relatively high degrees of inbreeding, such as the ones discussed here, the reliability of 'r' as a predictor of individual behaviour would be in the general range of $1.000 > r > 0.0325$.

Summary

1. A peculiar feature of human sociality, ethnographically and presumably historically, is that individuals arrange the marriages of their offspring. Male offspring in particular have difficulty acquiring mates due to the effects of polygyny, and therefore require kinship investments and cooperation more than females.

2. Mortality patterns, differences in ages of males and females at marriage, divorce and other sociodemographic features of tribal populations indicate that individuals can expect very little support from biological parents beyond adolescence, and must actively solicit support from non-parental kin through individual strategies that entail manipulations of kinship information and choosing to remain with and support particular kin.

3. Physiological changes due to ontogeny and the cultural attributes attached to them create a social milieu in which the individual must facultatively adjust to an ever-changing milieu while pursuing strategies which maximise inclusive fitness.

4. Variations in the reproductive accomplishments of ascending generation kin set into motion inequalities among individuals in the size and structure of the kinship network. Individuals can, through manipulation and calculated strategies of alliance, improve their reproductive potentials at the local level, thus adding an earned component to the unearned kinship network inherited at birth.

5. Many practical and theoretical problems in the application of kin selection theory to humans can be made more tractable by focusing on the relative changes that individuals make in their reproductive strivings at the local level. Inclusive fitness measurements can be distinguished into an earned and an unearned component, relatable to the success of individual strategies at the local level.

6. The sociodemographic features of small populations and local traditions of arranged marriages create a situation in which genealogical relationships are always discrepant with kinship classifications, and individuals must chronically reclassify relatives to keep age and generation in synchrony. The social arena in which this occurs involves incestuous marriages and kinship reclassifications in which the manipulators attempt to improve their inclusive fitness by the reclassifications. Such manipulations suggest that the coefficient of relationship, 'r,' might be a marginally reliable predictor of behaviour in the range $0.2500 > r > 0.0325$.

The sociodemography of reproduction in human societies requires that Man be as much a rule breaker as he is a rule maker.

The research on which this paper is based was provided by the Harry Frank Guggenheim Foundation, to which I am greatly indebted. Earlier field research support, yielding the data discussed here, was provided by the National Institute of Mental Health, the National Science Foundation and the Harry Frank Guggenheim Foundation.

I would like to express my gratitude also to King's College, to the Department of Social Anthropology, Cambridge University, and to the participants in the King's College Research centre's project on sociobiology, who graciously and warmly served as my hosts at King's College during my sabbatical leave (January through July, 1980) when this paper was written. I am especially indebted to Dan Rubenstein, Richard Wrangham and Meyer Fortes for insights and perspectives they shared with me in numerous conversations and informal meetings.

I would like to thank a number of colleagues who read earlier drafts of this paper and who offered many useful and penetrating criticisms of it; I would also like to apologize to them as well, since the final draft differs substantially from the one they so thoughtfully criticized, in part a result of their comments and in part a result of emphases I decided to add. Dan Rubenstein, Richard Wrangham, William Irons, Elizabeth Thompson, Paul Sherman and Thomas Melancon all read and criticized the earlier draft, and I am grateful to them for their many useful comments, suggestions and criticisms. I hope the final draft is an improvement in their eyes.

References

Alexander, R.D. (1979). *Darwinism and Human Affairs*. Pitman Publishing Limited: London.

Chagnon, N.A. (1974). *Studying the Yąnomamö*. Holt, Rinehart and Winston: New York.

Chagnon, N.A. (1975). Genealogy, solidarity and relatedness: limits to local group size and patterns of fissioning in an expanding population. *Yearbook of Physical Anthropology*, **19**, 95–110. American Association of Physical Anthropologists: Washington.

Chagnon, N.A. (1977 [1968]). *Yąnomamö: The Fierce People*. Holt, Rinehart and Winston: New York.

Changnon, N.A. (1979*a*). Mate competition, favoring close kin, and village fissioning among the Yąnomamö Indians. In *Evolutionary Biology and Human Social Behavior: An Anthropological Perspective*, ed. N.A. Chagnon & W. Irons, pp. 86–132. Duxbury Press: North Scituate, Massachusetts.

Chagnon, N.A. (1979*b*). Is reproductive success equal in egalitarian societies? In *Evolutionary Biology and Human Social Behavior: An Anthropological Perspective*, ed. N.A. Chagnon & W. Irons, pp. 374–401. Duxbury Press: North Scituate, Massachusetts.

Chagnon, N.A. (1980). Kin-selection theory, kinship, marriage and fitness among the Yąnomamö Indians. In *Sociobiology: Beyond Nature/Nurture?*, ed. G.W. Barlow & J. Silverberg, pp. 545–71. AAAS Selected Symposium No. 35. Westview Press: Boulder.

Chagnon, N.A. (1981). Terminological kinship, genealogical relatedness and village fissioning among the Yąnomamö Indians. In *Natural Selection and Social Behavior: Recent Research and New Theory*. ed. R.D. Alexander & D.W. Tinkle, pp. 490–508. Chiron Press: New York.

Chagnon, N.A. & Bugos, P.E. Jr. (1979). Kin selection and conflict: an analysis of a Yąnomamö ax fight. In *Evolutionary Biology and Human Social Behavior: An Anthropological Perspective*, ed. N.A. Chagnon & W. Irons, pp. 213–38. Duxbury Press: North Scituate, Massachusetts.

Chagnon, N.A., Flinn, M.V. & Melancon, T.F. (1979). Sex-ratio variation among the Yąnomamö Indians. In *Evolutionary Biology and Human Social Behavior: An Anthropological Perspective*, ed. N.A. Chagnon & W. Irons, pp. 290–320. Duxbury Press: North Scituate, Massachusetts.

Fox, R. (1967). *Kinship and Marriage: An Anthropological Perspective*. Penguin: London.

Fox, R. (1979). Kinship categories as natural categories. In *Evolutionary Biology and Human Social Behavior: An Anthropological Perspective*, ed. N.A. Chagnon & W. Irons, pp. 132–44. Duxbury Press: North Scituate, Massachusetts.

Hamilton, W.D. (1964). The genetical evolution of social behaviour, parts I and II. *Journal of Theoretical Biology*, 7, 1–52.

Irons, W. (1979). Investment and primary social dyads. In *Evolutionary Biology and Human Social Behavior: An Anthropological Perspective*, ed. N.A. Chagnon & W. Irons, pp. 181–213. Duxbury Press: North Scituate, Massachusetts.

Irons, W. (1981). Why lineage exogamy? In *Natural Selection and Social Behavior: Recent Research and New Theory*, ed. R.D. Alexander & D.W. Tinkle, pp. 466–89. Chiron Press: New York.

MacCluer, J.W., Neel, J.V. & Chagnon, N.A. (1971). Demographic structure of a primitive population: a simulation. *American Journal of Physical Anthropology*, 35, 193–207.

Melancon, T.F. (1981). *Marriage and Reproduction Among the Yąnomamö Indians*. Ph.D. Thesis. Pennsylvania State University.

Murdock, G.P. (1949). *Social Structure*. MacMillan: New York.

Murdock, G.P. (1957). World ethnographic sample. *American Anthropologist*, 59, 664–87.

Sahlins, M.D. (1976). *The Use and Abuse of Biology: An Anthropological Critique of Sociobiology*. University of Michigan Press: Ann Arbor.

Service, E.R. (1971 [1962]). *Primitive Social Organization: An Evolutionary Perspective*, 2nd edn. Random House: New York.

Trivers, R.L. (1971). The evolution of reciprocal altruism. *Quarterly Review of Biology*, 46, 35–57.

Trivers, R.L. (1974). Parent-offspring conflict. *American Zoologist*, 14, 249–64.

West-Eberhard, M.J. (1975). The evolution of social behavior by kin selection. *Quarterly Review of Biology*, 50, 1–33.

V

The problems of comparison

Edited by
T.H. CLUTTON-BROCK

Introduction

The great majority of sociobiological arguments are initially based on comparisons of the behaviour of animals in different social or ecological environments. Their development usually follows much the same pattern: field observations show that behaviour varies with social or ecological circumstances; a generalisation is constructed concerning the relationship between specific behavioural and environmental parameters; an adaptive explanation is proposed; and the generalisation and explanations are tested by experiments or by further comparisons. Though this process is often similar, the level at which comparisons are made varies widely. Traditionally, species were most frequently compared but, more recently, comparisons between populations, between social groups, between age or sex categories, or between individuals of the same age and sex category have become increasingly common.

In the first chapter of this section, Peter Jarman discusses the use of the interspecific comparisons. These have yielded many important insights into the adaptive significance of particular aspects of social behaviour – as Jarman's own work on antelope shows (Jarman, 1974). They have two principal advantages: interspecific differences in social behaviour and ecology are often so pronounced that relationships between them are obvious even if behavioural and ecological measures are rudimentary, or are based on different methodologies; and, within many adaptive radiations, a sufficient number of species have been studied to allow generalisations to be subjected to formal statistical testing. However, as Jarman points out, they have many limitations: the absence of any currency in which to measure adaptation; the widespread danger of confounding variables; the tendency for phylogenetically different species to adapt to similar environmental circumstances in qualitatively different ways; and the frequent impossibility of determining the direction of causality. Quantitative comparisons at this level also face a wide variety of more specific problems, including the quality and comparability of the information they are forced to use, uneven distributions of data within particular radiations, nonlinear relationships between ecological and behavioural measures and the need to allow for the confounding effects of differences in body size on both ecological and behavioural variables.

If these problems are to be solved or reduced, improvements in the methodology of comparisons are needed. In the second chapter, Paul Harvey and Georgina Mace describe some of the statistical pitfalls likely to occur in comparisons between species and suggest ways of avoiding or minimizing them. In particular, they draw attention to the implausibility of the assumption that values drawn from closely related species can be regarded as independent points and outline methods for determining the level at which taxa can be treated as being formally independent. The second part of their chapter is principally concerned with problems of controlling for the effects of variation in body size. Since both anatomical and physiological parameters and many aspects of ecology are influenced by differences in body size, attempts to investigate relationships between particular traits and ecological variation often require controls for size effects (Clutton-Brock & Harvey, 1979). The commonest technique is to plot size-related variables against body size itself and to compare the deviations of species allocated to different ecological groups from the overall regression line. However, as Harvey and Mace argue, there are several statistical problems inherent in this approach which have been largely ignored – among them, the fact that, regression analysis can produce a biased estimate of the line of best fit, and the tendency for the slope of regression lines to change in relationship to the taxonomic level of the group of animals considered. Though Harvey and Mace principally consider anatomical traits, the same problems apply to comparisons involving behavioural characteristics, many of which are also affected by body size. Moreover, they are not confined to interspecific comparisons but are likely to recur whenever animals of different sizes are compared.

Some of the problems faced by interspecific comparisons can be avoided by investigating the effects of ecological differences on the social behaviour of different populations of the same species, and a growing number of studies – particularly those of primates – have adopted this approach (see Chalmers, 1979). Though inter-population comparisons have demonstrated the extent to which aspects of social behaviour can vary within species, they have (with some notable exceptions) produced few generalisations. One problem is that the number of populations which can be compared is usually small. In addition, the effects of particular environmental differences on social behaviour are often confounded with those of variation in population density.

Perhaps the most promising approach of all in investigating the adaptive significance of social behaviour is to compare different individuals belonging to the same population. At this level, it is possible to examine the effects of differences in behaviour on variation in reproductive success, the raw material on which natural selection operates. In the final chapter, Nick Davies reviews recent attempts to explain individual differences in social behaviour as alternative strategies for maximizing reproductive success. His paper provides a classification of the evolutionary processes likely to produce and maintain behavioural variation in the same population. These break down into two principal categories – cases where selection favours different strategies because individuals vary in competitive ability; and those where two or more alternative strategies are maintained in equilibrium because their benefits are negatively related to their frequency in the population. Differences of the first kind are widespread though, on account of their conceptual elegance, those of the second have attracted more attention. However, it is often difficult to tell which are which. In a stable situation, alternative strategies maintained by frequency-dependent selection should have the same pay-offs (Maynard Smith, 1979). But what kind of evidence is needed to show that the pay-offs of two strategies are identical? A recurrent difficulty in measuring pay-offs is that the costs of particular forms of behaviour will include changes in the frequency of rare events, such as attacks by predators, which can have important effects on the net benefits of strategies but are unlikely to be measured in short-term studies. Another problem is that particular strategies may have delayed costs – for example, wild rams that breed very energetically may suffer a reduction in their lifespan (Geist, 1971). The same problems can also apply to measurements of benefits, though perhaps they do so to a lesser extent, and are common to all attempts to measure the costs and benefits of behavioural differences in terms of reproductive success. However, as Davies argues, they are least likely to be confusing where it is possible to measure the lifetime reproductive output of individuals who behave in consistently different ways.

In the past, the great majority of studies have relied principally on comparisons at one level. In future, it seems likely that studies which can compare the pay-offs of particular strategies in different populations, or different species, and can relate these to variation in their frequency and distribution hold great promise.

References

Chalmers, N. (1979). *Social Behaviour in Primates*. Arnold: London.
Clutton-Brock, T.H. & Harvey, P.H. (1979). Comparison and adaptation. *Proceedings of the Royal Society*, B, **205**, 547–65.
Geist, V. (1971). *Mountain Sheep*. University of Chicago Press.
Jarman, P.J. (1974). The social organisation of antelope in relation to their ecology. *Behaviour*, **48**, 215–67.
Maynard Smith, J. (1979). Game theory and the evolution of behaviour. *Proceedings of the Royal Society*, B, **205**, 475–88.

15

Prospects for interspecific comparison in sociobiology

PETER JARMAN

Comparison in sociobiology

This paper discusses the ways in which interspecific comparison can help sociobiologists to synthesise evolutionarily plausible explanations of social behaviour from knowledge of a species' ecology, morphology, physiology and general biology. As in other evolutionary disciplines, the adaptiveness of social behaviour can be expressed only in relative, not absolute, terms. Comparison remains a fundamental investigative method in sociobiology, being used to investigate the evolutionary paths taken by taxa, the diversity of forms of behaviour coexisting in a population, or an individual's relative success when behaving in one manner rather than another.

These uses of comparison cover the range of both interindividual and interspecific comparative studies, and arise from rather different questions. If the question takes the form 'in these circumstances, would an individual benefit most by doing X, Y, or Z?', then the studied animals must be as alike as possible in all respects except their behaviour, so that the relative success of each form of behaviour can be seen without confounding effects of variations in context. The compared individuals should be matched for species, populations, sex, age, social class, experience, nutritional and reproductive state, and any other relevant variables, before being compared for success resulting from different forms of behaviour. Such close matching is not always achieved, but may be approached when the individuals match themselves. In many societies, individuals of carefully matched categories compete over limited resources, opportunity to mate providing good examples. If such individuals use contrasting tactics to achieve the same ends, the relative benefits, and sometimes the costs, of the behavioural variants can be directly compared.

Such interindividual comparison in effect hopes to catch evolution in action. If the contrasted individuals differed only in their variants of behaviour, and if those variants were genetically or culturally inherited, then, balancing costs with benefits, the success of one variant implies an evolutionary advantage for one individual's behaviour over the other's *in those circumstances*. On such data are evolutionary models built, but in reality the behavioural differences are frequently associated with differences in the individuals' condition, experience, or expectations. When this is so, comparison answers the much broader question 'In what circumstances should an individual do X, Y, or Z?' The question assumes that observed behaviour is adaptive in the context of the animal and its environment, and therefore that differences in behaviour will be found to arise from differences in context. Such differences of context may be slight within species: a matter of age, experience, bodily condition, or perhaps sex of the compared individuals. The results of such comparisons reveal the flexibility in behavioural strategies that has evolved in many species.

However, when species are compared, differences in context can be profound since the contrasted animals differ in morphology and physiology, and occupy distinct ecological niches if sympatric, and at least different habitats if allopatric. There is no common currency in which to measure relative success between compared species. Nor is one needed, since the primary purpose of interspecific comparison in sociobiology is not to evaluate success, but to describe the associations that occur, in a particular taxonomic group, between the species' ecological, morphological and physiological characteristics and their behavioural attributes. These descriptions may then be generalised into 'laws' of sociobiological expectation, which are predictions of associations between these variables. Rather than predicting the outcome of two behavioural tactics opposed over the same problem, interspecific comparison assumes that the considered sociobiological strategies are those that have proved competitively most appropriate for that species in the evolutionary past.

Interspecific comparison supports arguments about evolutionary causality by inference. Its explanations, while not strictly disprovable, gain credence as they are found to be widely applicable. They depend initially upon recognising patterns of associations between behavioural and ecological or other biological variables within arrays of related species. However, these patterns may be difficult to perceive within a matrix of many inter-relating variables. Some variables may obliterate the effects of others, and the same form of behaviour may arise from the associations of quite different sets of variables.

Despite such thorny problems, the pioneering interspecific studies in sociobiology attracted attention because they made a coherent picture from a miscellany of seemingly unrelated data on the behaviour and ecology of species. Hinde (1955–6, 1956), Cullen (1957) and von Haartmann (1957) had already shown that some aspects of bird behaviour could be viewed as adaptations to their environments, when Crook (1964) first postulated adaptive causes for all the diverse forms of social behaviour in a large subfamily of birds, the Ploceinae. He argued that bird populations were limited by food supply and not predation, that individuals survive only if they can compete effectively to find and exploit food, and that adaptation for food exploitation will therefore be paramount.

> 'The social organisation of a species within its environment must therefore be primarily an adaptation to its food supply while adaptations with respect to predation and other factors appear superimposed upon this primary organisation. The nature of a bird society is determined fundamentally by its food economy' (Crook, 1964, p. 4).

He later (Crook, 1965) generalised this argument to all bird species.

Crook's intuitive appreciation of the patterns of association between behaviour and ecological attributes of species was acute and revelatory, yet his quoted argument, like any other about evolutionary causes, could only be speculative. Other sociobiologists held contradictory views: Cullen (1960) felt that anti-predator behaviour determined the nesting behaviour of terns; Estes (1974) emphasised the role of cover density in the evolution of antelope social behaviour; while Rood (1972) felt that finding physical refuge from predators influenced social behaviour in cavies, for example. Each or any might be right, although none can be proved to be so.

Once the associations between behavioural and other variables have been established within several arrays of species, the stage is set for comparative investigations between arrays. Have the same associations between social behaviour and ecology evolved in separate taxa; are there sociobiological 'laws' which are generally applicable? Has each behavioural phenomenon evolved consistently under the same circumstances? To answer this last question, as many taxa as possible must be reviewed for the occurrence of the phenomenon, so that a commonly plausible account of its adaptiveness can be given.

Data and methods of interspecific comparison

The steps in interspecific comparison are simple in outline. An ecologist or ethologist, aquainted with a range of related species, recognises that several characteristics of the species, their environments and their behaviour tend to vary together. The most clearly associated variable characteristics are measured and their associations described for each species. A plausible evolutionary story is then offered to explain the associations. The first step in this process depends on experience and intuition, the second on good field, museum, and library work, and the third on imagination and a feel for what is probable in evolution. There are problems at each step.

The first problem is the premise that the compared species are closely related, so that 'the effects of discrepancies in natural genetic endowment can be minimised, and that the true adaptive nature of social behaviour will thus be revealed' (Barash, 1974); 'discrepancies' obviously meant genotypic differences thought to be irrelevant to the comparison. As nearly as possible, sociobiologists want to compare species differing only in comprehensible, associated variables of ecology, morphology, physiology or behaviour. This is difficult because of intrinsic properties of radiations of species (discussed below), but is a reasonable approximation for most coarse-grained reviews.

The ideal study group would consist of species that have diverged from each other at a similar rate over the same span of time, without selective extinction or convergence. This is most likely to be true for the genus, but the number of species and ranges of values for associated variables are likely to be small. In the Family or Order, large numbers of species can be compared, but secondary radiations or selective extinctions may distort the values of associations between variables, and convergence may produce heterogeneity in the origins of associations, i.e. the same sociobiological effect may arise in response to several different combinations of variables.

Comparative studies seek to associate the species' behaviour with species-typical values of variables that are: *extrinsic to the animals* (such as physical attributes of the habitat, climate, food availability, food item dispersion, or probability of variations in these factors); *intrinsic to the animals* (such as body weight, metabolic requirements, age at maturity, horn shape, colouring, or sexual dimorphism); or *instantaneous interactions between these* (such as selected diet, activity pattern, population density, longevity, or exposure to predators). Some values are averages for the behaviour of individuals (such as median size of home range or territory, mean frequency of actions, activity profiles, or typical mating system); others characterise the population (such as descriptions of social organisation, differences between male and female mortality rates, sex ratio, or population density).

Only a few of this heterogeneous array of types of data can be measured simply; several need long and intensive field studies; others can be only described, not quantified. Some of the technical problems of gathering and expressing them are listed by Clutton-Brock & Harvey (1978):

  (i) species may have been studied by different and incomparable methods;
  (ii) only gross behavioural and ecological traits can be compared;
  (iii) field research may be spread unevenly across the array of species;
  (iv) a representative average may be difficult to calculate if an attribute varies greatly within a species; and
  (v) relationships between variables may differ between subgroups within the range of compared species.

The first three problems can be resolved by improvement and standardisation of techniques, and planned proliferation of field studies; the other two are discussed later. Comparative studies are limited by the highest common level of quality in a measurement, and by the difficulties of devising widely applicable measurements of behaviour, ecology, and social organisation. Some of the attributes used have been superficial (but obvious) consequences of the selective evolutionary processes being investigated (e.g. dimorphism, group size), rather than the primary factors involved in the selection (see below). When comparing such consequences, heterogenous causes can easily be confounded within apparently homogenous consequences; analogous attributes may be mistaken as functionally and causally identical. When the analogous attributes themselves are to be explained, their heterogenous causes must be distinguished; yet the same attributes may be treated as homogenous in their effects upon other attributes. For example, females in a few vertebrate species are significantly larger than males, and species vary in the combinations of circumstances that make this adaptive (see Ralls, 1976). Yet that dimorphism will have similar effects (females being successfully aggressive towards males, for example) in most of those species.

Producing a plausible explanation of the observed associations becomes easier as other studies offer model arguments. In trying to explain an evolved, interactive system, such as that shown by Crook & Gartlan (1966, Fig. 1), there are many opportunities for circular arguments. To avoid these it may be prudent to assume that at least one major interaction goes only or predominantly in one direction. Clutton-Brock & Harvey (1977), for example, assumed that changes in feeding niche caused behavioural and consequent organisational changes during the evolution of primates. Barash (1974) argued that the length of growing season for vegetation dictated the evolution of growth rate, ages at independence and sexual maturity, persistence of parent–offspring ties, interindividual behaviour, and hence social organisation, in marmot species. These assumptions are justified by the plausibility they bring to the evolutionary explanations.

Although there may be doubts about which data to use, or the comparability of data from different studies, and dismay at having to discard data from one good study because no comparable data were obtained in poorer studies, the strengths of interspecific comparison come partly from its data. So many data can be used; so many aspects of animals, their behaviour and their environments need to be known that almost any study can still contribute substantially. There is room for amateurs and armchair-naturalists; and it matters as much to complete surveys of well-known arrays of species as to pioneer a study of the most exciting obscure group.

Intrinsic properties of radiations of species

In a monophyletic radiation of many species there are typically a few large species, catholic in their diet and habitat preferences, several or many medium-sized species, and many small species, often narrowly specialised in diet, feeding technique, and habitat. This tendency is seen, among land mammals, in the Dasyuridae, Phalangeridae, Macropodidae, Microchiroptera, Primates, sciuromorph, myomorph and hystricomorph rodents, Mustelidae, Canidae, Viverridae, Felidae, Cervidae and Bovidae. (It is no longer clear in Ursidae, Equidae, Suidae, Camelidae, Proboscidea, Rhinocerotidae, Vombatidae, and others where the few extant species are often medium to large-sized remnants of formerly broader radiations.) The same tendency appears among other animal classes. It is simply explained in terms of the relative advantages of narrow and broad niche dimensions for small and large competitors respectively, the more numerous opportunities for narrow niches, and the relatively greater chance of isolation for a specialist. The result can be seen in any sociobiologist's scattergram where sizes, or size-dependent attributes, of an array of species are plotted against another variable; the scatter is sparse towards the large-bodied end of the range. This unequal spread of points causes problems in some descriptions of the relationship between the variables.

The relationships between variables in arrays of species are commonly not rectilineal. Different specialisations of behaviour and ecology accompany being large or small, and thus the relationships between attributes are likely to be very different at the extremes of an array's range of body sizes. Among the African bovids, for example, the biggest species, eland *Taurotragus oryx* and buffalo *Syncerus caffer*, are large enough to be safe from all but a few predators, to feed very unselectively, to store and mobilise metabolites efficiently, and to move long distances cheaply. Their life is not dominated by maintaining a battery of tactics to combat all sorts of predators, nor by a painstaking search for individual food items, as is the life of very small antelopes like suni *Nesotragus moschatus* or dik-dik *Madoqua* spp. Such small species, vulnerable to a range of predators, must be always alert, concealed and cryptic; their rare, scattered food items must be individually sought (Jarman, 1974). The selection of food items and avoidance of detection by predators, so important at one end of the size range, are less critical at the other extreme. The relative 'importance' of some external factors might be linked to body size as in Fig. 15.1; others might behave as in Fig. 15.2.

A species evolves its position in a radiation by modifying a cluster of coadapted characteristics which may not vary as simple scaled versions of a basic model. A dik-dik is not just a small gazelle, nor an eland a large one. Departures from a scaled model emphasise the adaptations of animals' attributes to their different relationships with environmental constants such as distances between resources, or size of plants, or dimensions of

Fig. 15.1. Hypothetical relationships between the 'importance'-rating of two attributes and the body size of antelopes. These exemplify probable curvilinear relationships of attributes and their evolutionary importance in arrays of species. Both these attributes become less important as body size increases, but at different and varying rates.

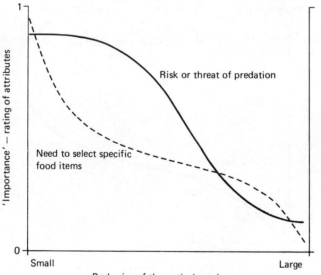
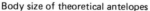

cover. One species may tolerate much greater variation in the availability of some less 'important' resource, or devote more time to obtaining some more 'important' resource, than does another species. As the importance-rating of factors varies, alteration in the cluster of coadapted characteristics will produce at the extremes of extensive radiations species which have evolved under quite different pressures. This makes it less likely that relationships between variables will be linear right across an array of species.

Trends in adaptation of attributes are often noticed because of the contrast between species at the extremes; indeed, Estes (1974) used several two-way classifications to analyse correlation of environmental and intrinsic attributes of African bovids. Such analyses lose information by forcing each continuously distributed variable into two classes (e.g. size large/small; inhabiting plains/forest; horns complex/simple), and discounting the evolutionary responses of the non-extreme species. Mid-radiation species may show great specialisation in one attribute coupled with catholicity in others, or general flexibility in their response to the environment. This flexibility is itself a most interesting sociobiological adaptation.

Fig. 15.2. Hypothetical relationship between the 'importance'-rating of two attributes and the body size of antelopes. These exemplify probable curvilinear relationships of attributes and their evolutionary importance in arrays of species. Both these attributes become more important as body size increases, but at different and varying rates.

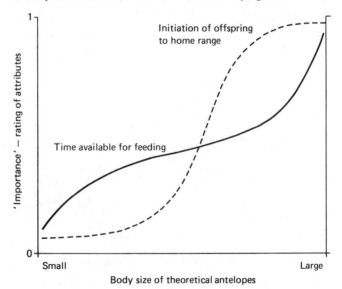

Comparisons between arrays of species

The sociobiologist's plausible explanation may explain the attributes of an array of related species, and may even predict successfully the attributes of additional, incompletely studied species in the same radiation. However, it often fails to predict details of the attributes of ecologically similar, but unrelated species. Yet a sound sociobiological argument ought to be generalisable; what goes wrong?

Arguments may not be generalisable because of incomplete and undisclosed premises typical of comparisons of small numbers of species. Orians (1961) argued, in socioecological terms, why two *Agelaius* blackbirds differed in their breeding systems; one species is territorial and monogamous, the other colonial and polygamous. He related these attributes to the dispersion and abundance of the species' food, and its predictability in time and space, during breeding. He did not discuss anti-predator behaviour, nor the adaptiveness of the highly gregarious roosting and feeding of both species outside the breeding season, since they appeared to differ little in these respects. Barash (1974), studying marmots, was able to ignore body size, the use of burrows, and diet and selectivity for food because they are similar enough in all *Marmota* species not to be causes or consequences of the differences he was trying to explain. In both studies the sociobiological arguments were essentially incomplete because they concerned differences, in a few attributes only, between closely similar species; the arguments could not be generalised for any species except other blackbirds or marmots.

Undisclosed premises show up when explanations that are plausible for one array of species fail to explain attributes in another radiation. For example, the arguments linking body size, avoidance of predators, and selection of diet, with choice of habitat and typical group size, in antelopes (Jarman, 1974) predict reasonably well the pattern of habitat use and grouping found in the Macropodidae; except that one of the smallest macropodids, which the generalised arguments predict should be solitary, is found in colonies – because it uses burrows. No antelope uses a burrow, and an undisclosed premise of the antelope arguments was that disappearing down a burrow was not a possible way of avoiding predators (neither was climbing a tree, or flying).

Sociobiological explanations concentrate upon the Aristotelian *differentia*, the attributes which distinguish between objects, accepting the *genus*, those attributes held in common. In comparing two arrays, characteristics of the *genus* of either may become *differentia* in need of explanation. Lack of burrowing, an unquestioned part of the *genus* of antelopeness, becomes an explorable difference within the class of objects 'all terrestrial, mammalian herbivores'.

Explanations which fail when transferred from one array to another need not be conceptually wrong; their terms may simply be too specific. For example, weaver birds may be classified dietarily as insectivore or granivore, antelopes as grades of grazer or browser, and primates as folivore, frugivore or insectivore, and intrinsic differences between these types of food for each radiation have been used to explain their ranges of species-typical grouping (Crook, 1964; Jarman, 1974; Clutton-Brock & Harvey, 1977). Although the types of food are different, the arguments are almost identical: species whose food items must be sought and processed individually and carefully are less likely to feed in groups than are those whose items are, at least locally, abundant and cheaply obtained. Generalised thus, the explanation is transferable between arrays; while couched in terms of actual foods, it was not.

Sociobiological 'laws' emerge when the association of attributes is similar in several arrays of species, and when the same explanation sounds plausible for each. Several recent comparative studies of Families or Orders have emphasised the determining effects of the same basic factors: the nature of the species' food (as quality, availability, dispersion, and processability of items), and their forms of avoidance of predators. Size is also frequently invoked, especially in studies of mammals. Some explanations take habitat as a determining variable, but many of its effects can be subsumed under nature of the food supply or measures to avoid predators. These basic factors are used to explain how species in arrays differ in the way their individuals distribute themselves in relation to resources and to each other; their mobility; their daily and seasonal pattern of activities; their rates of production of, and behaviour towards, offspring; and, above all, what sort and size of groups they form. As commonly expressed, the explanations are relative, applicable only within the array.

Although these relationships between attributes take the same form in several arrays, the relationships may be weak when sought across arrays. This is because there are conservative limits to the adaptations that are likely to arise in an array. For example, their basic morphology makes it most likely that the predator-avoidance strategy of ungulates and macropodids would include running or concealment, that of primates, climbing, and that of rodents, using holes; despite that, there will be a size-related trend in the precise form of avoidance of predation, and some species may not follow their array's typical strategy. The problem of extracting nutrients from low-quality plants has been solved by several mammalian arrays, sometimes by convergent means (see Geist, 1974; Janis, 1976; Hume, 1978; Jarman & Sinclair, 1979). Species in arrays tend to be all either fore-stomach fermenters, or hind-gut fermenters, or fore-and-hind-gut fermenters, or non-fermenters. Few arrays exhibit two solutions, even though there are wide variations in all arrays in degree of modification for fermentation, or rate of passage of ingesta, for example. There are similarly discrete levels of evolution in the encephalization quotient (Jerison, 1973), where within-array slopes are often less than between-array slopes (see, for example, Oboussier, 1979). These examples emphasise the obvious point that not all evolutionary solutions are equally available to all species. This makes it all the more encouraging when convergence between arrays in the relationships of their species' attributes is found.

However, comparisons between arrays show that some important aspects of social behaviour and organisation have yet to receive generalised explanations; these include mating strategies, social organisation, and sexual differentiation in morphology and environmental relationships. The relationships of these factors to sets of variables follow similar trends in some, but not all, compared arrays. Sexual dimorphism and socionomic sex ratio tend to be strongly associated in many mammal Families, for example; yet sexual dimorphism in colouring and socionomic sex ratio are very poorly related in passerines and many fishes. Such inconsistency in relationships makes these aspects appear secondary by contrast with the primarily related species-specific attributes like body size, nature of food supply, and avoidance of predators. This can be illustrated by antelopes, deer and macropods, three numerous modern radiations of herbivores occupying similar niches. The same plausible explanations, linking body size, food, and avoidance of predators, account adequately for choice of habitat, general mobility, and grouping in all three arrays. Yet the three arrays' ranges of social behaviour and organisation differ markedly. Most antelope societies are organised through some form of territoriality; this is not true for macropods, nor for many deer species. In many group-forming deer species, females are segregated from males for much of the year; this is not true of antelopes or macropods. Starting from similar bases of grouping and choice of habitats, species in the three radiations have tended towards different solutions to the male's problem of how to optimise his mating success. Male mating strategies, the related social behaviour, and the social organisation they induce are clearly secondary to grouping, habitat choice and mobility; the last three attributes themselves depend upon body size, nature of food, and avoidance of predators.

This implied hierarchy in the evolutionary determinants of social be-

haviour and organisation helps break the circularity in some sociobiological explanations of social behaviour ('animals form groups because of an
innate tendency to associate'). Parts of the hierarchy can sometimes be
tested. Impalas *Aepyceros melampus* form groups and move to chosen
habitats even when no territorial males are present; but without the organising behaviour of territorial males all sex and age classes mingle.
Therefore groupings, movement and use of habitat were not dependent on
territorial behaviour, while the stronger segregations in their social organisation were.

Animal-centred measurements

For broadly efficient hypotheses of the evolution of species-
specific social behaviour to be proposed, we need to measure attributes in
such a way that they may be validly compared within and between arrays.
The attributes must reflect how the different species use behaviour to
accommodate their morphology and physiology to the demands of their
realized niches. Although existing measurements still have a lot to contribute, especially in comparisons within arrays, they are sometimes too
coarse or array-specific for broad use.

Sociobiological studies easily reflect a human viewpoint in the measurement and description of attributes, sometimes making a species' behaviour
appear misleadingly complex. Topi *Damaliscus korrigum*, for example, in
Kenya inhabit tree-less plains, palm woodlands, grassy glades in evergreen
forest, and the shores of a desert-bound lake, at altitudes from sea level to
1700 m. These habitats, to us so different, are characterised by just a small
range of height and growth form of the grasses that the antelope eats
(Duncan, 1975; Jarman, 1977); the food-supplying fraction of the topis'
habitat is quite uniform, and their behaviour in selecting habitat thus
appears to be homogenous.

Conversely the human view of used habitat may be too general, sympatric
species being described as using the same habitat. From a human, bipedal
1.8-m viewpoint, an eland and a dik-dik may occupy a common habitat.
From their respective viewpoints the habitat is either sunlit, open *Acacia*
woodland with tall shade-trees, scattered *Salvadora* bushes and hock-high
grass, or shady, large *Salvadora* havens separated by deserts of dangerously
tall grass with rare and irrelevant tree trunks. In any comparison between
these species in which 'habitat' was a relevant attribute, a general biotope
term such as '*Acacia–Salvadora* savanna' or, worse, 'woodland', would
misleadingly imply common experience. Descriptions and measurements
are needed which reflect the experience of the individuals of each species.

Some antelope migrate to maintain the quality and availability of food; others take a diverse and varying diet and are sedentary; and other species mix these strategies. Many tolerate seasonal variations in the quality and availability of food, to which they may adjust by varying their gut morphology (Hofmann, 1973), digestive physiology, and use of metabolic reserves. How much of this flexibility can be shown in simple measurements which reflect the animal's, not the observer's, experiences?

Ideal measurements would compare the ease with which species' individuals feed themselves, and the risks they run in doing so. They could be approximated by identifying types of food items, measuring their field dispersions, calculating their potential contributions to the daily metabolic needs of an animal of that size, and similarly estimating the energetic costs of gathering them. However, the animals themselves can summarise their own experiences. Daily feeding time, bite or peck rates, steps per bite, ratios of searching to ingestion time, distance moved while feeding, and many other measures of activity and behaviour already in use are good indirect reflections of how the animal perceives its food environment. They obviate most adjustments for body size and metabolic differences between species, and are adequate where measurements need be only relative.

Other attributes which result from interaction between behaviour and environment should similarly be measured as experienced by the animal. Group size is an obvious example. The commonly measured mean group size reflects the perception of the external observer, not the social or ecological experience of the average animal being studied. For many sociobiological purposes the measure needed is the mean size of group in which the average individual finds itself; this is simple to derive (Table 15.1), and can be modified to describe the size of group experienced by the average member of a particular sex-and-age, or social, class. From this can be developed measures, such as profiles of change in social environment with age and development, for describing the complexity of social life experienced by individuals of each species. This has previously been approached via consequential attributes such as extent of repertoire of calls or signals (Brereton, 1971), or simply as the number of developmental or social stages in an individual's life.

Classes in a population which differ in social behaviour may also differ in their use of habitats, and behaviour when feeding and avoiding predators. Differential distribution of classes, a common phenomenon among vertebrates, arises from an individual's social position dictating how it uses habitats or resources. For example, subordinate males of many species escape aggression by avoiding the vicinity of dominant males. In con-

Table 15.1. *Examples of descriptions of the composition of groups of animals, illustrating the differences between conventional, observer-centred measurements, and measurements describing the experiences of the individual animal*

A. The individual's experience of group size, as distinct from the observer's. In a group of g_i animals, each individual experiences a group environment of g_i animals (including itself). Therefore in a sampled population the average individual experiences a group environment of

$$\bar{g} = \sum_{i=1}^{N} g_i^2 \Big/ \sum_{i=1}^{N} g_i \text{ animals, with a variance of}$$

$$s^2 = \left[\sum g_i^3 - \left(\sum g_i^2 \right)^2 \Big/ \sum g_i \right] \Big/ \left(\sum g_i - 1 \right)$$

where N is the number of sampled groups, and g_i the size of each. For some purposes the individual's experience is better rendered as $(\bar{g} - 1)$

B. To demonstrate how this differs from the observer-centred 'mean group size', as an expression of the animal's experience, consider this sample population.

Groups seen	Total
1 territorial ♂, 12 ♀♀, 8 juveniles	21
1 territorial ♂, 8 ♀♀, 5 juveniles	14
6 bachelor ♂♂	6
1 territorial ♂	1
1 territorial ♂	1
1 territorial ♂, 14 ♀♀, 10 juveniles	25
1 territorial ♂	1
8 bachelor ♂♂	8
1 territorial ♂	1
1 ♀, 1 juvenile	2

Total: 21 males, 35 females, 24 juveniles   80

C. Conventional analyses give descriptions such as the following
Mean group size = 8
Mean group composition = 2.1 ♂♂; 3.5 ♀♀; 2.4 juveniles
Mean number of females found together = 8.75
Adult sex ratio = 1 ♂ : 1.7 ♀♀

D. Descriptions of individual experience
Size of group in which the average individual is found = 17.1 (cf. mean group size = 8.0)
The average female is one of 11.6 females in her group (cf. mean number of females found together = 8.75)
The average bachelor is one of 7.1 males in his group
The average juvenile is one of 7.9 juveniles in his group
The average territorial male is the only such male in a group
The average female is in a group of 20.5 animals, as is the average juvenile; on average, a territorial male is in a group of 9.1 animals, and a bachelor in one of 7.1
The average female is in contact with 1 territorial male, 10.6 other females, 7.9 juveniles, and no bachelors.

sequence they may have to use different habitats and even different diets. Since an individual may grow through several social classes in a lifetime, a measure of the complexity of its lifetime's experience of some of these attributes could be a powerful comparative tool.

A step towards measurements typifying the animal's, rather than the observer's, experience has been taken in replacing 'adult sex ratio' by 'socionomic sex ratio'. This useful measure exemplifies the problems of defining an attribute with a particular analytical use in mind. Clutton-Brock *et al.* (1977) defined socionomic sex ratio as the number of adult females per adult male in breeding groups. For the mainly closed-membership groups of primates that they were discussing, the ratio defined thus describes both the instantaneous and the long-term experiences of adults of either sex in breeding groups (provided that the 'mean group size' trap is avoided; see above). However, socionomic sex ratio may not adequately describe each sex's experience of the other in other social systems. In many antelope species, for example, females wander, between solitary territorial males, in open-membership groups. The typical female instantaneously experiences one male and as many females as the group momentarily contains; long-term, she experiences several males and all the females whose home-ranges overlap her own. The average breeding male is instantaneously accompanying no females or the number in the average group (for once the mean group size is appropriate); long-term, he experiences all females whose ranges overlap his territory. Socionomic sex ratios are even more difficult to define for lek-forming species, and those in which males compete to consort only with oestrous females (Table 15.2).

Refinement of measurements to suit advanced analyses is a part of progress in any science. Sociobiology has grown out of comparisons of the simplest observable traits, such as adult sex ratio and mean group size, on which successful evolutionary hypotheses have been built. Much can be gained by extending those simple measurements to unstudied species and arrays; but many current hypotheses require for their testing new measurements, based on the animal-centred approach advocated here.

Interspecific and interpopulation comparisons

Sociobiological attributes of several species vary regionally, seasonally, or after a perturbation. Comparisons between populations, or the same population in different circumstances, are an attractive way of testing some sociobiological 'laws' without the masking effects of profound genetic differences implicit in interspecific comparisons. Populations in different parts of a species' range have been compared to see whether

Table 15.2. *Descriptions of one adult's contact with individuals of the other sex in different mating systems.*

	The number of opposite-sex individuals contacted by individual adults of breeding status	
Breeding system	instantaneously	in whole breeding life
A. One adult male with a fixed-membership group of females, in an exclusive range.	♂: G ♀: 1	$G(1 + R_f S_m)$ $1 + R_m S_f$
B. Open-membership groups of ♀♀ wander between territories held by single ♂♂; two groups in the same territory will amalgamate. Female remains in her home range. *Imagine* there is constant group size and perennial territoriality.	♂: either G or zero, these occurring in the approximate ratio F/GM : $1 - (F/GM)$ ♀: 1	$H(1 + R_f S_m)$ where $H = F(Z_f + Z_m)^2 \pi$ $T(1 + R_m S_f)$ where $T = M(Z_f + Z_m)^2 \pi$
C. (i) Oestrous ♀♀ visit breeding ♂♂ gathered on leks. *Imagine* a small lek used simultaneously by all males of breeding status.	♂: $FLOe$ ♀: in oestrus, P in anoestrus, zero	$FL(1 + R_f S_m)$ $P(1 + R_m S_f)$
(ii) As above, but *imagine* breeding-status ♂♂ are only intermittently on the lek. Proportion of time on lek $= p$; off lek $= 1 - p$	♂: on lek, $FLOe$ off lek, zero ♀: Pp	$FLOep(1 + R_f S_m)$ $POep(1 + R_m S_f)$
D. Males and females live in overlapping individual home ranges. Males associate only with oestrous females. *Imagine* that a male detects oestrus of all females in his home range.	♂: $OeF(Z_{oe} + Z_m)^2 \pi$ ♀: in anoestrus, zero in oestrus, $M(Z_{oe} + Z_m)^2 \pi$	$F(Z_{oe} + Z_m)^2 \pi (1 + R_f S_m)$ $M(Z_{oe} + Z_m)^2 \pi (1 + R_m S_f)$

Key

G, mean size of female group

R_f, rate of turnover of population (assumed stable) of adult, breeding females i.e. the proportion of individual females entering, or leaving the population of breeding adults per unit time.

differing environmental factors affect their sociobiological attributes. Examples are provided by: the effects of elevation and thus growing season on reproductive and social biology of yellow-bellied marmot *Marmota flaviventris* populations (Barash, 1974); the effects of difference in food item and habitat densities on grouping, and in seasonality of breeding, female group size and movements on territoriality and social organisation in impala (Jarman & Jarman, 1974; Jarman, M.V., 1979); and the effects of different structures and densities of habitat on song repertoire in great tits *Parus major* (Hunter & Krebs, 1979).

Similar comparisons can be made between attributes of one population measured under different circumstances which may even be experimentally contrived. Care must be taken in interpreting seasonal variations in attributes, since, as well as changes in the environment, major seasonal events such as breeding or migration may influence the species' sociobiology. Similar caution is needed in interpreting changes after perturbation, when the structure of the population may be altered through differential mortality or genotypic changes (Myers & Krebs, 1971). However, seasonal and longer-term changes within populations demonstrate the dynamic nature of some sociobiological attributes. They also provide the data on tolerable ranges in values of attributes which will be needed if a systems approach to sociobiology is to develop. Unfortunately there is a major drawback to interpopulation comparisons: only a small proportion of species, usually generalist or ecologically flexible in character, has populations living in environments different enough to have induced detectable socioecological differences.

Key to Table 15.2 (*cont.*)
R_m, the equivalent for males.
S_f, mean span of life as adult, breeding female.
S_m, mean span of life as adult, breeding male, or span as territorial male.
F, density of adult, breeding females.
M, density of adult, breeding males, or territorial males.
T, the number of territories, or male home ranges, wholly or partly overlapped by the average female's home range.
H, the number of female home ranges wholly or partly overlapped by the average male's territory or home range.
L, area occupied by the female population visiting a lek; the 'catchment' of the lek.
Oe, proportion of the year spent in oestrus by the average female.
P, number of lek-using males associated with a lek.
Z_f, radius of female home range (taken as circular).
Z_m, radius of male home range or territory.
Z_{oe}, radius of female range while in oestrus.

Interspecific comparison may have been tarnished by a too-eager look-ing for similarities and overlooking of differences, by occasional group-selectionism in its expression, and a lack of well planned research. Despite these faults, it has a leading part to play in demonstrating the existence of consistent relationships between species-typical behaviour and ecological attributes. Once those relationships are known, other approaches can be taken in investigating them.

Summary

1. Unlike comparisons between individuals, comparisons between populations, species, or genera cannot demonstrate that one be-havioural or ecological strategy is adaptively superior to another; they can show that groups of sociobiological attributes tend to be associated in species, and that these associations recur in unrelated radiations of species.

2. The diverse attributes considered in such studies are difficult to measure consistently amongst all species in a widely radiated group. In many radiations there are fewer large than small species, and this masks associations between some attributes; moreover evolutionary pressures may differ across an array of species; each environmental factor will not be equally important to all species so that values of association between attributes will differ between points in an array of species.

3. A study of one array may produce sociobiological explanations inadequate to account for the associations of attributes in another, comparable array, because the first set of explanations either considered too few species, took too incomplete a set of premises, or described attributes too restrictively, to be generalisable.

4. The plausible explanations offered by studies of unrelated arrays often run parallel, suggesting that evolutionary, sociobiological 'laws' do exist. A present barrier to revealing them is the anthro-pocentric nature of many descriptions of attributes, especially environmental ones: we need measurements which reflect the ex-perience of individual animals in the populations, not of the human observer.

5. Comparison within a species, between populations living in dif-ferent environments, or the same population in different circum-stances, can test some of the emerging sociobiological 'laws': such comparisons avoid the problems of major differences between species masking subtle responses to environmental variation.

6. Broad comparative surveys of many related species are still needed to reveal the full extent of the evolved relationships between species' environments, ecology, morphology, and behaviour.

I would like to thank the King's College sociobiology group for the stimulation and ideas which I got during six happy months spent at the Research Centre. My thanks also go to T. Clutton-Brock, H. Kruuk, M. Murray, K. Rasmussen and R. Underwood for constructively criticising earlier versions of this paper.

References

Barash, D.P. (1974). The evolution of marmot societies: a general theory. *Science*, **185**, 415–20.

Brereton, J. Le G. (1971). A self-regulation to density-independent continuum in Australian parrots, and its implication for ecological management, pp. 207–21 in *The Scientific Management of Animal and Plant Communities for Conservation. 11th Symposium of the British Ecological Society*, ed. E. Duffey, & A.S. Watt. Blackwells: Oxford.

Clutton-Brock, T.H. & Harvey, P.H. (1977). Primate ecology and social organisation. *Journal of Zoology*, **183**, 1–39.

Clutton-Brock, T.H. & Harvey, P.H. (1978). Species differences in feeding and ranging behaviour in primates. In *Primate Ecology: Studies of Feeding and Ranging Behaviour in Lemurs, Monkeys and Apes*, ed. T.H. Clutton-Brock, pp. 557–84. Academic Press: London.

Clutton-Brock, T.H., Harvey, P.H. & Rudder, B. (1977). Sexual dimorphism, socionomic sex ratio and body weight in primates. *Nature*, **269**, 797–800.

Crook, J.H. (1964). The evolution of social organisation and visual communication in the weaver birds (Ploceinae). *Behaviour Supplement*, **10**, 1–178.

Crook, J.H. (1965). The adaptive significance of avian social organizations. *Symposium of the Zoological Society of London*, **14**, 181–218.

Crook, J.H. & Gartlan, J.S. (1966). Evolution of primate societies. *Nature*, **210**, 1200–3.

Cullen, E. (1957). Adaptations in the kittiwake to cliff-nesting. *Ibis*, **99**, 275–302.

Cullen, J.M. (1960). Some adaptations in the nesting behaviour of terns. *Proceedings of XII International Ornithological Congress. Helsinki, 1958*, pp. 153–7.

Duncan, P. (1975). *Topi and Their Food Supply*. Ph.D. dissertation, University of Nairobi.

Estes, R.D. (1974). Social organization of the African Bovidae. In *The Behaviour of Ungulates and its relation to management*. ed. V. Geist & F. Walther, pp. 166–205. IUCN new series No. 24. Morges.

Geist, V. (1974). On the relationship of social evolution and ecology in ungulates. *American Zoologist*, **14**, 205–20.

Hinde, R.A. (1955–56). A comparative study of the courtship of certain finches (Fringillidae). *Ibis*, **97**, 706–54; **98**, 16–23.

Hinde, R.A. (1956). The biological significance of the territories of birds. *Ibis*, **98**, 340–69.

Hofmann, R.R. (1973). *The Ruminant Stomach. Stomach Structure and Feeding Habits of East African Game Ruminants. East African Monographs in Biology*, vol. 2. East African Literature Bureau: Nairobi.

Hume, I.D. (1978). Evolution of the Macropodidae digestive system. *Australian Mammalogy*, **2**, 37–42.

Hunter, M.L. Jnr. & Krebs, J.R. (1979). Geographical variation in the song of the great tit (*Parus major*) in relation to ecological factors. *Journal of Animal Ecology*, **48**, 759–85.

Janis, C. (1976). The evolutionary strategy of the Equidae and the origins of rumen and cecal digestion. *Evolution*, **30**, 757–74.

Jarman, M.V. (1979). *Impala Social Behaviour: Territory, Hierarchy, Mating, and the Use of Space. Advances in Ethology 21*. Paul Parey: Hamburg.

Jarman, P.J. (1974). The social organisation of antelope in relation to their ecology. *Behaviour*, **48**, 215–67.

Jarman, P.J. (1977). Behaviour of topi in a shadeless environment. *Zoologica Africana*, **12**, 101–11.

Jarman, P.J. & Jarman, M.V. (1974). Impala behaviour and its relevance to management. In *The Behaviour of Ungulates and its Relation to Management*, ed. V. Geist & F. Walther, pp. 871–81. IUCN new series No. 24. Morges.

Jarman, P.J. & Sinclair, A.R.E. (1979). Feeding strategy and the pattern of resource-partitioning in ungulates. In *Serengeti. Dynamics of an Ecosystem*, ed. A.R.E. Sinclair & M. Norton-Griffiths, pp. 130–63. University of Chicago Press: Chicago.

Jerison, H.J. (1973). *Evolution of the Brain and Intelligence*. Academic Press: New York.

Myers, J.H. & Krebs, C.J. (1971). Genetic, behavioural and reproductive attributes of dispersing field voles *Microtus pennsylvanicus* and *Microtus ochrogaster*. *Ecological Monographs*, **41**, 53–78.

Oboussier, H. (1979). Evolution of the brain and phylogenetic development of African Bovidae. *South African Journal of Zoology*, **14**, 119–24.

Orians, G.H. (1961). The ecology of blackbird (*Agelaius*) social system. *Ecological Monographs*, **31**, 285–312.

Ralls, K. (1976). Mammals in which females are larger than males. *Quarterly Review of Biology*, **51**, 245–76.

Rood, J.P. (1972). Ecological and behavioural comparisons of three genera of Argentine cavies. *Animal Behaviour Monographs*, **5**, 1–83.

von Haartmann, L. (1957). Adaptations in hole-nesting birds. *Evolution*, **11**, 339–47.

16

Comparisons between taxa and adaptive trends: problems of methodology

PAUL H. HARVEY AND GEORGINA M. MACE

Introduction

Many morphological and behavioural characters vary between taxa in similar ways. Some associations are not at all surprising, such as that between warning coloration and toxicity in the insects. Others are more perplexing, such as the repeated correlation shown between sexual dimorphism in body size and body size itself across many animal groups from insects to mammals (Rensch, 1959). Comparisons between traits which vary among taxa has been a useful tool for both generating and testing hypotheses about the functional or adaptive significance of morphological and behavioural variation (see Clutton-Brock & Harvey, 1979). However, such comparisons face methodological problems that are often ignored, or barely mentioned in passing. In this chapter, we shall be concerned with those problems, together with some possible solutions to them. We restrict our discussion to bivariate analyses of continuously distributed variables; as will be apparent, multivariate analyses face all the difficulties discussed here, plus some additional ones to which we allude at the end of the chapter.

The quantitative methods used will depend upon the purpose of the analysis, and in the first section we outline various uses of comparative studies in biological investigations. We then present some criteria to help determine a suitable taxonomic level at which to analyse the available data.

Once the purpose of the analysis is decided, and the appropriate taxonomic level selected, we must turn to the analysis itself. Three underlying statistical models are generally used for dealing with linear comparisons between normalised variables. However, the frequency with which they are used is not closely related to their suitabilites. We present a simple data set and use it to demonstrate differences in outcome between the three techniques. Finally, we discuss additional methodological problems (to some of which we can offer no solution) together with examples of recent papers that have encountered and sometimes fallen foul of such problems.

Hypothesis testing and hypothesis generation

Comparisons across taxa can be used in at least four ways. We deal briefly with each. First, they can be used to test general hypotheses; second, to test specific hypotheses; third, to describe new variables; and fourth, to identify the *form* of the relationship between variables. The first three may be used to test hypotheses and the latter two, as we shall see, are often useful for hypothesis generation.

Testing general hypotheses

As a science moves towards quantification, hypotheses to be tested often have only a general form. Biologists may forsee the outcome of general hypotheses before more precise engineering or energetic predictions can be formulated. An example can be drawn from the theory of sexual selection. We know that, across a variety of taxa, larger animals are more likely to win fights than smaller conspecifics. We also know that there are metabolic costs associated with increasing body size. The trade off between the two is likely to result in some optimal body size, given genetic and physiological constraints. Sexual selection theory predicts that the sex with the higher variance in reproductive success will compete among itself for access to mates. We therefore expect the divergence in body size between the sexes to increase with the difference in variance of reproductive success between the sexes. As a consèquence, we predict that (within some vertebrate groups) sexual dimorphism in body size will increase with the degree of polygyny, males becoming larger relative to females. But, we can make no precise predictions about the nature of the relationship because we can measure neither the costs associated with increasing body size nor the benefits of being larger, and because the degree of polygyny does not necessarily reflect the difference in variance of reproductive success between the sexes. At best, we can expect a positive correlation between the degree of polygyny and the extent of sexual dimorphism (Alexander *et al.*, 1979). Other examples of this kind are legion and illustrate the generality of the approach – the relationship between island size and numbers of species (MacArthur & Wilson, 1967), the positive correlation between prey size and some aspect of predator size (Hespenheide, 1973) and between territory quality and degree of polygyny in some birds (Verner, 1964).

Testing specific hypotheses

Hypotheses vary in their predictive power. If we are examining a linear relationship between two variables we may have some idea of the expected slope. Hypothesis testing then involves producing a line of best fit and examining whether the estimated confidence limits of the slope embrace the predicted value.

For example, Gould (1975*a*) predicted that in a number of vertebrate groups the logarithm of tooth area would increase with the logarithm of body size producing a slope of 0.75 (scaling at the same rate as metabolic costs) rather than 0.66 (scaling with surface area). Similarly, many of the scaling costs of locomotion can be formulated in precise terms from mechanical and energetic considerations and the actual performances may be compared with predicted values (Alexander, 1977).

Alternatively, hypotheses may be insufficiently formulated to predict the form of the relationship (in terms of slope or slope and elevation) but differences in slope or elevation between groups with different characteristics might be expected. For example, home range area relates to body size with the same exponent in mammalian 'browsers' and 'grazers' and we can predict a higher elevation for 'browsers' which depend on a less-abundant food supply. Mechanical arguments predict that the costs of running at different speeds scale differently with body size in quadrupeds and bipeds (Taylor, 1977).

Describing new variables

One of the all pervading problems facing cross-taxonomic comparisons is that of confounding variables (Clutton-Brock & Harvey, 1979). We are often interested in the relationship between two variables after the effects of a third have been removed. When that third variable is (body) size, as it often is, then we are dealing with deviations from an allometric relationship (Gould, 1966). The deviations either from an empirical line of best fit, or from some hypothetical relationship can be treated as measures of a new variable for further quantitative investigation. The relationship of these deviations to other scalar or ordinal measures can be used for both hypothesis generation and hypothesis testing.

A commonly used variable of this kind is the *encephalisation quotient*. Deviations from a best-fit line of the logarithmic plot of brain weight against body weight measure the brain size of an animal when the effects of the underlying relationship with body size have been removed. Encephalisation quotients have been used to test predictions about the differences in relative brain size between predators and prey (Jerison, 1973), and about ecological and behavioural correlates of relative brain size (Bauchot & Stephan, 1969; Pirlot & Stephan, 1970; Clutton-Brock & Harvey, 1980; Mace, Harvey & Clutton-Brock, 1981). Another example is *relative male canine size* (Harvey, Kavanagh & Clutton-Brock, 1978). It was predicted that once the effects of body size had been removed, the canine size typical of males from different primate species should be related to both breeding system (a sexual selection hypothesis) and mate defence strategies (an anti-predator hypothesis). Treating the measure of relative male canine size as a newly defined normal variate, tests of both hypotheses could be made using cross-species comparisons.

Identifying the form of a relationship

The scaling of one variable on another may provide important clues about the underlying cause of the relationship. For example, it is now widely acknowledged that in warm-blooded animals metabolic costs scale against body weight to the power of 0.75 (Kleiber, 1961). Thus the classical 'surface law' whereby the total energetic costs incurred by an animal should be proportional to it's surface area (i.e. to the power of 0.66) has had to be discarded (Gould, 1966) and, based on necessary distortions from geometric similarity between different sized animals, other testable causes for the relationship have been suggested (McMahon, 1973; Wilkie, 1977).

Choosing the taxonomic level for analysis

If we employ quantitative methods for comparative studies, we are bound by assumptions associated with statistical analysis and we have to make certain decisions about the validity of taxonomic groupings. Transcending taxonomic levels is unusual in biometry and as a consequence statistical assumptions may be unwittingly violated. In this section we mention some pitfalls and discuss ways to avoid them. An initial assumption is that the same taxonomic level is equivalent in different groups. While this may not be reasonable across very different phyla, the assumption is generally justified in more closely knit groups. For example, in a study of inter-family differences among the mammals, we would assume that the Hyaenidae are equivalent to the Muridae. We are then faced with two problems. First, the choice of taxon used to produce statistically independent points (e.g. species, genus, family); and second, the range of forms over which to collect the data. We refer to these as the choice of lower and upper taxonomic level respectively.

Choice of lower taxonomic level

The main problem here is the independence of data points. If our upper limit of analysis was the order, then we might use species, generic or family estimates for comparing relationships between variables within the order. When we are dealing with real data, species are not evenly distributed across genera, nor genera across families. If species within a genus tend to have similar characteristics due to phylogenetic constraints, then the analysis of species data will be statistically biased by those genera containing large numbers of species. An example may illustrate this point more clearly. Harestad & Bunnell (1979) undertook a study of home-range size and body size in mammals. They used species data, and compared relationships between dietetic groups. The four largest species in their herbivore sample were all from the genus *Odocoileus* and had similar body weights and home ranges sizes to each other, but smaller home ranges than other similar-sized species. Because of this single genus, the slope of the herbivore line was considerably reduced. Now, if these four congeneric species have similar characteristics due to phylogenetic constraints, they are not statistically independent and the analysis is biased by their presence – they really represent only one point. It is arguable, however, that they have similar body sizes and home ranges due to selection and convergence because they live in similar habitats; we cannot conclude *a priori* that similarity results from phylogenetic inertia. But, since we rarely have any external evidence to justify the latter interpretation, we should use the lowest taxonomic level that can be justified on statistical grounds, i.e. the lowest taxonomic level at which maximum variance is exhibited in our measured variable after the data have been normalized. Clutton-Brock & Harvey (1977a) suggest the use of nested analysis of variance to identify that level: in an analysis of primates, they were able to use genera as their lower taxonomic level for analysing seven of nine variables since no additional variance was revealed in comparisons among families over that found among genera within families.

It is not easy to produce hard and fast rules over this matter. Taking the practice of statistical conservatism to its extremes may only lead to other problems: sample sizes may become prohibitively small or analyses may become blurred through inclusion of very diverse groups. In general, the pitfalls encountered by taking too low a taxonomic level are serious enough to justify statistical safety. And subspecific points should not be combined with data from higher levels. The two are qualitatively different since subspecies or populations generally share the same gene pool.

Choice of upper taxonomic level

Relationships found within one taxon may be of a different form in other taxa. For instance, in species plots of brain weight against body weight, the elevations of best fit lines differ among genera, and the slopes of best fit lines vary among taxonomic levels (Gould, 1975*b*). Before amalgamating successive taxonomic levels for analysis, statistical tests should always be employed to ensure that no such differences exist.

Methods of comparison

Normality and linearity

For some models of best fit we assume that the data are normally distributed on both axes and that relationships are linear; standard tests of both assumptions are available from statistical texts. If correlation coefficients are low and normalising the data (by transformation) results in non-linearity, then serious problems can arise in attempting to describe the form of the relationship. We shall return to these and other problems after we have considered the methods available for establishing lines of best fit.

The line of best fit

Three models are generally used to estimate straight lines of best fit. They are regression analysis, major axis (= principal axis = principal component) analysis and reduced major axis analysis. It was claimed by Kermack & Haldane (1950) that reduced major axis is the technique most suitable for estimating lines of 'organic correlation', but for the historical reason that regression analysis is applicable to various models of experimental design, where one of the variables is measured without error, regression analysis has often and erroneously been used for comparative studies.

Before we distinguish among the three models, we should emphasise the distinction between the *strength* (i.e. correlation) and the *form* (i.e. parameters of the best fit line) of a relationship. As an increasing amount of statistical error variance is incorporated into measures on the two axes, so the correlation coefficient will decrease. The correlation coefficient (or its squared value, the coefficient of determination) is a useful adjunct to bivariate analysis and should usually be quoted. However, there is no *a priori* reason why the correlation coefficient should be a component variable in the calculation of the best fit line, despite the protestations of Jolicoeur (1968) and Jolicoeur & Mosimann (1968).

Each method of producing a line of best fit minimises some measure of the deviation of points around the line, Fig. 16.1 illustrates the quantity minimised in each case.

Fig. 16.1. Lines of best fit produced by a set of data (points are the black dots). Lines drawn from the points A1 and A2 show the distances minimised for regression analysis and major axis analysis, and the areas minimised for reduced major axis analysis. Imbrie (1956) gives a similar figure. For details see text.

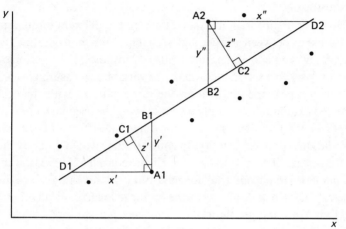

Regression of y on x produces that line which minimises the sum of squared distances of points from the line, when those distances are measured perpendicular to the x axis (Fig. 16.1: y' and y''), whereas the regression of x on y minimises the sum of squared distances measured perpendicular to the y axis (x' and x'').

Major axis analysis minimises the sum of squared distances of points from the line when the distances are measured perpendicular to the line of best fit (z' and z''). This line of best fit, therefore, is that which has the minimum variance of points about itself and consequently accounts for the maximum amount of variance in the data.

Reduced major axis analysis minimises the sum of the areas of triangles bounded by the line of best fit and lines drawn from it to the data points and parallel with the two original axes ($A_1 B_1 D_1$ and $A_2 B_2 D_2$ on Fig. 16.1; see also Imbrie, 1956).

Regression analysis only produces an unbiased estimate of the line of best fit when variables are without error* on the abscissa. As error is

---

*The error referred to throughout this chapter, unless qualified, has two possible sources. First, error due to inaccurate measurement. Second, error resulting from lack of dependence. If two variables are each, in part, determined by a third variable but not by each other, then they cannot be said to be independent and dependent variables. And, if one variable determines a second, but only in part, then the second will have error resulting from a lack of total dependence on the first. The hypothesized sources of error may determine the best-fit analysis performed.

introduced into the values on the x axis, so the slope becomes shallower when y is regressed on x. The regression of y on x is not affected when error is introduced onto the y axis. So long as the error variances on the two axes are equal, major axis and reduced major axis analyses do not suffer from this problem.

However, major axis analysis suffers from a different disadvantage: the relationship between the variables changes in a non-intuitive way with changes in the scale of measurement. For instance, if we perform a major axis analysis on a set of data where one variable is measured in centimetres and then repeat the analysis on the same data set with the centimetres changed to millimetres simply by multiplying the original values by ten, the slopes in the two analyses will not differ by a factor of ten, unless the correlation coefficient is unity. In contrast, they would differ by the scaling factor of ten if the analyses were by either reduced major axis or regression techniques. Under one transformation this disadvantage does not occur: when changes in scale are performed prior to logarithmically transforming the data for analysis, the slope is not affected (Jolicoeur & Mosimann, 1968). This caveat is important because logarithmically transformed axes are often used in comparative studies and tests for heterogeneity among more than two slopes are available for major axis but not for reduced major axis (see below).

In order to demonstrate these points as clearly as possible, we give the results of a simple simulation study that was designed to demonstrate the different outcomes from the three types of analysis.

An example

Three arrays of 100 numbers were each taken randomly from a normal distribution with a mean of zero and a variance of one. Data set A consisted of the first array, data set B of the first plus the second array, and data set C of the first plus the third array. Sets B and C are therefore correlated both with each other and with A, but have some added error variance which is equal in both data sets. The 'underlying' relationship between all three data sets is a slope of one when each is plotted against any other since there is a one : one correspondence through data set A.

Table 16.1 gives the results of comparing set A (without error) with set B (with error), and of comparing set B with set C (also with error). Clearly, the correlation between B and C is less than that between A and B because of the additional error variance associated with the first comparison.

Regression analysis of B on A reveals the 'correct' slope of one since A is without error. The other regression slopes are influenced by the error terms in B and C and underestimate the slope of one.

Reduced major axis and major axis analysis give similar answers to each other and give the 'correct' slope of about one when the error variance is equal on both axes (comparing sets B and C). However, the use of set A, because it is without error, renders both techniques inappropriate.

We now introduce data set D which is the same as set B, but with each value multiplied by ten. We use this set to demonstrate that major axis analysis results in a slope that is 'not invariant under changes of scale' (Kermack & Haldane, 1950). Depending on which data set is used to create the y axis, we would expect the slopes of D plotted against C to be either one-tenth or ten times greater than the slopes of C plotted against B. This is so for both regression analysis and for reduced major axis analysis, but not for major axis analysis where the scaling factor is not ten but about sixteen (Table 16.2). But if B were a data set that had been logarithmically

Table 16.1. *Slopes of best-fit lines relating pairs of data sets*

Ordinate	Abscissa	Regression	Reduced major axis	Major axis	Correlation coefficient
A	B	0.57	0.72	0.67	0.79
B	A	1.09	1.38	1.50	
B	C	0.67	1.04	1.07	0.64
C	B	0.62	0.96	0.94	

Data set A has no error variance while B and C have equal error variance which is the same as the total variance in A (see text). Comparisons giving the 'expected' slope of 1 are underlined.

Table 16.2. *Slopes of best-fit lines relating pairs of data sets*

Ordinate	Abscissa	Regression	Reduced major axis	Major axis	Correlation coefficient
D	C	6.71	10.44	16.14	0.64
C	D	0.06	0.10	0.61	
E	C	0.67	1.04	1.04	0.64
C	E	0.62	0.96	0.96	

Data sets B and C are as in Table 16.1, D is the same as B with all the values multiplied by 10 and E is B after the transformation $\log_e(e^B \times 10)$. Comparisons producing the 'expected' slopes are underlined.

transformed, then changing the scale before the transformation would not have influenced the slope. We can see this by examining the relationship between E and C, where the values of E are the natural exponents (i.e. antilogarithms) of the values of B multiplied by ten and then logged (Table 16.2).

Finally, we demonstrate the effects of unequal error variance on the two axes. We use data set F which consists of the first array plus the values of the second array adjusted so that their variance is halved while their mean remains the same. F is therefore data set B with less (one half) error variance. In the comparisons between C and F, even reduced major axis produces unsuitable results (Table 16.3). The variance of B is 2 while that of F is 1.5. Therefore, reduced major axis gives us a slope approximately equal to $(2)^{\frac{1}{2}}/(1.5)^{\frac{1}{2}}$, that is the ratio of the standard deviations. In this case we know the error variances of B and F to be 1 and 0.5 respectively, therefore we could have subtracted these prior to calculating the reduced major axis slope and establishing the underlying slope of one. In practice, we do occasionally have estimates of the error variance in our data and these can be similarly incorporated into our analysis to give a more reliable result (see Kermack, 1954, for a biological example).

In summary, when there is a perfect underlying relationship between two variables but error is present on both axes and of equal magnitude, then reduced major axis analysis produces the most satisfactory line of best fit. Regression is only appropriate when values on the abscissa are without error, and major axis analysis is only suitable for use on logarithmically transformed data because otherwise the line of best fit so produced changes unpredictably under changes of scale.

Additional problems

Before amalgamating taxonomic levels for analysis, it is always advisable to test whether the relationships have the same form in different taxa, or in different groups under test. Assuming normality and linearity of

Table 16.3. *Slope of best-fit lines relating data sets B and F*

Ordinate	Abscissa	Regression	Reduced major axis	Major axis	Correlation coefficient
B	F	0.83	1.17	1.25	0.71
F	B	0.60	0.85	0.80	

F is the same as C in Table 16.1 but with only one half the error variance.

relationships *within* taxa, two parameters – the slope and the elevation – may vary *between* taxa. If slopes differ between taxa, there is little value in comparing elevations, although techniques are available for doing so for a small overlap range between two empirical distributions (Imbrie, 1956). We shall concentrate on methods for comparing slopes, and then elevations for cases where slopes are assumed to be equal.

Comparing slopes. The slope of the reduced major axis is calculated as the ratio of the standard deviations of points measured on the y axis and on the x axis. If the standard deviation on the ordinate is greater than that on the abscissa then the slope is larger than one, and if it is less then the slope is below one. The value given (a ratio of square roots) is, however, always positive and the sign of the slope can only be found by examining the sign of the sum of cross-products (or the correlation coefficient). Comparing pairs of slopes (where the total sample size of the combined data is above 35) is straightforward: since standard errors of reduced major axes are the same as those of the corresponding regression coefficients (Tessier, 1948), simple z-tests can be employed (Imbrie, 1956).

Testing for heterogeneity between more than two slopes is not easy. We can suggest two approaches. First, the analogue of the analysis of covariance used to compare slopes in regression analysis (Snedecor, 1956). Analysis of covariance measures squared deviations from three types of regression line: within sample lines, the overall line ('total') going through all sample points, and the 'common' regression whose slope is a weighted average of within sample slopes (geometrically, it transforms each sample to have the same mean on both axes, leaves their variances unaltered, and calculates another 'total' line). The analogue of squared deviations in reduced major axis analysis is the sum of the areas of the triangles described above (see Fig. 16.1). Calculation of slopes presents no problem since the same variances can be used as in covariance analysis (see Snedecor, 1956), nor does the calculation of the summed triangle area, but statistical testing is difficult. Covariance analysis utilises variance ratio (F) tests, calculated from the F distribution, whereas using our suggested method produces a statistic whose underlying distribution is unknown (at least to us). Nevertheless, simple simulations which incorporate the relevant means, variances and covariances of our observed data set can provide a reliable statistic in any particular case. Clearly, a set of tables would be useful.

Second, since the disadvantage of the major axis technique which results from changes of scale disappears when we use logarithmically transformed data (Jolicoeur & Mosimann, 1968; see above), it is often possible to use major axis analysis to calculate lines of best fit for biological data. Commonly, logarithmic transformations are necessary to normalise the data, and the resulting transformations are linear. Statistical determination of heterogeneity among two or more samples is possible and we suggest using a maximum likelihood method (see Appendix).

Comparing elevations. If we are persuaded that slopes do not differ between taxa, then we may wish to test for differences in elevation. This entails the calculation of a 'common' reduced major axis slope (see above). Within samples, sums of squares are calculated and summed, and the ratio of the square roots of these values for the ordinate and the abscissa provides us with a common slope. Alternatively, when using major axis analysis on logarithmically transformed data, the common slope is determined during the procedure for testing slope heterogeneity (see Appendix). For convenience, a line can then be imposed which goes through the total sample mean on each axis, and deviations from the line can be compared using standard analysis of variance. The form of deviations used depends on the type of analysis involved in producing the line of best fit (see Fig. 16.1), and possibly on the reason for the analysis in the first place. If we were attempting to remove the effects of a particular variable, we might be justified in using deviations perpendicular to that axis *after* we had produced a line of best fit.

Discussion

In a methodological paper of this sort it is all too easy to highlight trivial errors in the work of others. That is not our intention. Rather, we wish to emphasise that the errors discussed above are widespread. Where possible, we cite our own work, or alternatively major papers which have been or can be expected to be widely quoted in the field of behavioural ecology or sociobiology. For convenience, we focus on certain topics (social behaviour, ranging behaviour and allometric relationships) to which we return as we develop our discussion in terms of the methodological framework outlined above. Our choice of topic is idiosyncratic, but the interested reader will identify parallel papers in other areas of comparative study.

Choice of taxonomic level

We have already mentioned how a limitation on the quantity of available data can tempt workers to inflate sample sizes by incorporating data from taxonomic levels below that at which the comparison contains statistically independent points. We discussed one example from the home range and body-size literature, but there are many others. We have chosen another example from a different kind of study to discuss here because it clearly illustrates the problem, and therefore it can be used to suggest a solution. Sherman (1979) demonstrates an association between chromosome number and eusociality in the Hymenoptera. He presents data from 382 species across 20 families. Three of the families are primarily eusocial and, treating species within families as independent points for analysis, he 'statistically compares' chromosome numbers between families. As Sherman himself notes, if there are phylogenetic constraints, (see above) on chromosome number then this procedure is clearly invalid. And there may be such constraints, so we should justify *statistical* independence of species data in the absence of any biological information. Nested analysis of variance (Sokal & Rohlf, 1969) reveals heterogeneity as high as the superfamily level within suborders, with no additional variation among suborders (both the within and among superfamily variances are greater than the additional variance between suborders).

If we were to be reasonably sure of the effect being examined, data such as Sherman's should be used only for comparisons within the taxonomic level immediately above that being employed for analysis. That is, interfamily comparisons must be restricted within a superfamily, and species should not be used as independent points to compare families within an order.

Another example comes from the allometric relationship between brain size and body size among mammals. It is well established that brain size increases to about the 0.67 to 0.75 power of body weight among adult mammals from diverse taxa. However, in lower-level taxa the exponent is smaller (see Gould, 1971, 1975*b*) so that within genera it lies between 0.2 and 0.4 (Lande, 1979). If we were comparing deviations from some line of best fit (as when producing the encephalisation quotients discussed above), quite different estimates would result from measuring species deviations from the generic or from the family line. Again, we suggest using the taxonomic level immediately above the one in question; thus, species deviations should be measured from the generic lines, and generic deviations from the family lines. If lines of best fit for brain-weight against body-weight relationships were being compared across different families, then slopes set by generic points should be used since the uneven distribution of species among genera can produce quite irrelevant differences in slope or elevation.

The line of best fit

As the variable on the abscissa is measured with increasing error, regression analysis produces a progressively lower slope. Usually, variables in comparative studies are measured with considerable error and correlation coefficients are far from unity. Regression then provides an unsuitable model and any estimate of slope calculated by regression analysis will be too low. Nevertheless, regression analysis has been used repeatedly in such studies and the error variances on the abscissas have been conveniently ignored. For example, since McNab (1963) first used regression analysis on logarithmically transformed data to investigate the relationship between home range size and body size in small mammals, the technique has been routinely used by later workers studying other groups (e.g. birds: Schoener (1968); lizards: Turner, Jeinrich & Weintraub (1969); primates: Milton & May (1976), Clutton-Brock & Harvey (1977a); these and other vertebrate and invertebrate groups: G.E. Belovsky & J.B. Slade (in preparation)). The slopes involved have been the subject of both discussion and controversy, but although it has been widely acknowledged that body weights have considerable error variance (e.g. see Turner *et al.*, 1969) it has apparently never been appreciated that the slopes underestimate the true values since correlations tend to be of the order 0.5 to 0.8. For example, Turner *et al.* (1969) quote a regression slope of 0.88 for the logarithm of home range regressed on the logarithm of body weight across female lizard species, but the correlation is 0.71 and a reduced major axis estimate of the slope would be 1.23. (We are not arguing that reduced major axis is the correct model for analysis here. Clearly, since home range size probably depends on body size (via metabolic needs), a regression model *that incorporates measurement error on the abscissa* would be more appropriate (Sokal and Rohlf, 1969).) The authors were interested in comparing the slope to that relating metabolic costs to body weight, but in the absence of any information on the extent of the error variances in the two analyses, the comparison becomes meaningless. Discussion of the biological interpretation of regression slopes (e.g. Clutton-Brock & Harvey, 1977a) now seems to us to be rather a vacuous exercise because they may have little biological relevance. The message is that when a perfect underlying relationship is postulated (as in the simulations), reduced major axis should be used wherever possible after removing estimates of the error variance from both variables (see above and Kermack, 1954).

Another disadvantage of regression is its ability, through extrapolation, to produce artificial differences in elevation of relationships measured across different taxa. Fig. 16.2 provides a hypothetical example; reduced major axis analysis would reveal no differences in elevation between the two data sets while regression analysis would indicate a difference. Imbrie (1956) provides a more detailed discussion of this point, together with an example taken from allometric relationships in brachiopod morphology. Those readers familiar with the brain : body size literature will recognise Fig. 16.2 as very similar to that found when brain size is plotted against body size on logarithmically transformed axes. In fact, in that case the differences in elevation still exist when major axis analysis is used (Clutton-Brock & Harvey, 1980; Mace *et al.*, 1981). As more data become available, and groups of animals are compared by plots of life history variables on body weight analysed by regression techniques (e.g. Western, 1979; Millar, 1977), we caution against uncritical acceptance of apparent slope or elevation differences when correlation coefficients are low.

The effect of changes of scale on slopes when major axis analysis is used on data that have not been logarithmically transformed is a source of serious potential error, and we need only turn to one of the major textbooks in the biological sciences (Sokal & Rohlf, 1969) to find an example of the technique being used incorrectly.

In a comment on the study of allometry, Gould (1975*b*) argued that the

Fig. 16.2. Lines of best fit produced by two data sets A and B. Regression lines are broken, and reduced major axis lines unbroken. The range of values in each data set lies between the ends of the lines on the *x*-axis. Intercepts for the two regression lines from data sets A and B are shown by points *ra* and *rb* respectively. The intercept for both lines produced by reduced major axis analysis is shown by the point *rma*.

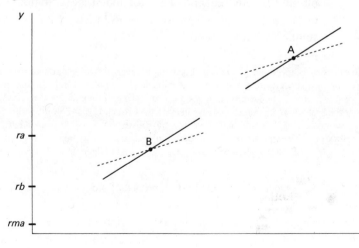

analysis of simple bivariate or double logarithmic plots would be relegated to 'minor significance if not historical oblivion' as 'multivariate techniques supercede bivariate studies'. That, hopefully, will be so. But as more independent variables are incorporated into regression equations so that we deal with a multiple regression model, then the problems concerning error discussed above are compounded. In addition, further bias as well as difficulties of interpretation are introduced when there is correlation between the independent variables (see Post, 1981). Nevertheless, papers in behavioural ecology employ multiple regression without considering the problems of error and correlation (e.g. Jorde & Spuhler, 1974; Baker & Parker, 1979). In some cases, the procedures used are so questionable that any conclusions drawn should either be discarded or treated with extreme caution. The problem does not end with regression models: principal component (major axis) analysis is commonplace nowadays, yet even the simple bivariate case has, as we have shown, problems of interpretation associated with it. How much more so for a multivariate analysis?

Summary

1. Behavioural and morphological variation across taxa provides a rich source of comparative data for both generating and testing adaptationist hypotheses.
2. Such comparative studies face a variety of problems that are often ignored. Choosing a suitable taxonomic level for study and the correct statistical technique for analysis are cases in point.
3. This chapter discusses a variety of methodological problems and pitfalls that are frequently encountered in the sociobiological literature. Solutions to several of these problems are illustrated with a simple simulation study.

This chapter is affectionately dedicated to King's College Sociobiology Group. We wish to take this opportunity to thank everyone associated with the Group for the hospitality, encouragement and academic stimulation shown during our numerous visits to Cambridge over the past few years. We should also like to thank John Maynard Smith for his continued encouragement at Sussex. Finally, we are grateful to those people from King's College, Cambridge, The University of Sussex, Harvard University, and The University of Washington at Seattle who helped at various stages during the preparation of this chapter.

Appendix. To test for heterogeneity of slopes using major axis analysis

The test depends on major axis analysis rotating the original axes through angle θ so that $(x, y) \rightarrow (x^*, y^*)$ and the correlation of points in the new coordinates (r_i for group i of size n_i) is zero. If we have g sets of data (groups), we investigate whether the covariance matrices of each group are diagonal (whether by roating we have removed all correlation). Morrison (1967, pp. 111 onwards) gives such a test for a single group. It computes the likelihood ratio

$$\lambda = |\hat{R}|^{\frac{1}{2}n}$$

where $\hat{R}$ is the observed correlation matrix. We perform g such tests so that

$$\lambda = g_{i=1} \prod |\hat{R}_i|^{\frac{1}{2}n_i}$$

(where for group i the observed correlation matrix is $\hat{R}_i$, so $|\hat{R}_i| = 1 - r_i^2$).

The degrees of freedom will be $gp(p - 1)/2$ which, since the number of variables p is 2, reduces to g. However, if we iterate on a common estimate of θ for all groups so as to minimise the likelihood ratio, this removes one further degree of freedom.

We can look up $-2\ln\lambda$ on a χ^2 table with $g-1$ degrees of freedom. Morrison points out that Bartlett suggests the use of

$$\chi^2 = -\sum_{i=1}^{g} (n_i - 15/6)\ln|\hat{R}_i|$$

rather than

$$\chi^2 = -\sum_{i=1}^{g} (n_i)\ln|\hat{R}_i|$$

as an improved value which converges to a true χ^2 distribution more quickly as all the n_i approach ∞.

If χ^2 is significant, we reject the null hypothesis that slopes are equal. If χ^2 is not significant, we use sine θ as our estimate of a common slope.

We thank Professor J. Felsenstein for developing this test.

References

Alexander, R.D., Hoogland, J.L., Howard, R., Noonan, K.M. & Sherman, P.W. (1979). Sexual dimorphism and breeding systems in pinnipeds, ungulates, primates and humans. In *Evolutionary Biology and Human Social Behavior*, ed. N.A. Chagnon & W.D. Irons, pp. 402–35. Duxbury Press: North Scituate, Mass.

Alexander, R.M. (1977). Mechanics and scaling of terrestrial locomotion. In *Scale Effects in Animal Locomotion*, ed. T.J. Pedley, pp. 93–110. Academic Press: London.

Baker, R.R. & Parker, G.A. (1979). The evolution of bird colouration. *Philosophical Transactions of the Royal Society of London*, B, **287**, 63–130.

Bauchot, R. & Stephan, H. (1969). Encephalisation et niveau évolutif chez les Simiens. *Mammalia*, **33**, 225–75.

Belovsky, G.E. & Slade, J.B. (in preparation). Body size – home range area patterns and an energy maximising explanation.

Clutton-Brock, T.H. & Harvey, P.H. (1977a). Primate ecology and social organisation. *Journal of Zoology, London*, **183**, 1–39.

Clutton-Brock, T.H. & Harvey, P.H. (1977b). Species differences in feeding and ranging behaviour in primates. In *Primate Ecology: Studies of Feeding and Ranging Behaviour in Lemurs, Monkeys and Apes*, ed. T.H. Clutton-Brock, pp. 557–84. Academic Press: London.

Clutton-Brock, T.H. & Harvey, P.H. (1979). Comparison and adaptation. *Proceedings of the Royal Society*, B, **205**, 547–65.

Clutton-Brock, T.H. & Harvey, P.H. (1980). Primates, brains and ecology. *Journal of Zoology, London*, **190**, 309–23.

Gould, S.J. (1966). Allometry and size in ontogeny and phylogeny. *Biological Reviews*, **41**, 587–640.

Gould, S.J. (1971). Geometric similarity in allometric growth: a contribution to the problem of scaling in the evolution of size. *American Naturalist*, **105**, 113–36.

Gould, S.J. (1975a). On scaling of tooth size in mammals. *American Zoologist*, **15**, 351–62.

Gould, S.J. (1975b). Allometry in primates with an emphasis on the scaling and evolution of the brain. In *Approaches to Primate Paleobiology*, ed. F. Szalay, pp. 244–92. Karger: Basel.

Harestad, A.S. & Bunnell, F.L. (1979). Home range and body weight – a re-evaluation. *Ecology*, **60**, 389–402.

Harvey, P.H., Kavanagh, M. & Clutton-Brock, T.H. (1978). Sexual dimorphism in primate teeth. *Journal of Zoology, London*, **186**, 475–86.

Hespenheide, H.A. (1973). Ecological inferences from morphological data. *Annual Review of Ecology and Systematics*, **4**, 213–29.

Imbrie, J. (1956). Biometrical methods in the study of invertebrate fossils. *Bulletin of the American Museum of Natural History*, **108**, 217–52.

Jerison, H.J. (1973). *Evolution of the Brain and Intelligence*. Academic Press: New York.

Jolicoeur, P. (1968). Interval estimation of the slope of the major axis of a bivariate normal distribution in the case of a small sample. *Biometrics*, **24**, 679–82.

Jolicoeur, P. & Mosimann, J.E. (1968). Intervalles de confiance pour la pente de l'axe majeur d'une distribution bidimensionelle. *Biometrie-Praximetrie*, **9**, 121–40.

Jorde, L.B. & Spuhler, J.N. (1974). A statistical analysis of selected aspects of primate demography, ecology and social behaviour. *Journal of Anthropological Research*, **30**, 199–224.

Kermack, K.A. (1954). Biometrical study of *Micraster coranguinum* and *M. (Isomicraster) senonensis*. *Proceedings of the Royal Society of London*, B, **237**, 375–428.

Kermack, K.A. & Haldane, J.B.S. (1950). Organic correlation and allometry. *Biometrika*, **37**, 30–41.

Kleiber, M. (1961). *The Fire of Life: an Introduction to Animal Energetics*. Wiley: New York.

Lande, R. (1979). Quantitative genetic analysis of multivariate evolution applied to brain : body size allometry. *Evolution*, **33**, 402–16.

MacArthur, R.H. & Wilson, E.O. (1967). *The Theory of Island Biogeography*. Princeton University Press: New Jersey.

Mace, G.M., Harvey, P.H. & Clutton-Brock, T.H. (1981). Brain size and ecology in small mammals. *Journal of Zoology, London*, **193**, 333–54.

McMahon, T. (1973). Size and shape in biology. *Science*, **179**, 1201–4.

McNab, B.W. (1963). Bioenergetics and the determination of home range size. *American Naturalist*, **97**, 133–40.

Millar J.S. (1977). Body size and reproduction in terrestrial eutherian mammals. *Evolution*, **31**, 370–86.

Milton, K. & May, M.L. (1976). Body weight, diet and home range area in primates. *Nature*, **259**, 459–62.

Morrison, D.F. (1967). *Multivariate Statistical Methods*. McGraw Hill: New York.

Pirlot, P. & Stephan, H. (1970). Encephalisation in Chiroptera. *Canadian Journal of Zoology*, **48**, 433–44.

Post, D.G. (1981). Sexual dimorphism in the anthropoid primates: some thoughts on causes, correlates and the relationship to body size. In *Sexual Dimorphism in Primates*, ed. C. Eastman & P. Heisler. Garland Press: New York. (In press.)

Rensch, B. (1959). *Evolution Above the Species Level*. Methuen: London.

Schoener, T.W. (1968). Sizes of feeding territories among birds. *Ecology*, **49**, 123–41.

Sherman, P.W. (1979). Insect chromosome number and eusociality. *American Naturalist*, **113**, 925–35.

Snedecor, G.W. (1956). *Statistical Methods*. State University Press: Iowa.

Sokal, R.R. & Rohlf, F.J. (1969). *Biometry*. Freeman: San Francisco.

Taylor, C.R. (1977). The energetics of terrestrial locomotion and body size of the vertebrates. In *Scale Effects in Animal Locomotion*, ed. T.J. Pedley, pp. 127–41. Academic Press: London.

Tessier, G. (1948). La relation d'allometrie: sa signification statistique et biologique. *Biometrics*, **4**, 14–53.

Turner, F.B., Jeinrich, R.I. & Weintraub, J.D. (1969). Home ranges and body size of lizards. *Ecology*, **50**, 1076–81.

Verner, J. (1964). Evolution of polygyny in the long billed marsh wren. *Evolution*, **18**, 252–61.

Western, D. (1979). Life history and ecological implications of size in mammals. *African Journal of Ecology*, **17**, 185–204.

Wilkie, D.R. (1977). Metabolism and body size. In *Scale Effects in Animal Locomotion*, ed. T.J. Pedley pp. 23–36. Academic Press: London.

17

Behaviour and competition for scarce resources

N.B. DAVIES

During the last thirty years the pioneering studies of MacArthur (1958), Tinbergen (1959) and Crook (1964) have inspired an enormous amount of interest in species differences in ecology and behaviour. This comparative approach has given rise to detailed descriptions of differences between species in their feeding, displays and mating behaviour. Every species is said to have a characteristic foraging niche, a mating system and a catalogue of specific behaviour, or ethogram. Differences between species can then be related to environmental parameters such as the abundance and distribution of food supplies and predators (Lack, 1968; Clutton-Brock & Harvey, 1978).

Little attention was given to individual differences within a species. Indeed, if some individuals behaved in a different way from the majority they were often thought to be abnormal. Male ducks that raped females instead of courting them in the fashion typical of the species were said to be behaving abnormally due to overcrowding. Male fish which behaved like females and deceived other males into courting them were described as abnormal; the function of this homosexual behaviour was considered to be an outlet for sexual frustration (Morris, 1952). Male frogs which remained silent during the croaking of other males in a chorus would, perhaps, have been regarded as ill or resting.

During the last decade, however, there has been a surge of interest in differences between individuals within a species; whenever we now see an individual doing something different we are tempted to label it as a strategy. Male fish that court other males are no longer considered queer; they are employing transvestite strategies. Male frogs that are silent are no longer tired or ill; they are adopting sneaky strategies.

There are probably three main reasons for this change of approach.

First, and most important, is the framing of evolutionary explanations in terms of advantage to the individual or gene rather than advantage to the group or species (Williams, 1966; Dawkins, 1976). The emphasis is now on selfish individuals competing to maximise their gene contribution to future generations. If some males are attracting females by calling, then we now expect to find other males parasiting their efforts and behaving as satellites. Secondly, the application of game theory to the study of behaviour has shown that it is possible to have stable equilibria with individuals behaving in different ways (Maynard Smith, 1976, 1979). Finally, an increase in the number of field studies with individually marked animals has shown empirically that individuals do differ in their behaviour.

In this paper I shall examine, from the field worker's point of view, some of the problems inherent in this new approach. It is undoubtedly important to study individual differences in order to understand the evolution of the strategies that animals adopt to compete for scarce resources such as food, mates or territories. However in practice, when we go into the field, problems of measurements mean that it will always be difficult to discover why individuals are different.

A classification of alternative strategies

The following classification is derived from Maynard Smith & Parker (1976), Dawkins (1980) and Dunbar (1983).

Conditional on environment

Different behaviour may be advantageous in different places or at different times. For example, on cloudy days male speckled wood butterflies, *Pararge aegeria*, search for females by patrolling in the tree canopy whereas on sunny days they sally out from favourite perches in sunspot territories on the woodland floor (Davies, 1978). Their strategy is thus, 'if cloudy, patrol; if sunny, perch'.

Conditional on phenotype

One of the most important sources of differences between individuals is that an animal's behaviour is often conditional on its size and strength, or what Parker (1974a) refers to as resource-holding potential. The largest and strongest individuals command the most resources, often by fighting, and the small, weak individuals have to 'make the best of a bad job' by sneaking or satellite behaviour. The strategy is, therefore, 'if large, fight; if small, sneak'.

Body size may be fixed throughout adult life and reflect feeding conditions experienced when immature. For example, male dung flies, *Scatophaga stercoraria*, which have poor food supplies as larvae grow into small adults that are not very good at fighting and so spend more time searching for females in the grass around the edge of cowpats while the larger males fight for mates on the pat itself (P.A. Arak, in preparation; Sigurjonsdottir, 1980). Similarly, small male bees, *Centris pallida*, hover above emergence areas waiting to copulate with airborn virgin females while larger males fight for females as they emerge from the ground (Alcock, Jones & Buchmann, 1977). In these cases small individuals will have to make the best of a bad job throughout their whole lifetime.

Alternatively, body size may be age dependent, in which case an individual will change its behaviour as it gets older and grows larger. Old male elephant seals, *Mirounga angustirostris* (Le Boeuf, 1974), and red deer, *Cervus elaphus* (Clutton-Brock, Albon, Gibson & Guinness, 1979) are strong and can fight successfully to defend groups of females while younger, smaller males hang around the edge of the harems and attempt to sneak copulations. Similarly, young bullfrogs, *Rana catesbeiana*, are small and not strong enough to fight for possession of a good territory; instead they behave as satellites, sitting silently in a large calling male's territory and attempting to intercept the females he attracts (Howard, 1978).

In all these examples measurements have shown that the large individuals do much better than the small ones.

Frequency-dependent equilibrium

Sometimes the term 'best strategy' has no meaning because the payoffs for behaving in a particular way depend on what others in the population are doing. Often a strategy does best when rare and we would expect frequency-dependent selection to stabilise the frequency of the different strategies so that each, on average, enjoyed equal success. The equilibrium can come about in three main ways.

Genetic polymorphism. The population may be polymorphic with different individuals programmed genetically to play different pure strategies. For example, we could regard male and female as different strategies whose payoffs are frequency dependent. Each does better when rare in the population and so we would expect frequency-dependent selection to bring about an equilibrium, or evolutionarily stable state, where the average success of the two strategies is equal (Fisher, 1930). Another possible example is male dimorphism in the ruff, *Philomachus pugnax*, where dark individuals are territory residents and pale individuals are satellites

(Hogan-Warburg, 1966; van Rhijn, 1973). If these were genetically alternative strategies whose success was frequency dependent then we might
expect individuals who are residents to enjoy, on average, equal success to
that of the satellites.

Individuals play a genetically fixed mixed strategy (mixed ESS). In this case
each individual plays a mixed strategy. A good example is provided by the
behaviour of the digger wasp, *Sphex ichneumoneus* (Brockmann & Dawkins, 1979; Brockmann, Grafen & Dawkins, 1979). Females either 'dig'
their own burrow or they 'enter' an already dug burrow in which case they
might be lucky and get a burrow for free or they may end up sharing an
occupied burrow. In the latter case there is a fight when the two females
eventually meet and the result is that only one succeeds in laying eggs in the
burrow.

It is easy to see that the payoffs for digging and entering could be
frequency dependent. If all the females were digging then there would be
plenty of empty (old and abandoned) burrows and entering would be a
highly successful strategy. If all the wasps were entering, on the other hand,
then more and more sharing and fighting would take place and it would be
better to dig. There would, however, be an equilibrium when digging and
entering were equally successful. In one population of wasps the success of
the two behaviours was indeed equal. Furthermore a female's decision
whether to dig or enter was not dependent on the environment (e.g. time of
the breeding season) nor on her phenotype (e.g. body size, age). Therefore
digging and entering seem to be alternative strategies whose frequencies are
maintained in an evolutionarily stable equilibrium. Individual females are
apparently genetically programmed with a fixed rule such as 'dig with
probability p, enter with probability $(1 - p)$'. The value of p has been fixed
by frequency-dependent selection so the success of the two decisions is
equal. We can refer to the females as playing a mixed evolutionarily stable
strategy (mixed ESS).

Behavioural assessment. Equilibria can also come about by individuals
assessing what others in the population are doing rather than by inflexible
genetic rules or polymorphisms. In supermarkets the customers are quick
to assess the lengths of the lines at each service counter and join the line
with the shortest waiting time. Provided all the serving clerks are equally
efficient and all customers have equal amounts of shopping to be processed
then the stable equilibrium will be for all the lines to be of the same length.
Fretwell (1972) refers to this kind of stable distribution as 'ideal free' and
Parker (1978) calls it a 'spatial ESS'.

A good example is the experiments of David Harper (1982) who threw pieces of bread to the ducks on a garden pond. The bread was thrown in at two places and the profitability of each was varied. The best place for one duck to feed obviously depends on where all the other ducks go. Population counts showed that they quickly adopted an ideal free distribution, with the number of ducks in each place reflecting their relative profitabilities (Fig. 17.1*a*). This is the stable state because with any other distribution it would pay some ducks to move between the feeding sites.

Fig. 17.1. (*a*) Feeding experiments with 33 ducks on a pond. (i) When site A is twice as profitable as site B, ideal free theory predicts that 22 of the 33 ducks should go to site A. (ii) When site A is only half as profitable as site B, 11 ducks should go to site A. The observed distributions (solid line) are close to the predicted (dashed line) in each case. However, individuals do not all achieve equal gain. (*b*) In both cases, a few dominant ducks snatch most of the food. (From D.G.C. Harper, 1982.)

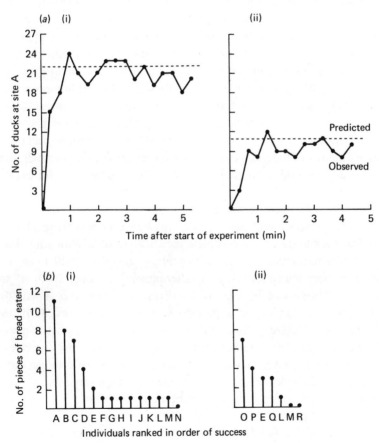

Behavioural assessment is also involved in bringing about equilibria of profitabilities in different searching areas of feeding shoals of sticklebacks, *Gasterosteus aculeatus*, (Milinski, 1979) and mating aggregations of toads, *Bufo bufo*, (Davies & Halliday, 1979). The stable distribution could come about by each individual duck, fish or toad sampling the various habitats and choosing the most profitable one, which will depend on where the other individuals have decided to go. Alternatively an individual could decide where to search by observing the amount of resources in each habitat and also the number of other competitors. The strategy would therefore be something like, 'if most of the population are at A, go to B'.

Stable distributions from population counts do not necessarily mean that all individuals will achieve equal rewards. Even though dungflies distribute themselves in an ideal free way around cowpats (Parker, 1974b) large males achieve more matings than small males (P.A. Arak, in preparation). In the duck experiments described above (Harper, 1982) one or two dominant ducks snatched most of the food at each feeding site (Fig. 17.1b). The apparent ideal free distribution from population counts probably came about because the subordinate ducks arranged themselves in relation to where the dominant ducks went. In effect, the dominant individuals are part of the habitat to which the subordinates respond. Similarly, when a small male bullfrog makes the best of a bad job by residing on a large calling male's territory as a satellite, the best territory to parasitise will depend on where all the other satellites have decided to go. We might expect the satellites to arrange themselves in an ideal free way with respect to the territory quality of the callers. If they do so then the number of satellites in each territory should be such that the profitability is the same for each.

The definition of a strategy

The word strategy has been used in two senses. Strictly speaking, it should be used to describe a complete specification of how an animal will behave in a particular situation. A strategy, therefore, will refer to a genetically determined behavioural alternative (Dawkins, 1980). If the difference in behaviour between two individuals is due to a genetic difference then we can say that they have different strategies. With this definition we can refer to 'resident' and 'satellite' male ruffs as two strategies because the difference between them is genetic. However we cannot call sneaking in young elephant seals or red deer a separate strategy; rather it is part of one conditional strategy 'if small, sneak; if large, fight'.

Strategy has also been used to describe a component of what an animal will do in a particular situation. Thus perching and patrolling in butterflies have been referred to as different strategies, as have sneaking and fighting in deer. There is probably a lot to be said for using the word strategy in this looser sense, partly because it is already commonly used like this in the literature, but mainly because problems of measurement mean that it is always difficult to say which of the categories in the classification above applies to any particular example.

Problems of measurement

Measuring costs

Most studies simply record the benefits obtained by individuals behaving in different ways, such as food intake, number of copulations or number of eggs, and measurements are often made over a short period like a day or a breeding season. The problem here is that different strategies may have different costs and therefore different effects on survival.

Ragland & Sohal (1973, personal communication) have found that both body size and activity influence survival in house flies, *Musca domestica*. Large individuals live for a shorter time than small ones and intense competition for mates also decreases the lifespan. Therefore some caution may be needed before it can be safely concluded that large individuals who are good at fighting have greater success when only short-term benefits have been measured (e.g. *Centris* bees).

High-benefit strategies, like fighting and calling, may also entail greater costs through attracting predators and parasites. Calling male bullfrogs not only attract females but also predatory snapping turtles in search of an easy meal (Howard, 1979). In the field cricket, *Gryllus integer*, there are also calling males and satellites. A caller attracts females but a parasitic fly also homes in on the calls and lays live larvae in the caller's body; when the young parasites emerge the cricket dies (Cade, 1979). Without good data on both the costs and benefits of calling it will be impossible to say which of the categories in the classification above applies to the alternative strategies of the cricket. Both calling and satellite behaviour may persist because each does better in a different environment; calling may be best at times and in places where parasites are scarce while satellite behaviour may be better when parasites are abundant. The strategies could also be conditional on phenotype; maybe only the largest males or those with the most energy reserves call? Finally they could coexist as a frequency-dependent equilibrium each enjoying, on average, equal success.

Sample size

It is impossible to demonstrate statistically that two strategies have exactly equal success. All we can do is infer equality if we fail to find a significant difference. The problem here is that the smaller our sample size the less likely we are to find a significant difference. Twenty years ago if someone returned from the field and announced that he had failed to find a difference between individuals behaving in different ways, he would probably have been encouraged to go back and collect more data. Nowadays, when we have a theory that predicts equality, he may be congratulated on discovering a mixed ESS! As Maynard Smith remarked, one of the great services made by the theoreticians to the field worker today is that fewer data are needed to support the new theories!

An example of the difficulties of interpretation of the data is provided by the experiments of Perrill, Gerhardt & Daniel (1978) who studied callers and satellites in the treefrog *Hyla cinerea*. Unlike Howard's bullfrogs described above, there was no clear size difference between the callers and satellites so the satellites were not simply young males who were making the best of a bad job because they did not have very fine voices or the strength to defend a calling site. In fact some male treefrogs were seen adopting both strategies. Furthermore the experiments showed that satellites could enjoy considerable success. When females were released near a caller and its satellite the calling male amplexed with the female on 17 occasions while the satellite did so on 13 occasions, which is not significantly different from a 1 : 1 ratio of success. The safest conclusion would be to say that this result is at least consistent with the idea of a frequency-dependent equilibrium, but then to go out into the field again and collect more data on the costs and benefits of the two strategies and the factors influencing a male's decision whether to behave as a caller or as a satellite.

Lifetime success or decisions?

To compare the success of two strategies when there is a polymorphism, like resident and satellite in the ruff, we would ideally like to know the lifetime reproductive success of individuals who are residents and those who are satellites. Short-term measurements, for example success scored during a breeding season, would not be good enough for three main reasons. First, individuals might improve with age and experience and so differences between individuals in one season may simply be due to age differences. Second, individuals that were very successful in one season might not achieve a higher lifetime success because they could live for a shorter time. Gadgil (1972) made this point when he suggested that there may be selection for two types of male in a population, those with a 'fast and furious' lifestyle which were very successful but only lived for a few seasons and others which were 'slow but sure', breeding at a lower rate but living for a longer time. In the ruffs, for example, satellites could live for longer than residents because they do not suffer the costs of territory defence. The third problem with short-term measures is that the success of a strategy may vary with the environment. For example the relative success of resident and satellite ruffs varies seasonally and on different size leks (Hogan Warburg, 1966; van Rhijn, 1973). Therefore it may sometimes be difficult with short term measurements to distinguish strategies that are making the best of a bad job from those that are suffering a temporary disadvantage because of a changing environment (Dunbar, 1983).

So far there have been no field studies that have measured lifetime success, so it is too early to say whether short-term observations are going to be useful or hopelessly inaccurate. In red deer stags there appear to be consistent individual differences in success over successive seasons and so short-term measurements may after all give a reasonable indication of lifetime reproductive success (Gibson & Guinness, 1980).

When individuals employ several strategies, however, we cannot compare the success of different strategies by comparing different individuals. A female digger wasp both digs and enters. A male treefrog behaves both as a caller and as a satellite. In these cases we have to measure the success of the strategies themselves, or decisions. A decision is defined as a commitment of a period of time to a particular course of action (Brockmann *et al.*, 1979). Caller and satellite could be regarded as two decisions for a male treefrog and an individual may make many such decisions in its lifetime. We could imagine some males deciding mainly to call, others deciding mainly to be satellites and others playing both roles about equally often. If two alternative strategies, or decisions, are in frequency-dependent equilibrium then we would expect the success of the two decisions to be equal regardless of which individuals employed them.

Measuring the success of decisions presents many of the same problems as with lifetime success. One method is to score benefits per unit time. This was the measure used by Brockmann *et al.*, (1979) for comparing digging and entering in the digger wasps. It is also the measure used in many studies of foraging and territorial behaviour. Using time as a common currency assumes that the different strategies (or different foraging methods and territory defence) are equally costly. This may not always be so; calling may be a more costly decision for a treefrog than satellite because of the greater energy expenditure and increased risk of predation. It is only recently that attempts have been made to measure the energetic costs of different activities (e.g. Bryant, 1979) or how animals behave when the costs of different activities, such as foraging and predation, are varied (e.g. Caraco, Martindale & Pulliam, 1980).

Flexible versus fixed rules

As mentioned above, frequency-dependent equilibria can come about either through individuals playing a genetically fixed mixed ESS (e.g. digger wasps) or through behavioural assessment (e.g. Harper's ducks). A good method for distinguishing between these is to do a perturbation experiment. If individuals were removed from one habitat then, with behavioural assessment, the remaining competitors should quickly redistribute themselves so as to achieve the equilibrium once more. In the treefrogs, if caller and satellite were maintained as a frequency-dependent equilibrium by behavioural assessment then individuals would play strategies such as, 'if most of the other frogs are calling, be a satellite'. Experimental removal of callers in the population should result in some of the satellites becoming callers so as to bring about the equilibrium mixture once again.

If, on the other hand, the animals were playing the various strategies with fixed probabilities then the perturbation should have no effect on an individual's behaviour. The implication of the study of Brockmann *et al.* (1979) with the digger wasp is that a sudden alteration in the habitat or a sudden removal of all the individuals who were digging at the time would have no effect on the frequency with which females played 'dig' and 'enter'. They would carry on exactly as before, blindly playing the two strategies with the probabilities that previously satisfied the mixed ESS.

Until experiments have been done it will not be possible to say which of these two ways of achieving an equilibrium will be commoner in nature. Intuitively it seems likely that the flexibility of behavioural assessment will be favoured whenever animals live in environments which are unpredictable in space and time and where individuals have the opportunity to assess what others in the population are doing.

Unequal payoffs

The field worker will often find that the data show two strategies have unequal payoffs. A good example is Thornhill's (1979) work on the scorpionfly, *Hylobittacus apicalis*. If a male is to attract a female he must first of all capture a prey item on which she will feed while he copulates. Without a nuptial meal the female will refuse him. Individual males adopt a mixed strategy for obtaining prey. Sometimes they 'hunt' for the prey item themselves but sometimes they 'steal' a prey from another male, either by flying at him and knocking the prey forcibly out of his grasp, or by adopting a female-like posture and duping the other male into giving up his prize. Because individuals employ both strategies we have to measure the success of hunting and stealing decisions.

Thornhill (1979) measured success in terms of time between copulations. For hunting, intercopulation time was 26 min but for stealing it was only 17 min. It is clear from these data that stealing decisions were more successful because they resulted in the male obtaining a prey quicker and hence copulating more often. It is likely that stealing is also less costly in terms of the probability of becoming ensnared in spiders' webs while obtaining the nuptial prey.

The interpretation of this result illustrates the problem of applying the various categories of alternative strategies to quantitative field data. There are three possibilities.

(a) The payoffs for hunting and stealing could be frequency dependent. It is obvious that all males cannot steal all the time. However, if most males were hunters then stealing would be very profitable. If there were no phenotypic constraints (e.g. body size) on whether a male could hunt or steal then we might expect frequency-dependent selection to stabilise the success of the two strategies as equal. If this mixed ESS idea is correct then the data suggest that the system is not very stable. Our first possible interpretation is, therefore, that hunting and stealing represent a mixed ESS and that the data do not correctly represent the costs and benefits of the two strategies. Perhaps there is some other unmeasured cost to stealing?

(b) The second possibility is that the data are accurate reflections of the payoffs, in which case the idea that hunting and stealing are a mixed ESS must be wrong. Hunting and stealing may be part of a conditional strategy such as 'if large, steal; if small, hunt'. Maybe just as only the strongest bullfrogs defend territories, so only the best male scorpionflies go in for stealing.

(c) The third possibility is that the mixed ESS idea and the data are both correct but that the population has not yet reached a stable equilibrium. Perhaps in time the frequency of stealing will increase and the payoffs stabilise as equal. This interpretation must be considered especially as many data are now collected in habitats recently modified by man, such as polluted streams and suburban gardens. This means that some animals may be using rules adapted to different environments from the ones in which we study them.

Measuring constraints

In many cases where behaviour depends on size and strength, individuals of poor competitive ability do less well than others. However they may still be adopting the optimal strategy for their own particular constraints. For example when Lack (1966) studied clutch size in great tits, *Parus major*, he looked at natural variations and found that individuals laying a particular clutch size produced the most surviving young. A common interpretation would be that individuals producing smaller or larger clutches than this optimal size had, so to speak, laid the 'wrong' clutch size. However, experiments by Perrins & Moss (1975) showed that although individuals producing a small clutch left fewer surviving young, they were nevertheless laying the optimal clutch size for their own particular ability. When their brood size was increased artificially they did less well than birds which had naturally large broods.

This idea is presented graphically in Fig. 17.2. The horizontal axis is a range of possible strategies. Reading from left to right these may represent, for example, lay one egg to lay ten eggs; eat small prey to eat large prey; behave as a satellite to fight and defend a territory. The main curve indicates that individuals laying ten eggs, eating large prey or fighting for a territory all have greater success. Nevertheless, experiments may reveal that individuals employing less successful strategies are still adopting their own optima. Individuals eating small prey may do less well if given larger prey, individuals laying small clutches may do less well with larger clutches

Fig. 17.2. The horizontal axis represents a range of possible strategies, such as 'never fight' to 'always fight', or 'lay one egg' to 'lay ten eggs'. The heavy line, whose shape is arbitrary, indicates that success increases with, for example, more fighting or more eggs. However, even though individuals who fight less or lay fewer eggs do less well than others, they may be at the optimum for their own particular constraints. The thin curves suggest that if an individual changed its strategy it would do less well.

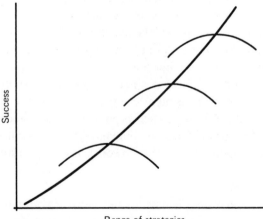

Range of strategies

and satellites may be too weak to defend their own territories. An individual may move to the right during development as its constraints change; birds may eat larger prey as their bills grow, frogs may fight more as they grow larger, and so on. Alternatively an individual may be fixed by its phenotype at one point on the continuum, for example small male dungflies whose adult size reflects poor feeding conditions as a larva. Therefore natural variation in behaviour may often arise because individuals have different constraints and thus different optimal strategies.

Theory and data

The main conclusion from the discussion above is that it is never going to be easy to measure the success of alternative strategies. Ideally we need long-term measurements of costs as well as benefits, of success at different times and in different places and of individual constraints. An important point is that we are not using the field data to 'test ESS theory'. What the theory helps us do is to identify truly alternative strategies. If we collect good data that show two strategies have different success, this does not mean that ESS theory is wrong. It simply means that the strategies we identified are not true ESS alternatives.

Interactions and conflict between strategies

Situations where territory owners associate with subordinates (satellites or helpers) provide a good illustration of how there may be a conflict of interests between individuals employing different strategies to compete for scarce resources.

Resident male ruffs sometimes allow a satellite male to reside on their territories. The presence of a satellite brings a benefit because it increases the number of females attracted. It also brings a cost because the satellite steals some of the copulations (van Rhijn, 1973). Breeding pairs of the pied kingfisher (*Ceryle rudis*) sometimes accept the presence of unrelated males at their nesting burrows. These extra birds bring a benefit to the breeders because they feed their nestlings but they may also inflict a cost because there is a chance that they will usurp the nest burrow for their own future use (Reyer, 1980). Finally, pied wagtail (*Motacilla alba*) territory owners sometimes tolerate juvenile birds on their winter feeding territories. These satellites bring a benefit in the form of help with territory defence but they also impose a cost because they deplete the owner's food supply (Davies & Houston, 1981).

In all these cases the satellites, or helpers, are sometimes tolerated and sometimes chased away. For the pied wagtail it can be shown that an owner will only tolerate a satellite on its territory when the benefits of the association to the owner outweigh the costs, benefits and costs being measured in terms of their effect on the owner's feeding rate. When an owner would achieve a higher feeding rate by being alone, it evicts the satellite from the territory (Davies & Houston, 1981). However, it is important to realise that there will often be conflicts of interest between owners and satellites. Under some circumstances a territory owner may well benefit from the presence of a satellite, but whether it pays the satellite to associate will all depend on the profitability of its alternative options.

An example of such conflict in pied wagtails is shown in Fig. 17.3. At low levels of food abundance the territory owner enjoys a higher feeding rate by being alone. As food abundance increases, there is a switching point above which the owner would do better by associating with a satellite. Below the

Fig. 17.3. An example of the influence of food abundance on a pied wagtail's winter feeding territory on the owner's feeding rate when it is alone (F_o) and when it shares its territory with a satellite (F_s). F_s also gives the feeding rate of the satellite. The owner will do better by sharing the territory when food abundance increases above point a, but the satellite will not want to come onto the territory until point z, when its feeding rate will be greater than it would achieve in a nearby flock. Details of the model and data are in Davies & Houston (1981).

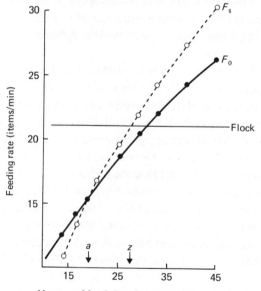

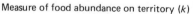

Measure of food abundance on territory (*k*)

switching point the costs of the satellite (sharing the food supply) outweigh the benefit (help with defence). Above the switching point the benefit outweighs the cost. One of the main reasons for the switch is that intruder pressure increases as food on the territory becomes more abundant. From the owner's point of view, therefore, we would expect tolerance of a satellite to occur after the switching point (point *a* in Fig. 17.3). However, whether the satellite will want to come onto the territory must depend on the feeding rate it could achieve elsewhere.

Field observations showed that owners, satellites and other wagtails often fed in a flock on a large flooded area not far from the territories (Davies, 1976). Owners continued to spend most of their time on territory even when the flock offered temporarily much greater rates of food intake. The territories were therefore a long-term investment concerned with the owners' survival over the whole winter and worth maintaining through periods of food scarcity.

Satellites, however, appeared to have no such long-term interest in a particular territory and they attempted to come onto the territories only when the feeding rate there was greater than that in the flock. The feeding rate in the flock varied during the winter and Fig. 17.3 gives an example when the rate was roughly constant during one month at 21 items per min. In this example the satellite will not want to associate with the owner until point *z*, even though the owner would benefit at point *a*. Between these points there will be a conflict of interest. The conflict would be in the opposite direction if the flock feeding rate was below that at the switching line, for example 12 items per min. In this case the satellite would want to come onto the territory before it is in the interests of the owner to accept it. Unless there is the unlikely event of the feeding rate in the flock being exactly equal to that of the owner at the switching point, there will always be a conflict of interest between owner and satellite.

The first point from this example is that there will often be conflicts of interest between individuals employing different strategies. It may not be sufficient to measure benefits from one individual's point of view in order to predict an association. Secondly, it is not going to be easy for the field worker to measure the costs and benefits because all alternative options have to be assessed (e.g. flock feeding) and long-term factors may be important.

Summary
1. The selfish gene approach to behaviour, the use of game theory and more detailed studies of wild populations with marked in-

dividuals have emphasised differences between individuals in the way they compete for scarce resources.

2. A classification of alternative strategies is presented; conditional on environment, conditioned on phenotype and frequency-dependent equilibria which can come about by a genetic polymorphism, by individuals playing a mixed ESS or by behavioural assessment.

3. The word strategy has been used to refer to a genetically determined behavioural alternative and also, in a looser sense, to describe any difference in behaviour. The advantage of a loose definition is that, in practice, it is difficult to categorise differences in behaviour in the classification because of problems of measurement.

4. Problems of measurement for the field worker include quantifying costs, sample size, measuring lifetime success, individual constraints, and what to conclude if measurements show unequal payoffs.

5. Conflicts of interest occur between individuals employing different strategies. An example is analysed where pied wagtail territory owners sometimes associate with satellites.

I thank Anthony Arak, Tim Clutton-Brock, Richard Dawkins, Robin Dunbar, John Maynard Smith and Dan Rubenstein for their comments and discussion, and David Harper for kindly allowing me to quote his unpublished experiments. I particularly acknowledge stimulating discussions with members of the symposium on 'Evolution and the theory of games' at the Zif, University of Bielefeld, Germany in 1978.

References

Alcock, J., Jones, C.E. & Buchmann, S.L. (1977). Male mating strategies in the bee *Centris pallida*, Fox (Anthophoridae: Hymenoptera). *American Naturalist*, **111**, 145–55.

Arak, P.A. (in preparation). The influence of body size on mate searching behaviour in male dung flies, *Scatophaga stercoraria*.

Brockmann, H.J. & Dawkins, R. (1979). Joint nesting in a digger wasp as an evolutionarily stable preadaptation to social life. *Behaviour*, **71**, 203–45.

Brockmann, H.J., Grafen, A. & Dawkins, R. (1979). Evolutionarily stable nesting strategy in a digger wasp. *Journal of Theoretical Biology*, **77**, 473–96.

Bryant, D.M. (1979). Reproductive costs in the house martin, *Delichon urbica*. *Journal of Animal Ecology*, **48**, 655–75.

Cade, W. (1979). The evolution of alternative male reproductive strategies in field crickets. In *Sexual Selection and Reproductive Competition in Insects*, ed. M. Blum & N.A. Blum, pp. 343–79. Academic Press: London.

Caraco, T., Martindale, S. & Pulliam, H.R. (1980). Avian flocking in the presence of a predator. *Nature*, **285**, 400–1.

Clutton-Brock, T.H. & Harvey, P.H. (1978). Mammals, resources and reproductive strategies. *Nature*, **273**, 191–5.

Clutton-Brock, T.H., Albon, S.D., Gibson, R.M. & Guinness, F.E. (1979). The logical stag: adaptive aspects of fighting in red deer (*Cervus elaphus*). *Animal Behaviour*, **27**, 211–25.

Crook, J.H. (1964). The evolution of social organisation and visual communication in the weaver birds (*Ploceinae*). *Behaviour* Supplement, 10.

Davies, N.B. (1976). Food, flocking and territorial behaviour of the pied wagtail *Motacilla alba* in winter. *Journal of Animal Ecology*, **45**, 235–54.

Davies, N.B. (1978). Territorial defence in the speckled wood butterfly (*Parage aegeria*): the resident always wins. *Animal behaviour*, **26**, 138–47.

Davies, N.B. & Halliday, T.R. (1979). Competitive mate searching in male common toads, *Bufo bufo*. *Animal Behaviour*, **27**, 1253–67.

Davies, N.B. & Houston, A.I. (1981). Owners and satellites: the economics of territory defence in the pied wagtail (*Motacilla alba*). *Journal of Animal Ecology*, **50**, 157–180.

Dawkins, R. (1976). *The Selfish Gene*. Oxford University Press: Oxford.

Dawkins, R. (1980). Good strategy or evolutionarily stable strategy? In *Sociobiology: Beyond Nature and Nurture*, ed. G.W. Barlow & J. Silverberg, pp. 331–67. Westview Press: Boulder, Colorado.

Dunbar, R.I.M. (1983). The logic of intra-specific variation in mating strategy. In *Perspectives in Ethology*, ed. P. Bateson & P. Klopfer. Plenum Press: New York.

Fisher, R.A. (1930). *The Genetical Theory of Natural Selection*. Clarendon Press: Oxford.

Fretwell, S.D. (1972). *Populations in a Seasonal Environment*. Princeton University Press: New Jersey.

Gadgil, M. (1972). Male dimorphism as a consequence of sexual selection. *American Naturalist*, **106**, 574–80.

Gibson, R.M. & Guinness, F.E. (1980). Differential reproduction among red deer (*Cervus elaphus*) stags on Rhum. *Journal of Animal Ecology*, **49**, 199–208.

Harper, D.G.C. (1982). Competitive foraging in mallards: ideal free ducks. *Animal Behaviour* (in press).

Hogan-Warburg, A.J. (1966). Social behaviour of the ruff, *Philomachus pugnax* (L.) *Ardea*, **54**, 109–229.

Howard, R.D. (1978). The evolution of mating strategies in bullfrogs, *Rana catesbeiana*. *Evolution*, **32**, 850–71.

Howard, R.D. (1979). Big bullfrogs in a little pond. *Natural History Magazine*, **88**, 30–6.

Lack, D. (1966). *Population Studies of Birds*. Clarendon Press: Oxford.

Lack, D. (1968). *Ecological Adaptations for Breeding in Birds*. Methuen: London.

Le Boeuf, B.J. (1974). Male–male competition and reproductive success in elephant seals, *American Zoologist*, **14**, 163–76.

MacArthur, R.H. (1958). Population ecology of some warblers of north-eastern coniferous forests. *Ecology*, **39**, 599–619.

Maynard Smith, J. (1976). Evolution and the theory of games. *American Scientist*, **64**, 41–5.

Maynard Smith, J. (1979). Game theory and the evolution of behaviour. *Proceedings of the Royal Society*, B, **205**, 475–88.

Maynard Smith, J. & Parker, G.A. (1976). The logic of asymmetric contests. *Animal Behaviour*, **24**, 159–75.

Morris, D. (1952). Homosexuality in the ten-spined stickleback. *Behaviour*, **4**, 233–61.

Milinski, M. (1979). An evolutionarily stable feeding strategy in sticklebacks. *Zeitschrift für Tierpsychologie*, **51**, 36–40.

Parker, G.A. (1974a). Assessment strategy and the evolution of fighting behaviour. *Journal of Theoretical Biology*, **47**, 223–43.

Parker, G.A. (1974*b*). The reproductive behaviour and the nature of sexual selection in *Scatophaga stercoraria. IX* Spatial distribution of fertilization rates and evolution of male search strategy within the reproductive area. *Evolution*, **28**, 93–108.

Parker, G.A. (1978). Selfish genes, evolutionary games, and the adaptiveness of behaviour. *Nature*, **274**, 849–55.

Perrill, S.A., Gerhardt, H.C. & Daniel, R. (1978). Sexual parasitism in the green tree frog, *Hyla cinerea. Science*, **200**, 1179–80.

Perrins, C.M. & Moss, D. (1975). Reproductive rates in the great tit. *Journal of Animal Ecology*, **44**, 695–706.

Ragland, S.S. & Sohal, R.S. (1973). Mating behaviour, physical activity and aging in the housefly, *Musca domestica. Experimental Gerontology*, **8**, 135–45.

Reyer, H.-U. (1980). Flexible helper structure as an ecological adaptation in the pied kingfisher, *Ceryle rudis rudis. Behavioural Ecology and Sociobiology*, **6**, 219–27.

Sigurjonsdottir, H. (1980). *Evolutionary Aspects of Sexual Dimorphism in Size: Studies on Dung Flies and Three Groups of Birds.* Ph.D. thesis, Liverpool University.

Thornhill, R. (1979). Adaptive female-mimicking behavior in a scorpionfly. *Science*, **205**, 412–14.

Tinbergen, N. (1959). Comparative studies of the behaviour of gulls (Laridae): a progress report. *Behaviour*, **15**, 1–70.

van Rhijn, J.G. (1973). Behavioural dimorphism in male ruffs *Philomachus pugnax. Behaviour*, **47**, 153–229.

Williams, G.C. (1966). *Adaptation and Natural Selection.* Princeton University Press: Princeton.

Index

Page numbers in italic type indicate references to tables or figures.
Species of animals are listed under English names only, and those having only a passing
reference are included under the general heading, birds, fish, insects, mammals, etc.